Synthetic Planet

Synthetic Planet
Chemical Politics and the Hazards of Modern Life

Edited by
Monica J. Casper

ROUTLEDGE
NEW YORK AND LONDON

Published in 2003 by
Routledge
29 West 35th Street
New York, NY 10001
www.routledge-ny.com

Published in Great Britain by
Routledge
11 New Fetter Lane
London EC4P 4EE
www.routledge.co.uk

10 9 8 7 6 5 4 3 2 1

Library of Congress Cataloging-in-Publication Data

Synthetic planet : chemical politics and the hazards of modern life /
edited by Monica J. Casper.
    p. cm.
  ISBN 0-415-93354-4 (hardcover : alk. paper) — ISBN 0-415-93355-2
(pbk. : alk. paper)
  1. Pollution—Environmental aspects. I. Casper, Monica J., 1966–

  TD196.C45S95 2003
  363.738—dc21

                      2002155821

For my daughter
Mason Olivia Casper
And all the world's children—
May you inherit a cleaner, safer planet

Then do let the devil take it for free, that wretched synthetic-made Chemistry.
—Wilhelm Koenigs (1912)

As the tide of chemicals born in the Industrial Age has risen to engulf our environment, a drastic change has come about in the nature of the most serious public health problems. Only yesterday mankind lived in fear of the scourges of smallpox, cholera, and plague that once swept nations before them . . . Today we are concerned with a different kind of hazard that lurks in our environment—a hazard we ourselves have introduced into our world as our modern way of life has evolved.
—Rachel Carson (1962)

From dry-cleaning fluids to DDT, harmful substances have trespassed the landscape and have also woven themselves, in trace amounts, into the fibers of our bodies. This much we know with certainty. It is not only reasonable but essential that we should understand the lifetime effects of these incremental accumulations.
—Sandra Steingraber (1997)

Without Chemicals, Life Itself Would Be Impossible.
—Monsanto corporate slogan, c. 1970

Contents

Preface and Acknowledgments

I have lived on Earth for more than thirty-five years. In those three and a half decades, I have breathed her air, ingested her food and water, bathed in her oceans and lakes, sifted and rearranged her pungent soil, and absorbed her loamy essence through my pores. I could write the history of my body through its relationship to the environment. As could we all, although our stories would differ considerably depending on our social and geographic locations. It is little wonder that the environmental memoir has emerged as a recent popular literary form.

As our planetary matriarch has been transformed by human interventions—chemical, nuclear, biological, industrial, sociopolitical—so too have we, her daughters and sons, *Homo sapiens* and the rest of the animal kingdom alike, been similarly refashioned. In the polluted air we inhale, in the toxic sludge that thickens our oceans, in the chemical residues that linger ash-like on crops, we are made anew. Hybrid creatures of modernity, beneficiaries and casualties of progress, we are poster children for the promises and pitfalls of industry and its applications. Our bodies are at risk and our communities in harm's way in a beautiful world that is also awash in noxious substances, however useful and alluring they may be to modern life.

Diseases are rampant, and we would be deluding ourselves if we believed they were not at least partly environmental in origin. Although the degree to which bodily ailments derive from pollutants is hugely contested, they are linked to industrial chemicals through both scientific findings and the popular imagination. Cancer—name the body part. Endocrine disorders. Leukemia, childhood and adult. Asthma. Genetic mutations. Birth defects. Infertility. Miscarriages. Our bodies are warped, twisted, damaged, dissolved, and made vacant by insidious intruders, many of which we cannot even identify. These substances are subtle, silent, and deadly effective corporeal terrorists.

In my own family, we are not strangers to environmental and occupational hazards. I come from hearty Midwest stock, thinned by arduous work in the steel mills of Chicago and the coal mines of rural downstate Illinois. My stepfather is a diesel mechanic with gnarled, oil-encrusted fingers who describes his eventual retirement, to which he should by all rights be looking forward, as the dismal time when most of the men in his line of work die from having been exposed repeatedly to solvents and to exhaust fumes in poorly ventilated garages, especially in the harsh winters when buildings must remain closed.

My mother, petite but strong, has chronic neck and back pain from moving heavy coils of steel in preparation for shipping to manufacturing clients. I have watched her struggle for years with the debilitating auto-immune diseases arthritis and asthma.

I have lost grandparents to lung and pancreatic cancer. For years, a paternal uncle was the human canary who descended into the coal mines ahead of the other workers to make sure they would be safe. And I have witnessed the illnesses and deaths from breast cancer of too many vibrant, lovely women.

Although I have been luckier than most—the life of an academic carries different sorts of risks than the work of my blue-collar kin—I have had my own painful skirmishes with contamination.

In 1994, I traveled to New Zealand to conduct research for a project on fetal surgery. A lush island paradise in hues of green and blue, it was astonishingly lovely from the air. I could not wait to disembark and set foot on the Southern Hemisphere, to dip my toes into the sparkling water of Hauraki Bay and to climb the island's volcanoes.

But upon landing in Auckland, we passengers were asked to remain on the plane while masked personnel came through to spray pesticides. An island country, New Zealand has been quite successful in using chemicals to keep its agriculture pristine, free from foreign pests. As the spacesuit-clad figures traversed the plane's center aisle spritzing insecticidal cocktails under and between our seats, a flight attendant assured us that we would be safe. However, she also recommended covering the noses and mouths of small children with a napkin or handkerchief.

In my excitement at being in New Zealand for the next five weeks, I did not make much of the spraying incident. I ignored the slight cold I seemed to be developing and launched myself into my research and explorations of Auckland. A few days later, however, when I began coughing scarlet drops onto my pillow, I was forced to reconsider what had happened on-board.

I became sicker within the next week than I had ever been in my life. I was fatigued, and I could not stop fluids spewing from my lungs. My hotel room was draped with handkerchiefs, increasingly rust-stained, that I kept washing out and hanging to dry like some mad chambermaid.

I did visit a doctor, a remarkably easy and inexpensive thing to do in a country with national health care. She assumed I had some sort of viral infection and prescribed antibiotics. The ensuing allergic reaction sent me back to bed for another two days, where I continued to paint my white cotton pillowcase in bright Jackson Pollack splashes.

Desperate and disappointed that I would not be able to continue my research, I phoned United Airlines to arrange an early flight home. Told that I would have to wait at least two weeks, I experienced a mind-numbing panic attack. In the throes of anxiety, I quickly packed my things, said a hasty good-bye to my colleagues in Auckland, and rushed to the airport. There, I registered for stand-by and then camped out near the United gate for 36 hours, utterly miserable.

I finally secured a flight, during which I slept most of the eleven-hour journey. As the plane approached Los Angeles, the descent was so painful to my assaulted respiratory system that I fainted in the aisle. The ENT specialist in San Francisco who I saw two days later was astonished I had been able to fly at all. She recommended fluids, rest, and no travel for at least six weeks. She was furious that the airline had permitted the spraying of potentially toxic chemicals in a closed space, and she believed that I had been poisoned by whatever pesticide had been in those tanks.

As I was recuperating, overcome with an exhaustion that stunned me, I wrote a letter to United Airlines complaining about my horrific adventure. In response, I received a free ticket voucher and a letter of apology stating that the company could not fly into New Zealand if it did not abide by that nation's rules about agricultural protection. Of course, the letter did not identify the chemicals I had been exposed to. I did a bit more research and discovered that New Zealand was at that time one of the fifteen or so nations that still practiced this form of global pest control.

Three months later, I returned to New Zealand to finish my work. This time, I was armed with a charcoal mask to filter out the pesticides on the airplane. Yet, as I hunkered safely behind my gear, I worried about everybody else on the plane without such protection and imagined the damage to their fragile mucous membranes.

The tiny volcanic country turned out to be as gorgeous and fecund as I had initially imagined. As I completed my work there and explored the North Island, I fell in love with the land and seascape surrounding me. But I speculated often about the price of that untamed yet carefully managed turquoise splendor.

A few years later, while living near Sacramento, California, in a rural area of dusty fields and tomato-splattered roads, I was diagnosed with adult-onset asthma (just as my mother and sister had been). On hot, dry summer nights, with temperatures spiking above 100 degrees, I would lie in bed gasping for each breath, afraid that I would suffocate. My eyes itched and burned, and my parched nose stung. The only relief I could find some nights was to sleep outside in the car, with the air conditioner running full-blast.

My then-partner, working as an agricultural consultant, was accidentally exposed to parathion one day in a client's field near Lodi. Ironically, part of his work was implementing integrated pest management (IPM) practices. The supposedly temporary illness he developed following this exposure so closely resembled what I had experienced in New Zealand that it sparked a long-term interest in the public health effects of pesticides. Clearly, we both had been victims of some type of chemical poisoning. After this incident, I pondered anew the origins of my asthma in California's Central Valley, where synthetic agriculture is king.

These are the kinds of bodily harms for which, say, a free airline ticket or a paycheck seem to be woefully inadequate compensation.

I wonder now, what lingers in my body? What man-made chemicals haunt my bloodstream like microscopic ghouls? What substances have taken root in my tissues like kudzu vine? What toxins reside like squatters in my breasts and other fatty, deposit-rich body parts?

I am pregnant, in my thirty-second week as I write this. I am filled with delight, awe, and infinite love for this writhing creature in my womb. I marvel at the morphing expansion of my abdomen created by the baby's exponential growth. I relish the labor involved in feeding and nurturing her, my little reproductive project, my future.

Yet, I am also more afraid than ever of what lurks in our environment. I live on an island in Puget Sound, north of Seattle. Surrounded by craggy snow-capped mountains and crystalline blue water, my habitat seems so pure and clean. It is the very picture of Nature. But local Orca whale pods are dying out, threatened by endocrine-disrupting synthetics in the food chain. Pollution from local paper mills, linked to an embattled but thriving timber industry, endangers our air quality. And the area has more than its fair share of military bases, recognized as among the worst polluters in the nation.

While I try to eat "all the right things," I fret that I can never fully know what chemicals lace my fruits and vegetables, or infiltrate my soy milk, or sequester themselves in my scrambled eggs. I eat fresh salmon from the local waters near my house, nervously imagining I can see actual PCB molecules clinging to the rosy flesh. I buy organic as often as I can, shopping at the Farmer's Market on Saturday mornings. But, I ask myself—aware of the middle-class privilege behind the question—are these activities enough? What else can and should I be doing to ensure healthy babies, my own and those of other women? Perhaps more important, what can society at large be doing?

As I lie in bed at night, restless and unable to sleep because there is no room for this rotund belly that I have sprouted, I envision the placenta within me. I imagine nutrient-rich blood flowing from my capillaries into those of my Lilliputian daughter, imbuing her with enzymes, antibodies, and with life itself. And I anxiously hope that my body is not also passing across that pulsating membrane other substances, such as those invisible compounds that do not bring good things to life.

* * * * *

In preparing this book, I have benefited from the help of many people. First and foremost, I wish to thank the authors for their provocative, insightful chapters. I gratefully acknowledge their considerable patience through the several years, iterations, and titles this volume required from start to finish. I have learned a great deal from reading their varied and fascinating research, and I am thrilled that they have chosen to be a part of *Synthetic Planet*.

I also wish to thank the amazing and intelligent Barbara Barnes. To label her simply my research assistant does not do justice to the intellectual gifts she has given me. Her help on this book was immeasurable; she offered me needed encouragement when my energy and attention were flagging in the post-baby months, as well as some fabulous suggestions for improvement of the collection. Her assistance in the final stages was invaluable. I look forward to working with her on many additional projects and to watching her certain professional ascendance. In addition, Barbara and I both are very grateful for the excellent and much-needed technical assistance provided by her husband, Eric Chesmar.

I owe a debt of gratitude to Ilene Kalish at Routledge for support, encouragement, good ideas, and friendship. This book certainly bears her creative imprint. And I would be remiss if I did not also thank the anonymous reviewers who offered terrific ideas for improving earlier versions of the manuscript. Finally, as always, thanks go to my family for believing in the "egghead" among them and loving me despite my chosen line of work.

Monica J. Casper
Whidbey Island, WA

Introduction
Chemical Matters

MONICA J. CASPER

Monsanto's corporate slogan declares, "Without Chemicals, Life Itself Would be Impossible." In *Synthetic Planet*, we explore the contradictions and ironies of such a universal claim, analyzing some of the ways that industrial chemicals have transformed environments, bodies, communities, and nations in the so-called modern age. This book is about the "impossible lives" and myriad consequences—material, ontological, corporeal, and political—ensuing from human use of and interaction with substances both inert and volatile. In one sense, the essays contained here explore tangible forms of matter, highly useful yet potentially lethal combinations of hydrogen, oxygen, nitrogen, carbon, and other building blocks. Yet in another and perhaps more important sense, this volume also articulates the contexts in which these elements have been used and their outcomes. Our intention here is to focus a critical lens on industrial chemistry and its products. We offer a chemical politics, if you will, tracing the multiple pathways by which synthetic chemicals migrate from their laboratories or factories of origin into environments and bodies and communities and nations, with considerable impact on ecosystem and human health, social organization, and political processes.

There are special ways, we suspect, that chemistry has been intimately tied to concepts of nation-building and civilization over the past century. As a thoroughly modern project, twentieth-century chemistry was invested with the hopes and dreams of Western and developing nations looking to a bright, prosperous future (Crone 1986; Meikle 1995). Synthetic chemicals were developed and widely used "to bring good things to life"—as DuPont so boldly promised in its catchy Jazz Age jingle—and, indeed, to show us what modernity was and could yet be. Jeffrey Meikle argues in his wonderful book on plastic that DuPont solicited advertisers' help in representing chemistry's unique contribution to modern civilization. He (1995, 134) writes, "The message reached a large audience through a new network radio program, *The Cavalcade of America*, which advanced DuPont's patriotism by dramatizing episodes from the nation's past, while its advertising celebrated present and future chemical wonders flowing from DuPont laboratories." Surely this message reached many of the nation's citizens, even its youngest inhabitants. After all, one of the most popular toys for children (at least boy children) in the West has been the ubiquitous chemistry set. DuPont, in miniature.

Bruno Latour (1991) has argued that "we have never been modern" but, if true, it was certainly not for lack of trying. Industry, fueled by two world wars and a booming post-war population, needed synthetic chemicals for an array of consumer goods such as cleaning products, solvents, machinery, tools, vehicles, and more chemicals—in short, the quotidian stuff of life in the contemporary West. Re-tooling after military research, chemists parlayed their wartime efforts into peacetime products; pesticides displaced chemical weapons, and processed chemicals moved from bunkers to kitchens (Aftalion 1991). Industrial chemicals have allowed major innovations in plastics, rubber, fuels, insecticides, pharmaceuticals, and weapons, among other areas, connecting techno-dreams of progress with nation-building activities such as design, transportation, agriculture, medicine, and militarism. Chemicals have also been key tools of globalization as Western nations pursue "development" activities in the Third World.

Yet, chemical activities have been articulated with nation-building in destructive as well as productive ways. For example, in his quest for a more perfect nation-state populated by Aryan bodies, Adolf Hitler, ghastly icon of twentieth-century excess, used Zyklon B—a poison akin to nerve gas—for genocidal purposes. This technical "innovation" facilitated vastly more deaths of "deviant" bodies—Jews, Gypsies, Catholics, homosexuals, and other targets of the Third Reich—than would have been possible with conventional munitions alone. Peter Hayes (2001) has shown that I. G. Farben and other industrial giants were fundamental to the rise and maintenance of the Third Reich. Certainly, Hitler's agenda of hate and power was profitable to chemical companies, many of whom were somewhat slow to grasp the full dimensions of their products' use while others had full knowledge. As Hayes (2001, 361) argues, "That the scales fell but slowly from the eyes of Farben's leaders may seem difficult to believe. After all, it was Zyklon B, a granular vaporizing pesticide, that asphyxiated the Jews of Auschwitz, and a subsidiary of IG, the Deutsche Gesellschaft für Schädlingsbekämpfung mbH (German Vermin-Combating Corporation), or Degesch, that controlled the manufacture and distribution of the Zyklon." Nation-building, indeed, but at whose expense?

As we embark on the twenty-first century, many chemical projects are in a state of flux. Developed as answers to hopeful dreams, industrial chemicals have instead become pressing social problems, articulated as environmental health risks (Greenberg 2001; Davis 2002). Consider, for example, the widespread concern about pesticides and consequent emergent organic and integrated pest management (IPM) practices (National Research Council 1989) in the West. Note that these concerns have not prevented the United States from exporting banned pesticides such as DDT to developing nations, at the rate of approximately nine tons per day (Steingraber 1997). The contributions to the current volume break new ground in showing how synthetic chemicals have been used as basic building blocks not only for a parade of material things, but also for new social and political arrangements. At the same time, the authors attend to the Janus-faced nature of synthetics as both beneficial and insidious, as often-invisible molecular tools for building and destroying worlds. Given this chemical schizophrenia, this volume is organized around the myriad "hazards" of industrial chemicals. As the renowned chemist Hugh Crone (1986, 2) has written, "we have adopted the chemical age without knowing its consequences." This book is concerned with both the historic promise and the ongoing pitfalls of synthetics and their accompanying social relations.

Given the great degree of attention devoted to environmental issues over the past few decades, synthetic chemicals have entered the popular lexicon as pollutants, toxins, poisons, and contaminants—in short, as rather villainous things. They are believed by many to be responsible for contaminating the planet and contributing to illness and death in humans and other species (Carson 1962; Steingraber 1997; Thornton 2000; Davis 2002). Indeed, environmental health controversies center on the complex but assumed role of industrial chemicals in causing disease and ecosystem damage (Crone 1986; Kroll-Smith, Brown and Gunter 2000; Kroll-Smith and Floyd 1997). Angry community activists and vulnerable citizens target industry, hoping to find some recompense for a world in which there is seemingly "no safe place" (Brown and Mikkelsen 1990). Moreover, since the mid-twentieth century, headlines around the globe have screamed news of yet another chemical disaster, branding into our collective consciousness names such as Agent Orange, thalidomide, Love Canal, Times Beach, Seveso, Bhopal, and other substances and places too numerous to name. These "incidents" and the decline of public faith in chemicals embody the multifarious nature of modernity, illustrating deepening contradictions in capitalism and sharp cleavages among Earth's 6 billion plus inhabitants.

Surprisingly, despite the rich and complex history of industrial chemicals, scholars outside of chemistry departments have paid scant attention to these substances. Synthetic chemicals have rarely been made into objects of analysis by sociologists, anthropologists, historians, and others. Even the interdisciplinary field of science and technology studies has tended to ignore the impact of industrial chemicals in favor of other, snazzier stories, such as physics and biotechnology. Where environmental health has been a focus, emphasis has often been on environmental justice issues, such as the location of toxic waste facilities. Chief concerns include, for example, people's experiences of environmental degradation (Kuletz 1998), political action and regulatory mechanisms (Szasz 1994), the stratified nature of pollution (Bullard 1993), and relations among industry, science, and the public (Markowitz and Rosner 2002; Davis 2002). While extremely valuable, most of these studies take industrial chemicals for granted in the sense that they are not "troubled" analytically; synthetics are background figures to the "real" story of community activism or government regulation.

While the contributors to this volume are also concerned with justice, activism, and the rules governments make (or fail to make), we hope our analytical lens is of sufficient scope to encompass the chemicals themselves. That means attending to more than just the harmful effects of synthetics; we attempt also to understand and locate industrial chemicals within their broader contexts of production and distribution. Rather than viewing them merely as a backdrop or spur to social action, we position chemicals themselves as a kind of material and symbolic "solution" flowing through, linking, and transforming environments, bodies, communities, and nations. The stories narrated here are as much about the substances—fluid, nimble, intricate, and potent— as they are about the consequences of their use.

Chemical Relativism, Chemical Realities

This is not a "how to" textbook. There are no complicated chemical formulas, no discussions of organic versus inorganic chemistry, no (or, rather, relatively few) unpronounceable words denoting matter. It is also not a treatise on the physiological aspects of chemical exposure. None of the authors are chemists or physicians, although several have a broad background in the liberal arts that includes the sciences. Those of us who research health and illness tend to do so from sociological, anthropological, historical, and public health perspectives. Yet, in examining environmental health controversies, we "outsiders" are thrust into a different world, one of Type I and Type II errors, risk assessments, dosage, toxicity, thresholds, synergistic effects, and toxic torts (Christensen 1999; Kroll-Smith, Brown and Gunter 2000). Not only must we make sense of the impact of industrial chemicals on human social life, but we must also attempt to understand how others—such as scientists, health professionals, and citizens—measure that impact at the level of environments, individual bodies, and whole populations. In doing so, we sometimes develop our own concepts, such as Phil Brown's (1992) very useful notion of *popular epidemiology*, for considering the numerous measurement disputes that plague the environmental health arena. What we often find upon entering into these worlds is that environmental health broadly, and the impact of industrial chemicals specifically as several contributions to this volume illustrate, are highly disputed and contested arenas (Kroll-Smith, Brown, and Gunter 2000).

Our task is further complicated by the recognition that chemicals are relative in multiple senses of that term. On the one hand, decades of research in social and cultural studies of science and technology have shown us that science is a social product, woven into the fabric of human society rather than existing outside in some pure, abstracted Nature (Biagioli 1999; Haraway 1991; Pickering 1992). Scientific knowledge does not merely reflect nature, but rather imbues it with meaning and indeed constructs it through a variety of concrete practices. Our knowledge of chemicals, and of chemistry as a discipline, is thus shaped by the social and political contexts in which that knowledge has developed. Because industrial chemicals so often have been linked to environmental illnesses, and because there are a variety of actors in these arenas with different, sometimes competing interests and agendas, knowledge about chemicals and their impacts is especially ambiguous. While many social actors, especially scientists and policy makers, strive to obtain "better" data, citizens and activists are more likely to contest the very grounds upon which that data is collected. This dynamic has significant implications for what we can know about the ways in which synthetic chemicals flow between industrial spaces and the bodies which inhabit them.

Another way in which chemicals are relative has to do with their toxicity, or capacity to affect environments and bodies. What makes industrial chemicals dangerous is not their mere existence on the planet—although some environmental activists might disagree. For example, a sealed container full of hydrogen cyanide is relatively harmless in terms of human or animal health. However, were that container to fall off of a laboratory bench and break, every living creature inhaling hydrogen cyanide vapors would likely die. Thus, chemicals become toxins, poisons, and contaminants only in relation to that which is being poisoned. As Hugh Crone (1986, 33) argues, "the term 'poisonous' is meaningless on its own. It assumes more and more meaning as the conditions under which it is harmful are more clearly and fully stated." And, we might add, experienced. Significant conditions include the dosage, the degree of toxicity to living organisms, the route of administration (e.g., oral, topical, intravenous), and whether or not an antidote exists. Some industrial chemicals may be quite innocuous to organic beings, while others can destroy tissue or cause death in a matter of seconds.

The degree to which industrial chemicals are perceived as dangerous and burdensome is determined, in part, by how willingly those affected assume such risks. Ulrich Beck (1992) argues that the concept of risk is central to late modern culture, and that we are all living in a "risk society." The risks associated with modern life are seen as an inevitable consequence of processes of modernization. Risks are increasingly global, and their presence seems to require the proliferation of advanced scientific techniques for measuring, calculating, and weighing their potentially harmful effects. The presence of these risks, and the institutions and discourses created to understand and control them, contribute to the creation of new subjectivities and selves, as Foucault (1978) might certainly have argued. We are, in short, a planet of at-risk subjects, forever calculating the degree to which our lives are imperiled.

When we willingly choose to participate in risky activities, such as smoking, drinking, "unsafe" sexual intercourse, or the ingestion of legal and illegal pharmaceuticals, we may embrace an autonomous, in-control subjectivity. However, when risks are thrust upon us, our sovereignty is threatened. It is one thing to pollute one's own body, and quite another matter to be poisoned. We are thus compelled to address the power relations that enable companies to pollute our neighborhoods or that prevent governments, especially but not only in capitalist nations, from regulating toxic substances. If we have cultural or economic capital, we may be able to resist; if we do not, we may suffer damage to vulnerable bodies and communities. Different subjectivities and responses are produced depending on whether we choose risk, or risk chooses us. In my own work on chemical weapons, I have found that workers in incinerators are far more likely to accept risk than citizens who live downwind of the smokestacks that, they fear, may contain unincinerated nerve agents.

Given this array of relativisms associated with industrial chemicals, what can we say about their realities? What do we actually know about how synthetics impact bodies and ecosystems? While knowledge about environmental illness is hotly debated (Kroll-Smith, Brown, and Gunter 2000), it seems clear that industrial chemicals can and do affect bodies. Indeed, certain substances such as chemical weapons and pesticides were developed and used precisely *because of* their toxic effects on organic tissue. Rachel Carson (1962), writing eloquently about pesticides developed in the shadow of World War II, described them as "elixirs of death." More recently, Edmund Russell (2001) has offered a superb history of the relationship between wartime chemicals and pesticides, focusing on the cultural and technical parallels between warfare against human enemies and the control of nature and its nonhuman "invaders." Pesticides are of course not the only chemicals in use, but they do make up a significant portion of the chemical armory—and we do not know as much about them as we should. Steingraber (1997, 99–100) notes that "between 45,000 and 100,000 chemicals are now in common commercial use; 75,000 is the most frequently cited estimate. Of these, only about 1.5 to 3 percent (1,200 to 1,500 chemicals) have been tested for carcinogenicity. . . . Only 10 percent of pesticides in common use have been adequately assessed for hazards; for 38 percent, nothing useful is known; the remaining 52 percent fall somewhere in between."

We do know some things. Crone describes the pathways through which chemicals enter into bodies, including by mouth (swallowing a substance), inhalation into the lungs, or skin permeation. He (Crone 1986, 42) writes, "The location of the target in the body varies depending on the nature of the chemical but, once the chemical reaches the bloodstream, it is carried round the body very rapidly so that in most, but not all cases, it is effectively then in contact with the target organ." Because bodies themselves are finely tuned biochemical organisms, the introduction of a foreign substance has the potential to drastically impact how the body functions. While humans and wildlife may be able to fight off some agents, others will be too toxic and will disrupt bodily systems (Colborn, Dumanoski, and Myers 1996; Christensen and Casper 2000). Cancer, birth defects, immune disorders, endocrine disruption, and a variety of other problems may all be caused by the introduction of a chemical intruder into the body.

And yet, even this knowledge does not necessarily help us to make sense of or to resolve environmental health problems. First, it is often very difficult to locate the exact origin of a chemical intruder. While living next door to a petrochemical plant may seem to make this determination easier, how do we account for the presence of toxic chemicals in our water sources, food chain, or air supply (Thornton 2000)? Even if we were able to precisely locate the beginning of a molecule's path, how can we measure the amount necessary to cause health problems? What if such problems take years to manifest in people's bodies, or do not show up until the next generation is born? As Steingraber (1997, 264–65) writes with respect to cancer research, "Within the scientific community, grand arguments have ensued from the attempt to classify and quantify cancer deaths due to specific causes. Traditionally, the final result of this task takes the visual form of a great cancer pie sliced to depict the relative importance of different risk factors . . . The quarreling begins immediately."

These questions become profoundly important, and potentially expensive, when we begin to assign blame and responsibility for damage to ecosystem and human health. In our Western legal framework of rights and responsibilities, in which the burden of proof is on the accuser, it is not enough to suggest fault. Rather, it must be proven, beyond a shadow of a doubt, that company A did indeed pollute the well that led to little Paco's leukemia or the damage to Mary Jane's reproductive organs. Science is enrolled in this litigious project, but even science is inexact. The environmental health field is characterized by an abundance of conflicting studies on a few widely used chemicals, no research on the vast majority of chemicals, and a highly polarized research community. Moreover, in its quest for objectivity and pure truth, science, like Western law, leaves little room for the anecdotal, the intuitive, and the gut-feeling sense that company A is responsible. While many environmental activists have become well versed in science, most ordinary folks have not.

Thus, knowing that a particular molecule can cause x-degree of damage to a living organism does us little good in determining the politics of accountability for ecosystem and health damage. We must look instead to the broader contexts within which these biochemical interactions take place. While we can surround ourselves with the very latest epidemiological and scientific data on hazardous exposures, we need to look beyond these data—themselves often quite contested—to environments, bodies, communities, and nations. In short, we need to follow the molecule from its point of origin, if that can be calculated, through all the other places and spaces that it travels. The information we gather can help to shed light on how bodies and whole ecosystems might be affected. Certainly, this is an important task for ecologists—and a highly charged political one (Carson 1962; Thornton 2000). As Steingraber (1997, 268) asserts, "In full possession of our ecological roots, we can begin to survey our present situation. This requires a human rights approach."

But there may be an equally important task for social scientists in conducting analyses of environmental health issues. We can tell stories about why these data are so contested, highlighting the flexible social processes through which truth and reality are negotiated and produced. We can investigate both the symbolic and material journeys of molecules, and the impacts they have in and across different social spaces. We can offer different interpretations of how knowledge is constructed, and why objectivity and "pure truth" may not solve certain pressing problems. We can, in other words, examine the relationships among industrial chemicals, the ecosystems they inhabit, the bodies they affect, the communities that care about them, and the national agendas that either foster or prohibit their migration. In this, we offer ourselves as partners to ecologists, public health experts, and others seeking to amplify our collective knowledge of the chemical hazards of modern life.

Follow That Molecule! Environments, Bodies, Communities, and Nations

Contributors to this volume were asked to "follow the molecule"—that is, to consider industrial chemicals in and across many of the sites where they matter. In part, the notion of following the molecule comes from science and technology studies, particularly actor-network theory that has encouraged consideration of the role of nonhuman entities in the development of sociotechnical worlds (Callon 1985; Latour 1988). Yet this perspective has an unfortunate tendency, despite its claims to analytical symmetry in treatment of humans and nonhumans, to follow scientists and engineers as the most important actors (Latour 1987). Susan Leigh Star (1991) has critiqued this as the "executive approach" to studying science and technology. Adele Clarke and I similarly argued that in following scientists and engineers around, other human actors remain outside the frame; plus, by demanding symmetry between humans and nonhumans, the distinctive role of human action and meaning may be lost (Casper and Clarke 1998).

Following the molecule, then, in both theory and method involves building on and extending science and technology studies approaches, while recognizing their limitations. Our collective approach in this volume, despite some important methodological and disciplinary differences, is to attend to the presence of industrial chemicals as nonhuman agents in a variety of social worlds where human action also matters extensively. It is, for example, to be aware of the fact that without industrial chemicals there would be no chemistry—and to be equally aware that without chemistry, there would be no industrial chemicals. Of course, without chemists, there would be neither synthetic chemicals nor chemistry, and it is interesting to note that chemists have higher than average rates of cancer (Steingraber 1997). Material entities are very much a part of our built worlds, including scientific specialties. We thus attend in this book to the ways in which chemical agents migrate, materially and symbolically, through and between different worlds, entering into and transforming environments, bodies, communities, and nations.

As such, in following the molecule, the contributors to this volume also problematize an additional set of concepts, namely what constitutes an environment, a body, a community, and a nation. Just as we take seriously the constructed yet significant role of industrial chemicals, we also recognize the shifting meanings of the other terms of which we speak. Indeed, in following the molecule we position industrial chemicals at the porous boundary between "nature" and "culture," attempting to understand how these substances shape our understanding of both domains as well as the ways in which we live as embodied natural *and* cultural subjects. As biochemical organisms inhabiting the planet, we, too, populate these border zones (Haraway 1985, 1997).

First, there is no standard meaning of the term *environment*. To some degree, the environment refers to that which surrounds us. While environment is often equated with nature or ecology, as in environmental movements, it can also refer to the built worlds in which we live or the industrial settings in which we work. Both "environment" and "nature" are human constructs, given shape and meaning by people who care about these spaces and concepts. William Cronon (1996, 20) argues that nature "is a human idea, with a long and complicated history which has led different beings to conceive of the natural world in very different ways. Far from inhabiting a realm that stands completely apart from humanity, the objects and creatures and landscapes we label as 'natural' are in fact deeply entangled with the words and images we use to describe them." Thus certain natural spaces become cultural icons, invoking a range of emotions in people who visit and experience them, while other, equally beautiful spaces become careless dumping grounds for hazardous waste (e.g., Kuletz 1998). What is clear is that environments, and nature itself, are deeply contested entities, continually shaped and reshaped by human action and intervention (such as pollution) and by the symbolic meanings assigned to them.

The chapters in this volume theorize the environment in a number of ways. There is a wide recognition that environments have been substantially transformed by industrial activities, with whole ecosystems being threatened and damaged by the impact of noxious substances (Colborn, Dumanoski, and Myers 1996). In this sense, the authors are following the molecule through natural and built worlds, in part because of our own intellectual and political concerns about threats to "the environment." Yet they also acknowledge that environments are shaped by responses to industrial pollution, such as environmental justice movements or government intervention. In this sense, environments are continually in flux, with industrial chemicals seeping into and out of them as communities and governments respond to perceived threats. Just as there is no settled meaning of nature or environment, neither is there consensus on what should be done about threats to these special places in the social imaginary. This volume attends, then, to the ways in which environments are affected, contested, transformed, and rebuilt, at both material and symbolic levels. Authors pose the following questions: Which environments? Under what conditions are they affected? And, with what consequences?

Bodies, too, are subject to critical analysis in this volume, with the recognition that human (and increasingly nonhuman) bodies live and die at the boundaries between nature and culture. Environmental health issues are important to us precisely because of the material realities of human embodiment. In one important sense, our bodies are internal environments that are ecologically linked to broader environments (Steingraber 1997). People are afraid of hazardous waste because they do not want to get sick and die, to give birth to a deformed or ailing baby, or to watch a loved one wither away from cancer, leukemia, skin diseases, respiratory ailments, or a host of other problems thought to be related to toxins in our air, food, and water supplies.

Fortunately, with some prodding by feminist scholars, in recent years the body has been given a great deal of attention by social scientists. Rather than seeing embodiment as peripheral to social life and human action, bodies and embodiment have come to be seen as central to how people live, act, and die in the world. As Bryan Turner (1991, 4) argues, "human embodiment creates a set of constraints . . . but equally important the body is also a potential which can be elaborated by sociocultural development." This is not to reduce human existence to a kind of biological bedrock, but rather to recognize that embodiment is a crucial feature of the social landscape, and that bodies are a ubiquitous feature of environments.

Several years ago, Arthur Frank (1991) wrote an insightful analytical review of the body in sociology. He posited four different categories of bodies: medicalized, sexual, disciplined, and talking. Nowhere in his scheme was there room for the vulnerable body, at risk for a host of invasions ranging from infection by contagious microbes to migrating toxic substances that do not recognize corporeal borders. Maren Klawiter (1999a), building on Robert Proctor's (1995) notions of "body machismo" and "body victimology," has argued that bodies, especially vulnerable bodies, need to be incorporated more fully into analysis of social movements. In her work on breast cancer, she attends to "the ways in which bodies figure not only as sites of disease, but as the vehicles and products of social movements, and as anchors and signifiers of contested meanings." Nancy Scheper-Hughes (1992) and Diane Nelson (1999) both have articulated notions of vulnerable bodies—especially but not exclusively those of women and children—in relation to broader contexts of poverty, hunger, racism, neo-colonialism, and so on. Most of the chapters herein feature a version of the body disrupted, made vulnerable by exposure to potentially toxic substances.

In focusing on bodily risk, the volume brings the topic of industrial chemicals firmly within the domain of human health and illness. Contributors pose a number of questions about bodies in relation to industrial chemicals. For example, in what ways is the vulnerable body a catalyst to social action? In what ways is it the corporeal and ontological link between the world of nature, with its microbes and toxic molecules, and the world of social organization? In what ways does it provide a kind of social/corporeal glue that links tiny molecules to people, communities, and nations? And lastly, how does corporeal vulnerability reflect broader social hierarchies of race, class, gender, geography, and political economy?

Social scientists think about *communities* in terms of social relationships that operate within certain boundaries, locations, or territories. Communities may be geographic or ideological, that is organized according to proximity or according to a shared set of beliefs and practices. In a popular sense, the term is also often associated with positive, progressive ideas about a sense of collectivity, spirit, or change. To have a sense of community is seen normatively as a social good, something to be encouraged and pursued. In terms of politics, community often provides the basis for civic action and intervention. Since people live in communities, it is not surprising that much activism, for example, begins at the community or "grassroots" level (Bullard 1993; Kuletz 1998).

The term is used in a number of ways in this book, ranging from groups of activists who care about a particular issue, to neighborhood conglomerations of people, to communities of practice in science and medicine, to specific spatial/geographic configurations. The chapters focus on several different communities variously defined, analyzing their connections and contentions. Each author has attempted to track the ways that their particular communities of interest—their objects of analysis—intersect with the other elements in this story, namely industrial chemicals (and thus industry), bodies, and nations or governments. Attention is also paid to how some communities become defined in the first place, through either a shared concern with environmental health issues or physical vulnerability due to proximity and/or embodiment.

Finally, the chapters in this volume attend to questions of *nation*, including but moving beyond government intervention. If, as cultural critic Benedict Anderson (1983) argues, a nation is an "imagined community," then this book, in part, advocates an assessment of the role of synthetic chemicals in fostering that imagination. The concept of imaginary refers to places where meaning-making happens, where, in the case of chemicals, synthetic worlds are creatively dreamed, hoped, built, challenged, and dismantled. These spaces might include advertising, film, music, dance, toys, literature, and of course science. Some examples include: Primo Levi's beautifully-crafted *The Periodic Table*, Rachel Carson's poetic *Silent Spring*, Don DeLillo's hilarious *White Noise*, folk and protest songs; Todd Haynes' film *Safe*, the witty British documentary *Good-bye Mrs. Ant*, Judith Helfand's acerbically droll *Healthy Baby Girl* and *Blue Vinyl*, the breast cancer documentary, *Rachel's Daughters*, the more recent popular films *A Civil Action* and *Erin Brockovich*, environmental memoirs such as *Body Toxic* (Antonetta 2001) and *Atomic Farmgirl* (Hein 2000), comic books featuring villains and superheroes made mutant by falling into vats of toxic sludge, and so on. From the mid-twentieth century on, these sites have increasingly reflected deep anxieties about industrial chemicals. More and more, synthetics both fascinate and repel us.

In addition to these symbolic elements, however, this volume is also concerned with more practical national and international issues, such as how and why governments intervene in environmental or health disputes, or other chemical matters. While there has been regulation of both areas in many parts of the world, a chief complaint of many environmental groups and concerned citizens is that governments have not done enough and are not currently doing enough to protect our natural resources and the health and well-being of the global citizenry. In each of the chapters in this book, there is some sense that what governments (local, state, national, and international) do, or refuse to do, can substantially impact the ways that industrial chemicals migrate, the communities that they migrate into, and the environments and bodies they affect—for better or worse. In other words, we ask, what can a molecule's trajectory tell us when it enters into the halls of decision making where such factors as political ideology, economy, and global context affect how much industrial waste will end up in our rivers and bloodstreams?

In following the molecule, then, this book attempts to cast a fresh analytical lens not only upon industrial chemicals, but also upon the environments, bodies, communities, and nations that they impact and that shape their movement. Authors have been asked to be theoretically bold in thinking in new ways about the relationships among migrating toxins, human bodies, social action, social organization, and public policy. At the heart of each chapter, whatever its substantive emphasis, is a recognition that the key elements of these stories are mutually constitutive; that industrial chemicals, environments, bodies, communities, and nations shape each other in the production of "impossible life."

It is our contention that this approach disrupts the linear notion that molecules move in only one direction. In following the molecules in these stories through all their transmigrations, and by attending to the places where they also do not appear, this volume attempts to provide broader understanding of what we might think of as "environmental health problems." In doing so, we hope to tell compelling stories about our synthetic planet and to provide tools for scholars, policy makers, and activists working to ameliorate ecological and social hazards. After all, however historically and socially constructed "the environment" may be, in another sense it is the only one we have. To jeopardize our "nature" is to continue to put ourselves and other living beings, and indeed Earth itself, in harm's way.

Organization of the Book

Attempting to organize the chapters in this book into a coherent whole proved to be challenging. The original schematic, with papers classified by theme, proved unstable. One reviewer suggested an organization based on the type or category of chemicals, such as those used in military contexts (there are three chapters on various wars and weapons), those used in industry, those used medically, and so on. This also proved unworkable as the kinds of chemicals discussed in this book are quite varied, and the resulting groups seemed chaotic. In some frustration, fearing that any organizational structure would seem random with such a diverse group of topics, I considered an alphabetical arrangement, preferring to let the chapters speak for themselves. This, however, seemed risky and too simplistic—I shuddered at the imagined reviews. Chemical terms—volatile, combustible, displaced, chain reaction, complex, buffer, catalyst—were mined for their classificatory utility, but abandoned as too self-consciously clever.

Then Barbara Barnes, my superb research assistant, brilliantly suggested a grouping of chapters along the four major spaces through which industrial chemicals are tracked in this book: environments, bodies, communities, and nations. What a bold idea, I thought, and proceeded accordingly. While all of the chapters take up some aspect of these categories and the traffic between them, each author also adopts a particular analytic valence. We have located chapters according to the dominant theme, recognizing that with a few alterations, they could just as easily have been placed elsewhere. Some of the disorder inherent to edited collections may remain, as the topics are diverse and the contributions original. But, if I might be permitted a chemical metaphor, there are no free radicals and the chapters taken together form a reasonably stable compound.

The first section, "Environments," begins with Peter Wynn Kirby's compelling tale of pollution and identity in two Tokyo enclaves. His story elegantly frames Japan's historical embrace of the chemical age, as well as its current dubious international supremacy in dioxin emissions. He shows not only how pollution impacts bodies, but also situates the link between environments and bodies in a distinctly Japanese context. That is, he is attentive to the ways that environmental problems, in this case hazardous waste, must necessarily be understood in terms of Japanese conceptions of nature. Thus, he connects the issue of environmental toxins to specific cultural perceptions of family, nature, and national identity. Drawing on rigorous ethnography, Kirby's account demonstrates that different meanings of environmental illness lead to different local and national responses, including expectations of the Japanese government and local communities.

Allison Shore focuses attention on the problem of indoor air pollution, considered by the Environmental Protection Agency to be a greater risk to human health than outdoor air pollution. Yet indoor pollution is less regulated, a discrepancy taken up by Shore's policy-centered account. She is particularly interested in VOCs (volatile organic compounds). Analyzing EPA documents and legislative testimony, she finds that not only have industrial interests blocked new legislation, but that policy makers have construed the problem as "voluntary" and "private." Current solutions thus emphasize information dissemination and market-based approaches, as well as individual behavioral changes, rather than regulation of harmful substances. The unintentional result is unequal protection; the less affluent remain unprotected inside, while those with class privilege are encouraged to avoid exposure. In this story, then, indoor air pollution has a great deal to do with questions of justice.

My chapter on chemical weapons disposal explores the mundane politics of air monitoring. In accordance with the international Chemical Weapons Convention, the U.S. government is incinerating its stockpile of approximately 30,000 tons of nerve agents, mustard, and other chemical munitions contained in millions of pounds of metal artillery. Each of the nine American stockpile sites is mired in controversy. Activists accuse the U.S. Army of practicing chemical weapons "dispersal" rather than disposal, suggesting that what is emitted from smokestacks may be dangerous. I trace the history of the chemical weapons program and examine air monitoring practices in Tooele, Utah. Drawing on ethnographic research, I outline the controversy associated with incineration and address the varied, often competing meanings of environment, risk, and safety that are held by different stakeholders in this arena. I suggest that chemical weapons qua migrating toxin—equal parts tangible material and potent symbol—disrupt and reorder corporeal, organizational, cultural, and political boundaries.

The second section of the book, "Bodies," opens with Diane Niblack Fox's disturbing account of the continuing legacy of Agent Orange in Vietnam. Containing the notorious molecule dioxin, Agent Orange was a catch-all term for the approximately 19 million gallons of toxic chemicals, mostly defoliants and herbicides, used by U.S. forces across wide swaths of Vietnamese landscape. Not only was an enormous amount of land and wildlife destroyed, as has been well documented, human health was also adversely affected. Yet, despite thousands of deaths and the haunting presence of people in Vietnam affected by Agent Orange, including younger generations who were disabled in utero or via reproductive damage to their parents, the "true" effects of the toxins on bodies are still being disputed. While the U.S. government ultimately made reparations to American soldiers, no such admission of responsibility has been forthcoming toward the Vietnamese. Drawing on years of fieldwork in Vietnam, Fox explores the politics of knowledge that imbue ongoing international struggles, illustrating that toxins know no national boundaries. In the process, she provides a glimpse into the illness experiences and everyday struggles of Vietnamese affected by Agent Orange.

Zsuzsa Gille takes us to Eastern Europe, a region she identifies as containing some of the worst environmental problems in the world. She examines chemical waste in Hungary as the material and metaphoric expression of post-socialism, following a repressive Soviet regime that was dominated by cultural ideologies of metallurgy. This transition from "hard" communism to "soft" post-communism reflects not only political economic transformations, but changing conceptions of bodies as well. With the ascendance of a chemical model, earlier waste-reduction measures based on the metallurgy model, in which solid wastes were recirculated into production processes, were weakened. Chemical waste became seen not as an environmental problem, but as one of the failures of communism. Materials, not bodies, were being wasted. Gille argues that the image of sickly and weak Hungarian bodies replaced dominant images of strong, metallic Soviet heroes, in a hegemonic move that played into industrial concerns opposed to democratic control of waste production. The chemical waste model and accompanying cultural ideologies prevented adequate analysis of an ongoing and quite serious problem with environmental hazards. Throughout her analysis, bodies, ideologies, and national agendas are seen to be complex and interwoven, with implications for policies on waste reduction.

Virginia Adams O'Connell delves into the world of childhood cancer, where she explores families' views about protecting their children from environmental risks. She finds that the families in her study see the environment as full of potential toxins, but also seem to accept that living in a toxic world is the price of modernity and progress. Such risks were not seen as problematic for these families until their children became ill with pediatric cancer. However, rather than finding fault with industry or government, many of the families blamed themselves for failing to take necessary precautions. Their own, local etiologic theories affected the cancer experience, especially when their children returned home after treatment. O'Connell shows that people struggle to maintain some sense of order and meaning in a world full of chaos and risk. Her chapter raises provocative questions about how safe our environments should be, who is responsible for ensuring that safety, and what kinds of knowledge will help us to make those evaluations. At issue in her analysis is a concern with the ultimate costs of modernity.

We turn next to the section on "Communities," which begins with Karen Hoffman's engaging portrayal of a committed group of activists on the eastern shore of a large bay in the United States who have been working to combat dioxin. Their main targets are the petrochemical companies that dot the shore like giant, squat, smoke-spewing drums. The chapter offers an array of important information about dioxin, surely one of the most insidious molecules of the twentieth century, as well as highlighting the impact of both community activism and government regulation on industrial pollution. Hoffman tracks the molecule through bodies as well as boardrooms, communities as well as industry, showing us some of its material and symbolic consequences. At the heart of her analysis is an assessment of what constitutes civic action and how communities might respond to environmental risk.

Maren Klawiter's chapter explores breast cancer activism in the context of environmental justice movements. She highlights two important, often contradictory ways of conceptualizing cancer: a biomedical model in which prevention is framed as "chemoprevention" and ill people are given toxic chemicals, and an environmental model in which toxic chemicals are suspect and prevention involves regulating or eliminating potential carcinogens before they can enter into bodies. Klawiter shows how both models have been woven into breast cancer activism, particularly that of major national advocacy groups backed, in part, by industry. She shows how various women's health groups began to more fully incorporate the environmental model as breast cancer activists collaborated with and borrowed from environmental justice movements. Yet the environmental wing of the breast cancer movement faced major challenges within groups with heavily entrenched biomedical agendas, including integration with the chemical and pharmaceutical industries. Klawiter uses the case studies in her chapter to argue for the wisdom of the precautionary principle.

Turning to communities of practice, E. J. Woodhouse chronicles the promising emergence of "green chemistry," a more environmentally benign or sustainable version of chemical science. Narrating the history of the discipline and the practice of organic chemistry, Woodhouse discusses the distinctions between "brown" and "green" chemistry, the technical potential of the newer approach, and the role of policy in fostering new and perhaps more democratic knowledge. Woodhouse not only follows the molecule, but also shows how molecules may be rearranged in line with changing social orders, especially communities of practice such as science and industry. His account raises fascinating questions about the relationship between expertise and social context, suggesting that changes in chemistry itself have a great deal to do with knowledge of the environment, the impact of industrial chemicals on human bodies, and social organization.

The fourth section of the book focuses on "Nations." In the first chapter, Susan Bell offers an insightful tale about chemical microbicides and international women's health activists. Unlike many of the other case studies in this book, which involve groups of people struggling to keep chemicals out of their bodies or to seek reparations for unwanted exposures, Bell chronicles a case in which women actively sought an industrial solution to health concerns. Here, certain groups of women wanted to bring chemicals into their bodies to prevent other, more pressing conditions such as pregnancy and HIV/AIDS or other sexually transmitted diseases. Two unlikely bedfellows, Women's Health Advocates on Microbicides (WHAM) and the Population Council came together to forge a collaboration despite previously quite different agendas. Bell's chapter showcases the ways in which molecules might form both the social and the technical glue holding together different embodied actors. Her work broadens our understanding of the place, or multiple places, of industrial chemicals in the twenty-first century. While on the surface this story may seem remotely connected to environmental health issues, we would do well to remember that population control politics are often intimately linked to environmental concerns, and not always in pro-feminist ways.

Phil Brown, Steve Zavestoski, Meadow Linder, Sabrina McCormick, and Brian Mayer narrate a timely tale of national security and environmental health: the ongoing dispute over Gulf War Illness. They argue that some 70,000 veterans of that conflict have sought treatment for illnesses related to toxic exposures in the Gulf. Yet there is widespread disagreement about the definition, etiology, and treatment of what are now called Gulf War–related illnesses (GWRIs). Drawing on a range of data, Brown et al. suggest that determining the cause of an environmental illness is far more complicated than simply tracing it to a particular chemical or molecule. Rather, they show how illness is socially constructed out of an array of factors. Pointing to the U.S. government's stress-based explanation of GWRIs as a dominant epidemiological paradigm, the authors suggest that the "nature" of an illness has as much to do with the social organization of science and medicine and with government interests as it does with molecules. They offer a rich, nuanced account of how illness definitions come into being, and why they are subject to dispute.

Finally, in closing, we return to Eastern Europe. Diana Mincyte examines the geopolitical processes by which a chemical facility in Lithuania became an agent of Sovietization in the 1960s. She documents the ways that the Kedainiai Chemical plant and its products came to symbolize the post-Stalinist, pro-science and technology version of the Soviet Union's cultural and political imperialism in Eastern Europe. Her account features fascinating details of the scope of this planned socialization, including the use of chemical products to transform landscapes, social practices, urban environments, and vulnerable Lithuanian bodies. However, the Soviet's national agenda was not unchallenged, and Mincyte's account features resistance by the local population to Soviet hegemony. In the end, she argues, the chemical plant did "modernize" the region and alienate local subjects, but in doing so, it spawned national resistance that eventually helped to topple the Soviet regime.

PART I

ENVIRONMENTS

1
Troubled Natures
Toxic Pollutants and Japanese Identity in Two Tokyo Communities

PETER WYNN KIRBY

Contemporary Japan and particularly its cities have embraced the chemical age as ardently as any society in the world. Plastics and other chemical products have become ubiquitous in nearly all spheres of social life, from household products to synthetic fabrics to high-tech industrial output. Japanese people in general, while not always forsaking traditional Chinese-influenced medical knowledge, depend also on Western-style medicine and technoscience to treat what ails them (Ohnuki-Tierney 1984; Lock 1980). And Japanese farmers, for their part, use more pesticides per hectare than those in other developed countries (OECD 1999). Yet Japan has begun to discover that, while the chemical age held great promise and provided remarkable convenience and sanitation, a downside exists as well. Chemicals, medicines, and chemical products such as plastics can bequeath side effects that gravely influence quality of life and, in doing so, penetrate discourses on health, family, nature, and national identity in Japan.

This is particularly the case with waste disposal. Japanese households and businesses in Tokyo, for example, churn out waste containing plastics and other synthetic materials at a rate that threatens to overwhelm local landfills and waste services (Waste Reduction Comprehensive Planning Office 1995; Institute for Global Environmental Studies 1999; cf. Eades 1998); this state of affairs has led the Japanese and metropolitan governments to devise aggressive strategies for waste disposal, some of which I address directly in this chapter. Japan has by far the developed world's highest emissions of dioxins, the planet's most lethal man-made family of substances (United Nations Environment Programme 1999; Institute for Global Environmental Studies 1999; World Health Organization 1999), predominantly as a result of the common practice of waste incineration there. In addition to waste incinerators, other state and industrial facilities yield chemical by-products that ravage the bodies of local residents and the environment. While the Japanese government has, by and large, taken great strides in reining in the worst of the environmental defilement that accompanied Japan's postwar surge of economic growth

(Broadbent 1998), it still has yet to grapple fully with the gravity of its waste predicament. Because the noxious effects of toxic pollution are often difficult to isolate from other environmental factors and defy easy detection (cf. Berglund 1998; Edelstein 1988), cases of toxic defilement are often fraught with ambiguities, nigh-impossible to "prove" and stubbornly resistant to successful resolution. More often than not, in Japan as elsewhere, denial is the knee-jerk reaction to this darker aspect of waste disposal. Yet toxic pollution intervenes in the lives of the Japanese I studied, affecting bodies and consciousness in a manner that profoundly influences the experience of life there.

In this chapter, I delve into the ways that toxic pollution, specifically that which results from the disposal of plastics and other appurtenances of the chemical age, negatively affects bodies as well as environments. I also examine how toxic pollution calls into question closely held tenets of Japanese identity that influence Japanese perceptions of family, nature, and national cohesion. First, I engage theoretically with links between bodies and environments, paying special attention to Japanese conceptions of nature and the body and their close relationship with national identity in Japan. Subsequently, I describe a nation/wide toxic pollution scare, largely created and exacerbated by the mass media, that brought some of these issues to the fore. I then, in turn, look at a toxic pollution protest involving a waste facility in a community not far from where I lived. An interesting comparison to the charged political atmosphere of the protest is the neighborhood community where I used to live, which received (and interpreted and sometimes distorted [cf. Thompson 1995]) information on dioxins transmitted largely through the mass media; I address the influence of this toxic pollution (that which was quantifiable and that which was perceived) on bodily health, national identity, and reproductive consciousness there. In doing so, I hope to elucidate the links between the local, the embodied, and larger discourses of "nature"[1] and nation.

Bodies and Environments: From Nature to National Identity

Embodiment scholarship engulfed the social sciences during the 1990s, partly as a result of reengagement with extant work; leaving aside the well-known work of Foucault (e.g., 1991, 1994),[2] problematizations of "the body" have been inspired by the theories of several influential twentieth-century thinkers, most notably those of Merleau-Ponty and Bourdieu. One coherent synthesis of these ideas can be found in the embodiment scholarship of anthropologist Thomas Csordas, who discerned that Merleau-Ponty's perceiving, phenomenological body needed to be supplemented with Bourdieu's socially-focused theories of practice and habitus in order to address the complexity of bodies in social contexts (Csordas 1993). This combining of Merleau-Ponty's "being-in-the-world" (Merleau-Ponty 1995) with Bourdieu's theories of habitus and practice makes possible an inclusion of the lived body in the analytical sights of the social sciences. With a topic as vast and complex as the body in society, it is perhaps not surprising that some work done under the rubric of "the body" falls short of its promise. Yet good embodiment scholarship has expanded this realm of theoretical and ethnographic inquiry, interrogating relations between body and spatial environment (e.g., Pandolfo 1989) and complex constructions of nature, culture, and gender, and the role of technologies in their negotiation (Franklin 1997; cf. Haraway 1991).

One fruitful arena for investigating the intersections between the body and its larger social milieu is the social scientific analysis of illness. A sustained focus on the somatic experience of health and illness in medical anthropology in particular has engaged with material well suited to the analysis of corporeal strategies, largely in marginalized socio-cultural settings (e.g. Desjarlais 1993; Scheper-Hughes 1992).[3] Yet there has been relatively less research done on the links between bodies and the insalubrity of "developed" environments, particularly with regard to the environmental blight of toxic pollution. Eeva Berglund's *Knowing Nature, Knowing Science* (1998) trenchantly analyzes a group of German activists' protest against a toxic waste dump near their community and the light it sheds on larger discourses surrounding global environmentalism and wieldings of the technoscientific knowledge on which the latter so often depends. Yet because Berglund's informants did not knowingly suffer from the ill effects of toxic pollution in any palpable sense, her ethnographic and theoretical work does not have the opportunity to probe into the somatic[4] experience of toxins and their symptoms.

The case of the Tokyo pollution protest I sketch out below proves informative in this regard, since most protesters were alerted to a previously-unknown toxic pollution problem when their bodies experienced debilitating symptoms of toxic poisoning; yet only a minority of the local population actually "felt" these symptoms, heightening the political register of disease poetics. This analysis has benefited from the work of Emily Martin (1994); for, in a setting not so dissimilar to the charged atmosphere of the AIDS crisis in the United States and the intensified consciousness surrounding HIV and immunity, a nationwide dioxin scare in Japan in early 1999 ushered in a political climate in which efficacious action could be taken on both local and national levels—and in which conceptions of national and cultural identity could fall into question to a greater extent than in more secure and quotidian circumstances.

Bodies and environments are closely wedded in cycles of consumption and production that blur the boundaries placed between them by socio-cultural conceptions of the two. Just as bodies take in sustenance and air from their surroundings and respond on a physiological level to variations in temperature, light, smell, and other sometimes more violent changes around them, environments to a marked extent bear the impress of manifold subtle and not so subtle human and animal interventions. It is interesting to note that, historically, Japanese society has made less of a distinction between the body and its

milieu (Kalland and Asquith 1997; Kyburz 1997; Berque 1997). Though it remains unclear to what extent contemporary, urban Japanese still conceive of
the body in this way, "nature" (i.e., the socio-cultural construct that helps societies domesticize "the environment")[5] has long been conceived as present also
in the body. Yet the Western human sciences have, historically, made sharp distinctions between the corporeal and the environmental. Edward Casey's text
Remembering (1987), well known to embodiment scholars in exploring "body
memory" and "place memory," is a revealing case. Our bodies remember place
in a very profound (and largely inarticulable) manner. This memory is often
manifested in habitual actions and other close, phenomenological engagement with milieus. While Casey enumerates ways that lived bodies respond on
cognitive and physical levels to attributes of their surroundings, his abrupt
separation of the corporeal and the environmental is problematic. Despite admitting that place and the body are bound together by mnemonic conflation
and physical fact (Casey 1987, 189), Casey still separates the two types of
memory for analytical convenience. This sort of Cartesian theoretical bias,
while on its own perhaps understandable, seems more serious when other
such traditional Western intellectual habits bleed through. For example, Casey
conceives of place, after Aristotle, as a "container" with "an internal and an external horizon" (Casey 1987, 212, 203): the singular qualities of each container,
such as landscape[6] or indoor spatial layout, are what influence the bodies contained within it. Lefebvre for his part, however, cautions against Cartesian, du-
alistic perspectives that treat space as empty, waiting to be filled. For "[s]ocial
spaces," which environments undoubtedly are "interpenetrate one another
and/or superimpose themselves upon one another" (Lefebvre 1994, 86–7, emphasis in original omitted). Writing in the seventies, Lefebvre prophetically
states that "what is overlooked is the body" in analyzing space and environment (Lefebvre 1994, 162). Yet he himself does not pursue this vector of research. In this chapter, particularly in the penultimate section, I examine the
interrelationship between bodies and environments as the former responds to
toxic chemical defilement that is, admittedly, the unintended by-product of
the progress and development that Japan has zealously embraced for over a
century.

Nationhood and national identity are interwoven with conceptions of the
natural milieu in many societies. America and Germany, for example, have
each in their own way revered wilderness as a source of strength and purity;
discourses on nature have greatly informed national identity and political
consciousness in these contexts (cf. Schama 1996; Daniels 1993). On the national level, nature and culture are both implicated in the construction of
"imagined communities" (Anderson 1983), as constructs of shared characteristics or shared history of social groups often incorporate ideas of race, place,
and distinctiveness that resonate with natural and cultural discourses. In this

vein, Marilyn Ivy indicates that "Japan" should be conceived of as a nation-culture, since ideas of culture are so intertwined with the homogeneity of the Japanese nation as a whole that the separation of these two ideas is artificial (Ivy 1995). And as constructions of nature comprise such an important component of Japanese culture and Japaneseness (Berque 1997), it is important to engage with discourses on nature, culture, and nation in order to do justice to the complexity of the Japanese milieu. While environmentalism on the national level does not command the attention and concern in Japan that it does in many Western countries (Broadbent 1998), rhetoric surrounding nature in Japan is vast and diffuse and has a profound (though subtle) influence on relations with natural surroundings (cf. Kalland and Asquith 1997). I believe this attention to and concern over "nature," though not always environmentalist or conservationist in character, contributes to a kind of environmental consciousness that can help social scientists interpret environmental issues in contemporary Japan. My evaluation of links between bodies and environments in Japan often makes reference to ideas of nature in this chapter as an acknowledgement of this relationship.

Urban Japan seems particularly apt as an example of a social milieu in which discourses on nation are politically leveraged on the twin fulcra of nature and the body. The idea of "Japan," of course, resonates on both individual and collective levels as the product of a pervasive cultural (and cultural nationalist) discourse on Japanese uniqueness. And *Japaneseness*, or the essence of being Japanese (*nihonrashisa*), exists as a multivalent, often retrospective, discursive skein of identity usually interwoven with nostalgia in present-day Japan (cf. Robertson 1998, 1991; Ivy 1995). Every citizen of Japan in his or her own way (and, too, a not inconsiderable number of systematically disenfranchised groups such as Japan-born and -schooled ethnic Koreans and other minority residents) carries ideas of what it is to be "Japanese" that inform their identity and behavior. This contested nature of identity is, of course, not exclusive to Japan—every culture plays host to this tension between competing conceptions of identity to a greater or lesser extent. What is particularly notable about Japan, however, is the extent to which the characteristics of collective Japaneseness tend to be agreed upon by otherwise disparate culture-bearers. For example, young informants, despite stressing the progressive aspects of what makes *them* contemporary Japanese, might describe collective Japaneseness according to a far more traditionalistic construct of characteristics typical of that of their elders. This rough consensus even among sometimes-polarized groups seems largely the result of the subtle yet powerful operations of tradition and nostalgia in a swiftly modernized nation, reflected in such influential conservative vehicles as nationally standardized textbooks in schools, for example—as well as ideologically biased educators (Yoshino 1992, 133–37, 143–56).[7] Notions of Japaneseness derive at least in part from the public diffusion of conservative scholarship in Japan, on which I elaborate below. One facet of Japaneseness that has an especially intriguing significance in this discussion is the fundamental importance of the idea of nature in Japanese culture.

"Nature" is a prevalent trope in contemporary Japanese society. Along with the pervasive notion that Japan is a homogeneous society with distinctive universal characteristics, such as groupism, and bearing a uniqueness that distinguishes Japan from all other nations, Japan resonates with the belief that the unique characteristics of Japanese culture derive from particularities of Japanese nature (Berque 1997; Dale 1986). This rendering of "Japanese nature" has thrived within the pseudo-scholarly genre of conservative, essentialist Japanese writing known as *nihonjinron* (or "discourses on the Japanese"), and has influenced many laypersons in a country known for collective introspection. Before delving into these highly political conceptions of nature, I give some background to the *nihonjinron* and their pervasive ideas in an attempt to sketch out one stratum of the intellectual topography of contemporary Japan.

The *nihonjinron* genre has been reviled repeatedly in Western texts for its skewed logic and facile conclusions, called "cultural essentialism" (Allison 1994, 80, 212), "crass determinism" (Berque 1997, 94), "cultural nationalism" (Yoshino 1992), and other epithets. While more visible in recent decades, "nativist" scholarship (Harootunian 1988) has operated in Japan since the Tokugawa period, when an ideology of ancient, indigenous agrarian culture was concocted by scholars in the eighteenth century in response to the looming presence and vast diffusion of Chinese culture in the institutions and language of Japan (Harootunian 1988; Ohnuki-Tierney 1993; Duus 1976). Later, pioneering ethnologist Yanagita Kunio was instrumental in creating an agrarian mythology in the first years of the twentieth century. Yanagita and his disciples turned to "native ethnology (*minzokugaku*)" (Harootunian 1998, 144)[8] in order to hunt for and preserve (and romanticize) the "pure" Japanese culture that, they perceived, was vanishing from a society bent on rapid modernization, urbanization, and adoption of Western technology and capitalism (Scheiner 1998, 67–68). These historical constructions of rural nostalgia continue to resonate in the current socio-cultural milieu of urban Japan. More than three-quarters of Japan's population now live in urban areas—this, coupled with sustained modernization and the persistent appropriation and assimilation of the Western, has led to a pining for a lost poetry of village life that has taken on vast dimensions (Robertson 1998, 1991; Ivy 1995). This affective realm, existing in the idealized precincts of cultural nostalgia, is always on the verge of "vanishing," but not quite—like Yanagita's *jōmin*, or common people, and their fragile, nature-ensconced village life, nostalgia for the countryside gains its poignancy from imagined ephemerality (Robertson 1998; Ivy 1995; Hashimoto 1998). Conservative writers (and the diffusion of their perspectives) keep these ideas of Japanese nature and Japanese uniqueness in the consciousness of a considerable number of Japanese.

This understanding of the history and political implications of constructions of the Japanese countryside is essential to the question of bodies and environments in Japan. For quasi-intellectual conservatives (and the Japanese to whom their opinions have diffused) have positioned the uniqueness of Japanese in these spatio-corporeal terms—though problematically so (cf. Dale 1986). *Nihonjinron* writers aver that the Japanese people's stereotypical traits stem from immersion in the sequestered Japanese natural milieu (Watsuji 1975; Berque 1997): for example, as the *nihonjinron* argument often goes, a history of benevolent (though changeable) climate[9] and abundance of natural resources predisposes the Japanese to lead a peaceful, nonaggressive collective agrarian existence in harmony with nature vis-a-vis carnivorous foreign peoples who slaughter livestock, fight internecine wars, and grapple with a harsh environment (Tsukuba 1969; Berque 1997, 92–93; Dale 1986, 41–46). This uniqueness of Japanese nature also resides in the Japanese body: in the face of evidence that Japanese and Koreans share ancestral roots and that even the Imperial House bears some foreign heredity (Dale 1986: 43), essentialist Japanese scholars argue that the Japanese people's heritage extends back through the millennia in an unadulterated line. This uniqueness is, not infrequently, characterized in terms of blood. *Nihonjin no chi,* or "Japanese blood," signifies the inherent Japaneseness of natives (and the undeniable otherness of foreigners) (Yoshino 1992, 118, 22–32). Thus, by extension, the Japanese gene pool (dimension of Japanese reproductive nature), sheltered in this island country (*shimaguni*), is positioned as utterly unique and pure when compared with the exogamous "alien 'horseriding nomads'" that allegedly comprise the blood mix of non-Japanese (Dale 1986, 43).

Though *nihonjinron* writings suffer from circular logic and a two-dimensional portrayal of the Western (not to mention the Japanese), these ideas about Japanese nature (and Japanese natures) do surface frequently in public discourse in the broadcast and print media. Perhaps equally as often, though, these politically charged ideas of Japaneseness come out in discussions with ordinary individuals,[10] having diffused into their thinking and behavior amid the ideological topography of the Japanese milieu. For example, more than a few of the residents of Horinouchi I interviewed brought to my attention, in almost conspiratorial tones, the fundamental difference between Europe, a hunting culture (*shuryō*), and Japan, a farming culture (*nōkō*)—thereby hinting at, in their opinion, the vast gulf between our worlds. Numerous times, informants have stressed the fact that Japan is unique in the world due to its having four distinct seasons; the four seasons (*shiki*) concept, though clearly erroneous when compared for instance to the climate of my home in Vermont, serves to emphasize the singularity of the Japanese climate (as mentioned earlier, a popular *nihonjinron* theme) and to explain the minute attention many Japanese pay (or imagine they pay) to the vicissitudes of the weather and the turn of the seasons. The much-bandied Japanese love of nature, as well as the Japanese *idea* of Japanese love of nature, reverberates throughout Japan despite the urban lifestyles of a high proportion of Japanese.

It is this incompatibility between the idealized and the concrete that makes incidents of toxic pollution in Japan a fascinating vector of inquiry regarding bodies, "nature," and nation. Such pollution interrogates closely held ideas about what it is to be Japanese and stimulates discourse on the subject that would otherwise likely lie embedded in the milieu. Furthermore, the problematic nature of the chemical age and its downside helps shed light on the promise and convenience that plastics and other chemical products were supposed to bring as well the predicament of communities that typically have to bear an unequal share of the environmental burden these synthetics generate. Inevitably, perhaps, failings in this regard are blamed as much on national and prefectural governments as on the swiftly changing times. I first sketch out the dimensions and implications of a nationwide toxic pollution scare in Japan before moving on to a specific toxic pollution protest that involves bodies, nature, environment, and the national-cultural discourses with which the former are imbued.

Toxic Anxiety: The Waste Predicament In Tokyo

News Synopsis:[11]

In February of 1999, TV Asahi's popular news program "News Station" aired a report on dioxin poisoning taking place in Saitama prefecture, a predominantly agricultural region just to the northwest of Tokyo. Citing independent sources, News Station's anchor reported that vegetables grown near the city of Tokorozawa had been found to contain a concentration of dioxins far higher than considered healthy by the government.[12] The television news report exposed a fact long known to locals in the city of Tokorozawa: that nearly sixty waste incinerators operated near the Tokorozawa area, producing dioxin-laden smoke that becomes embedded in the soil and vegetables grown nearby. As the Saitama region is well known for its spinach, among other agricultural products, this was a damning report— within days, major supermarket chains had withdrawn all Saitama vegetables from their shelves and prices had plummeted nationally. Yet soon after the broadcast, journalists and other commentators began to cast doubt on the validity of News Station's source, which turned out to be a private research institute commissioned by the program. The following week, News Station aired a retraction of sorts[13] over their choice of the word vegetable (yasai) over leafy produce (happamono), admitting that while all Saitama vegetables tested bore toxic levels somewhat above average, in fact the reported high level of dioxins was found only in tea.[14] This and subsequent reports were seized upon by TV Asahi's competitors and ricocheted between the domestic news media for a number of weeks.

The shock of the initial story (contaminated vegetables being sold and consumed all over Japan) proceeded to reports of Saitama prefecture vegetables being boycotted by supermarket chains. The following week, the Tokorozawa agricultural cooperative presented findings from a previous report showing vegetables to have relatively safe dioxin concentrations. This prompted TV Asahi to recant on some of the language of its initial report and, inevitably, very much called into question the validity of their coverage. Yet amid the fallout surrounding News Station's apparently intentional flouting of journalistic "integrity," newspapers and television stations also began to expose the wretchedly unhealthy quality of the air in Tokorozawa with its scores of reportedly unsafe incinerators in high density there. Tales of residents' struggles with dioxin pollution in the area over the years and the vast political difficulties of ameliorating the environmental situation mingled with reports from joint-ministerial government surveys of Tokorozawa's vegetables, soil, and air that proclaimed the area's agricultural produce safe for consumption. Along the way, as Japanese consumers and supermarkets hesitantly returned to buying and selling Tokorozawa produce, newspapers and television programs aired intermittent reports of the head of TV Asahi apologizing to Tokorozawa farmers and even explaining News Station's handling of the story in front of a critical Japanese parliament.

One fascinating, related turn of events developed over the following months. Prompted by the public outcry against such contamination, and almost certainly concerned that the widespread practice of incinerating waste in Japan would come under fire at a time when landfill space is fast running out in Tokyo especially,[15] the national government stepped into action. (This was an extraordinary move due to the fact that the Japanese government is typically quite inertial regarding administrative change, not to mention regarding intensification of environmental regulation of industry in a recessional climate.) An investigative commission was organized to assess the tolerable daily intake of dioxins. Ministries and agencies, in cooperation, set targets to regulate existing incinerators and limit the number of incinerators allowed to operate in close proximity to one another (a move seen as directly related to unhealthy conditions in Tokorozawa). During the course of the spring and summer, political parties agreed on a tolerable daily intake of dioxins 60 percent lower than the one previously urged by the Public Health and Welfare Ministry. They also vowed a 90 percent reduction of national dioxin emissions, at 1997 levels, by the year 2002.[16]

This ongoing dioxin news story and all manner of tangential rumor, allegation, and innuendo resonated for many months throughout my two field-sites. Though the data on which the first TV-Asahi report was based were later deemed to be less than reliable, dioxins had already been very much "in the air," so to speak, after intensive news coverage of a very real toxic pollution debacle at an incinerator outside of Osaka in 1997. Due to this and other well publicized cases, Tokyo-ites had already begun to regard the state and private incinerators within and near the capital region as necessary evils at best and at worst, a grave danger to local welfare. Therefore, the reception of information on the Tokorozawa dioxin problem, though initially based on flawed reporting, reacted with explosive information and attitudes that were already circulating within the milieu, though to a subdued, less articulated extent.

Dioxin pollution in particular commands a prominent position in the tension between the Japanese government, its waste policies, and Japan's many communities and their local health concerns. It must be said that Japan's domestic environmental situation has good points as well as bad points.[17] Yet much of Japan's daily production of more than 1 million tons of waste is incinerated. The preponderance of dioxins in the atmosphere, in soil, and in food sources such as seafood, fruit and vegetables, as well as its sometimes sensationalistic coverage by domestic news organs, helps to fan the flames of community ire and concern. Rather than evaluating these toxic anxieties in the abstract, I ground them below in the specifics of the following field-site and the articulations of informants there.

Neighborhood Tokyo

The case of the community where I lived speaks volumes in the context of an analysis of the pitfalls of the chemical age. Horinouchi[18] is a more or less middle-class residential neighborhood in southern Azuma ward, in western Tokyo. I began my ethnographic research in Horinouchi by investigating local residents' relations with the natural milieu, conceptions of nature, articulations of tradition, and environmental practices (including, for example, waste disposal and recycling, broadly defined). Soon, though, exploration of these topics progressed into discussions of the toxic perils that residents felt might (or in some cases, might not) endanger themselves and their families. Partly, this resulted from the fact that the TV Asahi/Tokorozawa dioxin pollution scare had literally seized the nation—this months-long saga caused even people living in reputedly "safe" areas far from incinerators to stop buying vegetables from Saitama prefecture and to ponder the contamination they might have unwittingly suffered up until the initial broadcast of the report. This, of course, is the value of the Tokorozawa dioxin scare for assessing the environmental consciousness of Japanese who are usually less concerned with abstract macro-environmental questions and more concerned with environmental issues that directly affect their lives, communities, and families.

In spite of Japan's reputation as a global environmental villain, relative lack of space and resources back home have forced cities like Tokyo to enforce strict waste protocols: residents divide household trash into "burnable" (*moeru/kanen gomi*) and "unburnable" (*moenai/funen gomi*) categories, as well as "bulky waste" (*sodai gomi*)—furniture, appliances, and the like. Burnable waste includes organic matter such as leftover food scraps, as well as paper products, and was typically collected two or three times a week. Unburnable waste was usually collected once a week and consists of plastics and other kinds of synthetic waste. Burnable waste is destined for Japan's many incinerators, while unburnable waste tends to end up in landfill sites. In theory, the former is organic while the latter is not. But in fact, all sorts of chlorine-based products reside in so-called "burnable" waste that can release dioxins and other chemicals into the atmosphere when incinerated.

In recent years, recycling has become a mantra of government sanitation agencies (cf. Kirby 2001: chapter 8). So in Horinouchi, for example, there is now a recyclables (*shigen*) collection day each week as well: old newspapers, plastic (PET) bottles, glass bottles, metal cans, and metal foil. Euphemistically dubbed "resources"—though, in one sense, in bulk these are relatively precious materials in a resource-poor nation—*shigen* are sometimes processed into other products of consumption like polyester shirts or fabrics, sports shoes, and so on. During the "Bubble" years, seemingly anything could be jettisoned onto the street on bulky waste day. Nowadays most desirable castaways are sold off to a new breed of companies (*risaikuru shoppu*) that have sprung up to refurbish and resell appliances and the like. Other bulky waste commands a steep charge from the government in a bid to reduce demands on landfill space.

With all the profuse Japanese rhetoric surrounding nature, against the backdrop of these waste protocols, it might seem that Tokyo-ites would be acutely sensitive to waste policies and their larger conservationist aims. But the vast majority of informants managed and sorted their trash output simply because the state enforced such behavior. Due to media exposure, however, in time toxins and the repercussions of their emission enjoyed a deeper absorption into the consciousness of residents.

Most of my informants[19] in Horinouchi mentioned dioxins in connection with questions regarding quality of life in Tokyo even before the first TV Asahi report aired; but certainly after, dioxins frequently became the subject of discussions surrounding health in the community. Of course, though informants had heard of dioxins via the mass media or the mechanisms of gossip and informal discourse, they often differed wildly in their understanding of the toxins, their dangers, and how they are produced—and this case stands as a vivid example of the permutations of mass-mediated knowledge in community settings. For example, though many residents knew that dioxins (*daiokishin*) were bad, they might have seized on different elements of news stories or hearsay that resonated with their own concerns. Many middle-aged mothers especially were worried about how the toxins can attack young children's immune, endocrine, and nervous systems (World Health Organization 1999). Reports that breast-feeding infants ingest an extremely high amount of dioxins through mother's milk were particularly unsettling.[20] Several women, like Fukushima-san, explained incidences of illness in the neighborhood in terms of dioxins: "That incinerator [nearby], right? The terrible thing is, people living around there talk about babies being born with only one arm, or fingers missing. There are miscarriages. Cancer. [. . .] I don't know what I'd do [if I were having another child]." Of course, birth defects, miscarriages, cancer—all these misfortunes befall families all over the world in every conceivable living environment. But the fact that they were being interpreted by some in terms of a newly recognized chemical poison known for attacking human reproductive systems reveals the power of toxic anxieties amid the barrage of media portrayals of environmental dangers. Particularly in a nation with a long-term declining birthrate, where increasing ages of marriage and procreation tend to crop up in conversations surrounding family and parenthood, the prospect of a toxic threat that might negatively affect a couple's ability to raise a healthy family was a poignant one.

One less publicly discussed dimension of dioxins was at first voiced indirectly by Japanese women in the neighborhood: Japanese described how, via media reports, they learned that dioxins allegedly affect the development of male genitalia. Though none of my male informants discussed this element of the effect of dioxins without prompting, their silence is telling. (One Public Health and Welfare Ministry official, who was reading aloud from a ministry report on dioxins during an interview and assumed I could not read scientific jargon in Japanese, actually skipped over a sentence mentioning this side effect of the toxin.) Japanese males' discomfort with the topic is hardly surprising— the belief that "bigger is better" is certainly not peculiar to Japanese men. (Revealingly, though technoscientific studies have determined that only testicle size is affected [e.g., Ohsako, Miyabara, et al. 2001], much of the discourse surrounding the issue mistakenly assumed that penis size was the casualty of dioxin exposure.) Though some men consented to discuss the issue, female informants were more candid. One woman in her forties, unmarried and working as an executive in a small fitness company, compared the speed with which the government reacted to the dioxin problem (touched on above) with the coterminous controversy surrounding Viagra and female oral contraceptives—at the time, while government approval for the pill had languished for twelve years, Viagra had been put on a fast track and was approved in six months. The woman put it this way: "The Japanese government is usually slow. When they do something fast, you have to be suspicious, don't you?" In male-centric Japan, these gendered dimensions of the toxic waste problem further indicate that some bodies "matter" more than others in the nation's politically fraught calculus of environmental health.[21]

Members of the community also criticized the government for not acting more resolutely in creating regulations that would rein in the production of dioxins and other environmental poisons. Many respondents explicitly lamented the use of cling-wrap or Styrofoam in grocery/packaging or take-away products. When discussions arose over dioxin emissions and waste incineration, my older informants in particular would often reminisce about the days when fish purchases at the market were wrapped in paper, rather than plastic, and when *bentō* box lunches were constructed of light wood, instead of Styrofoam. Though it is highly likely that any increase in the use of wood products would cause further serious depredation of Southeast Asian rain forests, for example (Dauvergne 1997), these informants were more concerned with avoiding the use of products that, when burned, launch dangerous toxins into the environment. As Furuhashi-san, a tavern owner in her sixties, commented:

> But I have no patience for dioxins and pollution. We're already seeing it. We can get rid of it person by person. Country by country. *Bentō* boxes and the like, we should stop using them. We should be making burnable (*moeru*) things. It's going to be the young people's world from here on. You can see it already. The earth is remembering, the air is remembering (*oboeteru*).

Like Furuhashi-san (who was more outspoken and opinionated than most), no one I interviewed, apart from active environmentalists in other parts of Tokyo, voiced any misgivings about increasing the amount of "burnable" waste. Their value judgments were, unsurprisingly, firmly anchored in the Japanese waste treatment context. In their minds, if dioxins were caused by the burning of chlorine products, including many plastics, that find their way into waste burned in Japan, then it would behoove Japan to burn products that do not contain dioxin-generating materials. A number of my informants believed that the only way to deal with the situation is for the government to step in and encourage the use of alternative materials in packaging. Though one entrepreneur, Mr. Murayama, who ran a food-catering business nearby, rejected the very notion that he would spend more money to provide eco-friendly take-away containers, more people like Mrs. Furuhashi were of the opinion that in order to avoid toxic pollution of the environment, policies should be enacted from above. (I explore the government's role in the dioxin problem more fully in the next section.) Phasing out the practice of burning millions of tons of waste annually was, for most, simply not a conceivable option. Not coincidentally, this was a sentiment shared by the Japanese and Tokyo metropolitan governments.

The gravity of the waste predicament in Tokyo is such that all efforts are being made to incinerate *more* waste, not less. Government policy promotional materials point out that landfill space in Tokyo is swiftly coming to an end (estimated to run out in the year 2001 [Waste Reduction Comprehensive Planning Office 1995]). Waste processing facilities attempt to winnow the burnable waste, mistakenly disposed of, out of the many loads of unburnable waste before sending the latter off to landfill sites in Tokyo or elsewhere. Another problem is, the more waste Tokyo carts off to waste processing sites and landfill sites in near or distant prefectures (Tokorozawa city, in Saitama prefecture, being a common and controversial destination), the more resentful citizens of these areas become toward Japan's capital. The complexity of these issues, and the economies of dealing with burnable waste at home, dictate that Tokyo's government lean in the direction of "safe" incineration at state-of-the-art "cleansing facilities" (*seisō kōjō*) within the confines of Tokyo. With this solution in mind, the Tokyo metropolitan government would like to construct additional high-tech incinerators within its twenty-three wards in order to deal with the increase of waste projected in coming years.

The proliferation of dioxins and other toxic chemical residue, detritus of an intensively consumer-driven society, points to links between living environments and the cycle of production, consumption, and waste that characterize the predicament of living in contemporary Japan. Nearly all my informants acknowledged that there had been a trade-off in developing Japan. Growth, or *seichō*, was an oft-spoken term, referring to the postwar economic prosperity that had irrevocably transformed many aspects of Japan. After Japan and its economy resurrected themselves from the rubble of the immediate postwar period, the nation enjoyed phenomenal economic growth that has widely been dubbed an "economic miracle." Unfortunately, this prosperous time also spawned the pollution debacles of the 1950s, 1960s, and early 1970s—"the world's worst health damage from industrial pollution" up until that time (Broadbent 1998: 14). The four most egregious pollution excesses that came to light during this period were the *itai-itai* disease in Tōyama, resulting from decades-long discharge of heavy metals and cadmium into a nearby river; petrochemical industrial pollution in the city of Yokkaichi, where fish became inedible and thousands of locals were exposed to severe air pollution, resulting in acute asthma problems; the notorious case of methylmercury poisoning in Minamata Bay during the 1950s and early 1960s, where hundreds were killed and thousands crippled for life; and in Nōgata prefecture, where another case of Minamata disease appeared in 1965 (Kalland and Asquith 1997, 6; Japan Environment Agency 1999). Kawasaki City, near Tokyo proper, also suffered from excessive air pollution, leading to the respiratory condition called Kawasaki disease. In addition to these more publicized problems, communities all over Japan, and urban Japan especially, complained of environmental degradation as a direct result of the headlong economic growth the nation pursued.

As a direct result of this widespread pollution, an inevitable by-product of the government's aggressive economic policies, citizens' groups rose up in protest against environmental defilement, culminating in a crescendo of activist politics in the early 1970s (Broadbent 1998, 114–23; Institute for Global Environmental Studies 1999, 1). In time, some powerful conservative LDP politicians became galvanized by the crusade as well and eventually oversaw an impressive turnaround in Japan's environmental situation by the late 1970s (Broadbent 1998, 126–27). However, as the public began to have fewer cases of extreme pollution in front of them (or broadcast to them), these activist environmental political movements lost momentum, falling far behind American and European counterparts during subsequent decades. In the absence of cases such as Minamata disease, with thousands of casualties horrifying the nation, national causes lost appeal, and Japan settled into politics as usual, though with better environmental conditions than in its recent past (Broadbent 1998, 282–95).

In the community of Horinouchi during the protest, the issue of toxic pollution called into question many deeply held notions of Japanese identity already perceived to be under threat in the complex cultural milieu that comprises Tokyo. Urban life in Tokyo hardly corresponds to the idealized construct of bucolic village life discussed above. Though this national-cultural ideal is still resonant in the urban context, it found itself under threat during the Tokorozawa scare. Dioxins' reported negative effect on the reproductive system (and thereby, their menace to idyllic social constructions of family), was a particularly worrying element. The slippage between reassuring abstract, affective ideas of nation and negative impressions of the Japanese state's earnestness in safeguarding the health of Japanese people led to tension between the local and the state that plays out more clearly in the next section.

While the overwhelming majority of Tokyo residents had no concrete physical ailment that could be tied directly to dioxin poisoning, and therefore was able to keep the subject at something of a psychological distance, one community near where I lived in Western Tokyo was riven by a toxic pollution protest involving dioxins and other chemical toxins. I first evaluate the embodied experience of common symptoms contracted soon after the commencement of operations of a new waste facility in the middle of the neighborhood. I then assess the effect of the above media event (and the strident national reaction it provoked) on relations between local and state "bodies" and the development of the protest.

The Poetics of Embodied Toxic Illness: "Azuma Disease" and Its Victims

One night in May 1996, Miyamoto Yōko awoke unable to breathe. Very frightened and basically incapacitated, she managed to call a neighbor who hurried over to help and look after her until the ambulance arrived shortly after to rush her to the hospital. Though Miyamoto-san was able, under care, to recover somewhat, she remained concerned because this was only the most acute episode of a condition that had been worsening for about a month. At the start, she had suffered from some headaches and breathing problems. But these symptoms had gradually worsened until she developed painful migraines and her respiration had become troublesome. Her eyes burned. Not long after, she was released back to her home to recuperate, and the symptoms recurred, increasing her sense of anxiety.

Miyamoto-san is a plucky woman in her sixties with a high-pitched voice that cracks and falters slightly while recounting her story. Modestly, she explains that while she had never enjoyed perfect health, she had probably been not so different from the norm, and the sudden decline in her health was dramatic and unusual. She insists that she suspected nothing when she began wondering whether some external factor might have brought about this change in her health.

Kimura-san, a soft-spoken man in his fifties who works as a playground monitor and self-styled nature and ecology instructor at the local middle school, tried to help his friend Miyamoto-san when he heard about her emergency room episode and her condition's inscrutable etiology. According to Kimura-san, he searched around the neighborhood looking for construction projects, businesses, and so on that might have been producing unhealthy fumes that could have affected the elderly woman. Some residents had complained over the years about a nearby highway that gives off copious exhaust fumes (*haiki-gasu*), especially during the near-gridlock of Tokyo's rush-hour traffic. But the highway had been there for some time, and Miyamoto-san's complaints had been relatively sudden. While Kimura-san felt no such symptoms himself, he felt obliged to investigate. He thought he might be able to discover something simply due to his long history of living in the neighborhood. He recounts:

> One morning, I went over to the [new] waste transfer facility (*gomi chūkeisho*). The facility isn't an incinerator, and I didn't really think there would be smoke or whatever that would have an effect on Miyamoto-san. But I went anyway, since there weren't really any other places [to check]. . . . I entered the park over there [under which the waste facility was built], sat under the exhaust ventilation tower, and waited awhile. About an hour later, my eyes started to hurt and water, and my throat began to get sore. . . . Not much later, I went home—the symptoms gradually subsided until I felt better again.

During this same period, a number of other members of the suburban community began to realize that they shared common symptoms: burning eyes, respiratory problems, skin outbreaks, headaches, loss of taste, acutely swollen lymph nodes, and so on.[22] One woman in her twenties, who had recently moved to the area, related her condition: "I just had a miscarriage. Lately, I've increasingly been having unexplained bodily illness. Lack of energy, weariness, dullness (*darusa*), but even when I get a [medical] examination, there's no abnormality [that they can find]." Another woman, in her thirties, stated: "In the past I've been prone to terrible allergies [. . .] during the summertime. But this year, worse than any time before, it's been so severe that I can't sleep at night

[...] I have two children, ages eleven and two, and both of them have slowly started becoming allergy-prone as well (nose and skin). I'm very worried, thinking that my children will inhale things that are even worse in the future." A woman approximately the same age said, "Since I moved here (it might just be the fault of aging), my dependence on headache medicine and other medicine has increased markedly. Since I have a small child and I am thinking about having another, I'm hoping we can live in an environment where we'll feel at ease (*anshin shite kuraseru kankyō*)."

Contrary to the criticisms of detractors in the neighborhood (who did not suffer symptoms, and who seemed to have ulterior motives in portraying their community, and their investments, in a favorable light), the epidemic was not limited only to women (in the critics' minds, hypochondriac women). For instance, one man in his twenties who had recently moved to the area reported: "From the beginning, I've had a weak stomach, but [these days] I've got terrible diarrhea. I often catch colds. There have been times when I've had a cough for two months. I always suffer from diarrhea and a throat that feels out of sorts (*fukaikan*) [...] Since I work at home all day long, I'm very worried about this." A man in his thirties, who had lived in the area only two years, reported these symptoms: "I tire easily, and I've become prone to lose my temper. I've lost eight kilos . . . I've also noticed that the trees in front of the facility's ventilation tower are withering." A man in his sixties who had lived in the area for thirty-five years, for his part, had this to say: "This year, it has become easier for me to catch cold, and moreover, it has gotten harder to get better. In particular, when I get a cough, it becomes extremely painful and hard. This August, I got sick three times. . . . In the morning when I open the window, a strange, bad smell comes from outside." Hundreds of residents within 500 meters of the facility reported grave symptoms along the lines of these responses. One woman showed me photographs of her and her family members' bodies: swollen lymph nodes, swollen joints, acute skin rashes, discolorations, and so on. Though seemingly of two minds about it at first, she then went on to display a picture of her breasts, with their distended lymph nodes. The act suggested that the disease had taken away all shame, and that no taboos remained (cf. Edelstein 1988, xv).

In the months after the facility commenced operations, residents began comparing symptoms amongst themselves, to their surprise finding commonalities in how their bodies were sensing and responding to the environment. Originally through these informal, personal networks, and by virtue of an extended discourse amongst the neighborhood that began largely through gossip and hearsay, the most seriously afflicted of the "victims" (*higaisha*) began to meet up and discuss their health problems. By July of 1996, they had organized into a formal protest group named the Group to End Azuma Disease (*Azuma-byō wo Nakusu-kai*, hereafter by the English acronym GEAD), an entity that began to lobby the ward and metropolitan governments to close down the waste facility in question. Though the exact cause of the illness was at first a mystery, residents began framing their discourse surrounding the disease in terms of dioxins, as well as other lesser-known toxic chemical substances (*kagaku bushitsu*), about the time when these began to garner exposure in the mass media. They also, two years later, commissioned a survey by a scientist who had performed tests for the Public Cleansing Bureau; he found scores of dangerous chemical substances in addition to dioxins in the atmosphere of the community, even after employees at the waste transfer facility had made attempts to filter its emissions (GEAD documents 1999).[23] I further examine these residents' embodied relationship to the illness below after describing the waste facility and delving into the state's role and motivations in introducing the facility into the community—and its reluctance to close the facility down.

The waste transfer facility was the result of a concerted Tokyo metropolitan effort to make the burgeoning waste problem more cost-effective and manageable. With the millions of tons of waste that the Tokyo area produces each year, one way to deal with "unburnable" waste more economically is to compress it together with extreme force and then either deposit it in local landfill or, more likely, transport it out of the city, where distant rural communities charge by the truckload. This, in a nutshell, explains the waste facility in Izawa. As a waste transfer facility, or *chūkeisho*, the Izawa facility served as a relay station between the relatively small trucks that navigate the labyrinthine byways of neighborhood Tokyo to collect community waste and the much larger container trucks that take the waste to its final destination. The smaller trucks dump the waste into enormous rectangular compressors within the facility that violently pound the refuse together before sliding the compacted mass into a container on the other side. These containers are then what is lifted onto waiting larger trucks to be transported away beyond the city limits. Recyclables such as plastic bottles, glass containers, and metal cans are also sorted and taken away for processing.

The mystery of this facility, and source of bitter controversy surrounding Azuma disease, was that because there was no *incineration* of waste there, it was difficult to explain how the toxins measured in the community were released into the atmosphere. The members of GEAD claimed that, *somehow*, toxins are released through the extremely forceful compression of plastics deep within the bowels of the Izawa waste facility. GEAD members reasoned that, as the air leaving the facility through the ventilation tower was from the beginning treated only to filter odors, rather than more dangerous substances, the alleged toxins had been discharged directly into the air and wafted away over the neighborhood on usually northerly-southerly winds. And as the facility was apparently the first of its kind in the world, the protesters went on to claim that science had not had a chance to verify the dangers of compressing plastic in order to protect such residents as themselves.

The other mystery in Izawa was that not everyone felt the symptoms of Azuma disease. A study commissioned by GEAD members in 1998 found that nearly 400 of the residents living within 500 meters of the waste facility (or roughly ten percent) had manifested aggravated symptoms common to Azuma disease since the facility became operational. Protesters explained this as the result of different *kagaku-bushitsu kabinshō*, or chemical sensitivity. According to the GEAD, some individuals—like Miyamoto-san—with a hypersensitivity to toxins fell prey to the alleged poisonous toxins almost immediately. Others carried on with their lives as though nothing had changed in their environment (though their health still suffered, GEAD protesters stressed, as a result of daily exposure). Most of the rest of the population, including the roughly 400 residents afflicted with varying symptoms of Azuma disease, fell somewhere between these two extremes. Due to the vicissitudes of chemical sensitivity, then, a facility might have a grave effect on a fraction of the population while seeming relatively innocuous to the majority—such was the case, protesters reasoned, in Izawa. To be sure, theirs was a controversial claim, one that was at first mocked and then more systematically attacked by government officials since the protesters' campaign began. (Due to constraints of space, and the stated aims of this chapter, I do not delve here into the saga of the years of wrangling between protesters and the state [cf. Kirby 2001; chapters 3 and 8].) Even in cases where more conventional arguments prevail, toxic pollution and the illnesses that result from it are extremely difficult to prove. Since most chemicals, even such lethal substances as dioxins, are statistically rather harmless in small amounts and perilous in larger amounts, the assessment of risk comes down to scientific analysis and shifting definitions, much of which are open to interpretation, influence and downright sabotage (e.g., Berglund 1998).

This brings up a key point of interest of the protest, and an important difference vis-à-vis Eeva Berglund's (1998) significant findings in Germany: the afflicted in Izawa *knew* that there was a toxic problem because they registered it with their bodies; they felt this was without question an "unnatural" state for their health to be in; and this was an embodied knowledge that came to override any other social logic, including the "scientific" data produced by the waste facility in the early stages attesting to the safety of the facility. While the GEAD might, as a group, have eventually taken recourse to technoscientific knowledge to give their claims legitimacy, they only sought under the raiments of science to persuade those who weren't chemically sensitive enough to contract debilitating symptoms about that which they, the protesters, already knew. This presents a very different model than that which Berglund puts forward with her German opponents against the toxic waste dump in Hessberg. Berglund makes the point repeatedly that one striking characteristic of toxic pollution is that it is discernible only through recourse to technoscientific discourse: "what defines the issue is language, since the source of danger is imperceptible to the senses" (Berglund 1998, 48). This is due to the fact that, "Often a substance is considered harmless in small quantities, and only high concentrations make it hazardous. However, exact boundaries between harmless and harmful concentrations are difficult to establish. . . . It depends on human judgment" (Berglund 1998, 46). Of course, I very much agree with her latter point as regards the difficulty of defining toxicity. But while definition of the issue through language alone might have been the case in Germany, due to the precise nature of the alleged toxic pollution in that setting, in my field-site there were immediate repercussions from the advent of toxic pollution. These were embodied repercussions that set the tone of the debate and brought the issue beyond mere rhetorical battles over definitions. Interestingly, the GEAD members used the verb "to feel"(*kanjiru*) when describing symptoms of Azuma disease. The use of this verb rather than some other more clinical term, like "contract" or "catch" (*kakeru*) leaves the impression (at least on the part of the GEAD faithful) that the "disease" is out there and, though some might not feel it, they are affected by the toxins involved (cf. Ohnuki-Tierney 1984, 54 on *taishitsu*, or types of bodily constitution and their associations in Japanese culture).

One complicating factor, however, was that most of the members who were afflicted with Azuma disease balanced their health against their desire to remain in their homes, and chose to leave Izawa. The GEAD was, therefore, a kind of long-distance network dedicated not only to the eradication of the alleged cause of their misfortune, but also to the nostalgic memory of what their lives had once been in their community. As Shinoda-san, a woman in her late fifties, related one day in a coffee shop in Kodaira City, her new home for two years at the time: "I was desperately lonely after leaving [Izawa]. Sometimes I go back for coffee and so on, but it's not the same." Though her health, like that of other self-exiled protesters (whose conflicted memories of Izawa invariably included the specter of the waste facility as a reviled landmark in their nostalgic articulation and conception of the erstwhile community [cf. Lynch 1960]), eventually started getting better once she'd left the toxic environs of the waste facility, it was a long time before her life returned to normal: "It took the better part of a year to get better once I'd left [*Izawa*]. In addition to the headaches and the skin rashes, these shooting pains used to go down my leg and I absolutely couldn't walk. Slowly, though, I began to feel [the disease] less and less."

In the end, it appears that it was the Tokorozawa dioxin scare in early 1999 and the exposure it lent to Japan's toxic predicament that sparked a heated public reaction to toxic defilement and gave a considerable boost to the Izawa protesters' fortunes. In such a political climate, informants and government officials explained, it became extremely difficult to cling to the status quo. Before dioxins had become big news, the GEAD had labored mightily for months to make their protest a success, but resistance in the bureaucracy had stalled their campaign for well over a year. Suddenly, during the spring and summer of 1999, the newly elected mayor[24] of Azuma ward opened the case and evaluated the GEAD environmental complaint for possible reference to the Tokyo metropolitan government. The waste facility is still in operation, though a government study is underway to determine its viability. In the meantime, those suffering from symptoms of toxic pollution are having their medical bills reimbursed by the government.

Conclusions

If there is anything to be learned from ethnographic fieldwork in Tokyo, it is that many Japanese informants are conflicted over whether the chemical lives they have chosen over recent decades have brought the much-vaunted promise that they anticipated. Narratives of informants—whether merely reflecting anxiety over toxic dangers (as was the case with my field-site in Horinouchi), or voicing toxic suffering and recovery (as with Izawa)—were characterized by the knowledge that life in Japan had changed since the post-war surge in economic growth. The bitter fruits of the chemical age, as evidenced by toxic pollution debacles either portrayed in the media or experienced in a community, led a not-inconsiderable number of Japanese to vociferous castigation of environmental degradation in a society bent on consumption of resources and generation of waste.

Though informants in both field-sites perpetuated (under specific circumstances, such as during local festivals or in other thematized domains of the leisure sphere) long-standing, idealized discourses on "nature" in Japan and the Japanese people's supposedly uniquely harmonious relations with the natural milieu, these were often phrased in ways that contrasted contemporary (often polluted) urban life with that in rural communities more in line with Japanese imaginings of national identity and traditional values. It is perhaps not surprising that those afflicted with what came to be called Azuma disease were considerably less likely to take recourse in idealized conceptions of Japanese nature—with the insalubrious consequences of Japan's contemporary chemical transformations so readily at hand, these afflicted found common imaginings of nature in Japan (and Japanese interactions with the natural milieu) far less satisfying against the backdrop of defilement of bodies and environments in Tokyo and Japan more generally.

In this sense, the protesters and residents suffering from Azuma disease voiced opinions very much informed by a Western environmentalist perspective. (For a more comprehensive mapping of this discursive shift, see also Kirby [forthcoming].) There was a palpable sense, among these informants, that Japan had gone astray and that the state needed to be enlightened from beyond national boundaries. (The recurring political significance in Japan of *gaiatsu*, or "pressure from the outside" [i.e., international pressure], is interesting with respect to these informants' perspectives.) There was also a much stronger sense (compared to my ethnographic findings before dioxins had mushroomed in the media) that idealized positionings of nature in Japan, and their integral relationship with the idea of nation, were less able to mitigate interrogations of state failures to safeguard the health of its citizenry. Government attempts in recent years to tackle the waste predicament in Japan, particularly through robust recycling initiatives, will perhaps go some way toward rehabilitating the state's Confucian image as benevolent protector of the common good.[25] Yet the Japanese state will have a difficult (if not impossible) task in coping with the bodily and environmental traumas, engendered by toxic pollution, that I witnessed during my research.

2
Indoor Air Pollution
Environmental Inequality Inside

ALLISON SHORE

Since World War II, we have experienced the rapid chemicalization of our daily lives. We come into contact with chemicals indoors in our homes, schools, and workplaces. They have become such a "normal" part of living that we often do not even notice them—while engaging in simple activities such as cleaning the house or taking a shower, we can expose our bodies to a wide range of synthetic formulations. Despite their invisibility, exposure to these substances can have short-term and long-term adverse effects on our health. While the public is largely unaware of the risks, researchers within the U.S. Environmental Protection Agency (EPA) are concerned about them.

From 1979 through the late 1980s, EPA Total Exposure Assessment Measurement (TEAM) Studies measured and compared individuals' exposure to toxics, specifically volatile organic chemicals [VOCs] and pesticides, from indoor and outdoor sources (Wallace 1991). Led by Dr. Lance Wallace, TEAM researchers conducted their studies in locations where outdoor air pollution was significant—in agricultural areas and near petrochemical plants in the United States. The findings were surprising. Indoor air pollution exceeded outdoor air pollution, sometimes quite dramatically:

> US Environmental Protection Agency (EPA) studies of human exposure to air pollutants indicate that indoor levels of pollutants may be 2–5 times, and occasionally more than 100 times, higher than outdoor levels. These levels of indoor air pollutants may be of particular concern because it is estimated that most people spend about 90 percent of their time indoors. (U.S. EPA 1995b, 1)

Although the TEAM studies made EPA more aware of the significance of indoor air pollution as a problem, regulation does not reflect these findings. As Wallace observed, EPA priorities do not reflect actual risks:

> All four TEAM Studies . . . made possible the discovery that, for nearly 50 or so targeted pollutants, personal exposures exceeded outdoor levels

by large margins. The conclusion . . . is that the major sources of exposure are personal activities and consumer products. This result is at odds with most existing environmental regulation which generally does not deal with products or with indoor air in homes, in favor of regulating "major" stationary and mobile sources. These sources, however, provide only between 2–25 percent of personal exposure to most of the two dozen or so toxic and carcinogenic VOCs and pesticides included in the TEAM studies. (Wallace 1993, 135)

Wallace's reports and publications were not the only ones that identified the need for more regulatory attention to indoor air. In 1987, EPA published the three-volume report *Unfinished Business: A Comparative Assessment of Environmental Problems.* In this now somewhat controversial[1] report, EPA experts ranked thirty environmental problems according to cancer risk, noncancer health risk, ecological risk, and welfare (economic) effects. The Cancer Work Group ranked "Indoor Air Pollutants other than Radon" and "Consumer Exposure to Chemicals"[2] as the fourth highest priorities (they tied for the number 4 slot). The report also ranked both categories as posing high noncancer health risks. As a result, the authors concluded:

The ranking by risk . . . does not correspond well with the EPA's current program priorities. Areas of relatively high risk but low EPA effort include: indoor radon; indoor air pollution; . . . consumer products; and worker exposures. (U.S. EPA 1987, xv)

Four years after the publication of *Unfinished Business,* attention to indoor air pollution was still not up to speed. In 1991, a GAO report to the U.S. Senate noted, "in fiscal year 1990 the research funding for the national air quality standards was $18.4 million, more than four times greater than the $4.3 million for indoor air research" (U.S. GAO 1991, 6).

If the goal of EPA is to minimize exposures to the most common sources of toxic chemicals, regulating sources of indoor air pollution should be given high priority—but it is not. This raises two questions: Why is there a discrepancy between risk and policy? And, what are the consequences of this discrepancy?

Beginning with background on the health risks associated with indoor air pollution from volatile organic compounds, I will review possible causes for the discrepancy between the risks posed and the lack of regulatory priority—including inadequacy of existing regulation, industry blockage of new legislation, and policy maker framing of indoor air pollution as a "private" problem. I will then examine the current form of EPA indoor air quality (IAQ) policy.

As I show, by analyzing EPA technical documents, policy statements, and brochures created specifically for public education, the current policy emphasizes mass education, consumer choice, and commodified responses rather than restricting production and use of substances the EPA classifies as harmful. The cornerstone of EPA indoor air quality (IAQ) policy is "informing" the U.S. public of the risks and hazards posed by indoor air polluting substances so that individuals can take action or "make informed decisions" to protect themselves and their loved ones. However, rather than protecting an undifferentiated public, this strategy can only protect middle-class, suburban homeowners—those who do not fit this description are unlikely to be empowered to enact the strategies EPA recommends.

This narrow focus for protection stands to exclude not only the economically marginalized, but also children, the elderly, women, renters and transient populations, and people of color (who disproportionately comprise the economically marginalized). Ironically, these groups do not inhabit the normative white adult male bodies upon which most environmental health risk research has been based, making it likely, especially in the case of children, that even greater protections are necessary for these populations. As a result, current IAQ policy promotes environmental inequality by differently protecting people based on race, class, gender, and age—leaving non-normative bodies at greater risk.[3]

Indoor Air Pollutants 101

Many of the objects and materials that compose indoor spaces, as well as many of the products we use inside those spaces can be potential sources of indoor air pollution.[4] Although I focus my analysis on chemicals, these are not the only sources of indoor air pollution.[5] Indoor air pollutants can be biological, such as molds, dust mites, or cat dander, or can be created as a by-product of combustion (for example, from cooking or heating).

The primary indoor chemical pollutants are VOCs. VOCs are compounds that become gases at room temperature. They can be emitted from either solids or liquids, for example from furniture or cleaning products (U.S. EPA et al. 1994, 12). Scientists generally refer to this process of emission as "outgassing." Almost all exposure to VOCs is through inhalation of gases, rather than through skin contact (U.S. EPA et al. 1991, 89).

As of 1991, researchers had identified over 900 kinds of VOCs in indoor air (U.S. EPA et al. 1991, 88). A few of the most prevalent include formaldehyde, benzene, p-dichlorobenzene, methylene chloride, and perchloroethylene (U.S. EPA et al. 1994; U.S. EPA et al. 1991; Wallace 1991). Specific examples of products that emit these VOCs include moth balls, air fresheners, toilet bowl deodorizers, disinfectants and degreasers, dry-cleaned goods, perma-pressed clothing or drapes, stored or applied paints and paint thinners, solvents, varnishes, perfumes, cosmetics, lead-based paints, white-out fluids, indelible ink pens, carpets, pesticides, and wood paneling (U.S. EPA et al. 1991, 94–95). In 1987, the EPA estimated formaldehyde, methylene chloride, p-dichlorobenzene and asbestos (not a VOC) in consumer products to cause 100–135 cases of cancer per year (U.S. EPA 1987, 89).

Surprisingly, taking a hot shower or washing dishes puts us into contact with yet another common VOC—chloroform. Part of a group of chemicals known as trihalomethanes (THM's), chloroform is a naturally produced by-product of the chlorination process. When water is heated, chloroform gas is released that we then inhale. In addition to chloroform, if other contaminants are present in the water (such as pesticides in well-water, or MTBE), these too can volatilize and form gases in the home. In 1987, EPA estimated disinfection by-products and radon in public drinking water to account for 400–1000 cases of cancer annually (U.S. EPA 1987, 72). As a result, the *Unfinished Business* report considered "drinking water as it arrives at the tap" a serious concern (U.S. EPA 1987).

In addition to cancer, VOCs can cause a variety of short-term and long-term health effects depending on the particular chemical and the dose. Short-term effects include "fatigue, headache, drowsiness, dizziness, weakness, joint pains, peripheral numbness or tingling, euphoria, tightness in the chest, un-steadiness, blurred vision, skin irritation, irritation of the eyes and respiratory tract, and cardiac arrythmias" (U.S. EPA et al. 1991, 90). VOCs can also act as a narcotic, depressing the central nervous system (Ibid.). Long-term effects include liver and kidney damage. Although carcinogenic chemicals generally cause more alarm, chemicals with immediate and acute effects can cause significant pain and suffering as well. After repeated exposures some people can become sensitized, causing them to become quite ill when exposed to even minute amounts of these substances.

While researchers have documented the potential health effects of a handful of the most common VOCs, no research to date has looked at the synergistic effects. In other words, in our daily lives we rarely encounter just one indoor pollutant or harmful substance at a time, rather we encounter them in hundreds of different combinations over our lifetimes. Both the long-term and short-term effects of combined exposures have been greatly understudied.[6] Also greatly understudied are the risks posed by these chemicals to so-called "vulnerable populations"—children and people with smaller-than-adult-male bodies, elderly, chronically ill, or others who fall outside the "normative" adult male population.[7] For example, the EPA Office of Children's Health Protection stresses how important differences between the bodies and behavior of children put them at potentially greater risk:

(Children) are not little adults. (They) breathe more air, drink more water, and eat more food, pound for pound, than adults. When (they) play, (they) crawl and put things in their mouths. This could increase (their) exposure to potential pollutants. (Their) body systems are still developing, and are less able to metabolize, detoxify, and excrete these pollutants compared to adults. As a result, (they) are more vulnerable to many toxic environmental pollutants. (U.S. EPA, Office of Children's Health Protection website 2002)

At the same time, EPA acknowledges that little if any existing risk data, upon which regulation is based, has included specific assessments on the impact to children.[8] As such, they conclude:

> The array of environmental threats facing children today—and the uncertainties in the adequacy of current protections derived principally to protect adults but that may not do enough to protect our children—will require great care and commitment to address. (U.S. EPA 1996, np)

Thus chemical-laden products and building materials literally surround us. In a sense, we live in a "chemical soup," with yet to be determined long-term consequences to our own bodies, and those of future generations. The pervasiveness of these chemicals is worrisome, as is our overall lack of awareness of them. Even more disturbing is the fact that policy makers, specifically at the EPA and the U.S. Consumer Product Safety Commission (CPSC), do know of the harmfulness of these chemicals, classifying many of them as "known" or "probable" human carcinogens or "hazardous air pollutants" (including benzene, formaldehyde, methylene chloride, and p-dicholorobenzene), yet they have not been able to ban or heavily restrict their use.[9] Instead, they have mounted a campaign of informing consumers, "dialoguing" with industry, and promoting commodified solutions. In the next section, I will explore the question of why EPA has not focused more regulatory attention on indoor air pollution, followed by an in-depth analysis of the agency's current approach to the problem.

Discrepancy Between Risk and Regulation—Why?

There are many possible ways to explain the discrepancy between EPA's knowledge about indoor air pollutants and the lack of regulatory attention it devotes them. In the past, the EPA itself has blamed lack of public interest in indoor air (U.S. EPA 1987, 93, 95–96) as well as lack of "legislative mandate"[10] (U.S. GAO 1991, 6) as primary causes of inattention. However, an examination of current statutory authority over toxic and hazardous substances, as well as of the history of four years of attempted but failed legislation, reveals that industry has largely shaped EPA's current approach.

Inadequacy of Current Regulation

Although no legislation currently exists that specifically addresses indoor air pollution, several agencies have regulatory power over VOCs through existing statutory authority. In fact, so many agencies have jurisdiction over some aspect of indoor air pollution that this in itself impedes action. Although EPA is the lead agency for indoor air pollution overall,[11] the Consumer Product Safety Commission (CPSC), Department of Energy (DOE), Department of Health and Human Services (DHHS), National Institute for Occupational Safety and Health (NIOSH), and Occupational Safety and Health Administration (OSHA) all regulate some aspect of indoor air pollution. For example, CPSC is the lead agency on consumer exposures to harmful substances, while OSHA and NIOSH handle worker exposures to the same substances. Although their efforts are supposed to be coordinated through an organization called the Interagency Committee on Indoor Air Quality (CIAQ), according to the GAO, CIAQ "lacks a clear charter that establishes the roles and responsibilities of all federal agencies and defines how the agencies will work together to address indoor air issues" (U.S. GAO 1991, 6–7). CIAQ's primary accomplishment as of 1991 was the publication of a list outlining each agency's IAQ problems activities (Ibid.). Since that time, they have focused their efforts on information brokerage—publishing brochures and resource lists, and creating an IAQ information clearinghouse.

Even within EPA, jurisdiction is split among a multitude of offices: the Office of Air and Radiation, Office of Research and Development, Office of Pollution Prevention and Toxics, and the Office of Pesticide Programs being just a few.

This fragmentation of responsibility across agencies and offices means that no one agency is making sure that progress is being made—and no agency is accountable for improving IAQ. Additionally, these regulatory bodies can come into conflict when they decide to take different approaches to the same chemical, as when the CPSC and EPA both tried to deal with formaldehyde (Fagin and Lavelle 1996).

In addition to fragmented authority, the statutory authorities that do exist have proven inadequate in addressing indoor air pollutants. It would seem that the 1976 Toxic Substances Control Act (TSCA) significantly empowers EPA to regulate or ban harmful indoor air polluting substances. According to EPA,

> TSCA grants EPA broad authority to control chemical substances and mixtures that present an unreasonable risk of injury to health and the environment. EPA has authority to require testing of chemical substances and mixtures by prohibiting or restricting their manufacture, processing, distribution and disposal; review new chemicals and their intended uses; and impose labeling or notification requirements. (U.S. EPA 1993)

However, in its first twenty years of existence, EPA successfully regulated only nine substances under TSCA (Fagin and Lavelle 1996, 138). In contrast, as of 1991, the GAO estimated 60,000 chemicals were available in U.S. commerce (U.S. GAO 1992). Regulators know very little about the vast majority of these substances (U.S. EPA 1987, 16).[12] Why hasn't EPA used TSCA to regulate more chemicals, especially those that it classifies as known, probable, or possible human carcinogens, which are common ingredients in consumer products?

One problem relates to the agency's need to rely on data supplied by the manufacturers themselves. TSCA permits EPA to demand such data from manufacturers, but does not require or allocate resources for EPA to conduct such studies itself. TSCA also allows manufacturers to produce and market chemicals while they are conducting the studies. Health and environmental studies routinely take years, and there is no incentive for the manufacturer to hurry—especially if it may show their product to be hazardous. In essence, TSCA assumes a substance to be harmless unless someone proves otherwise (Fagin and Lavelle 1996). In the end, TSCA places the burden of proof on the public and federal agencies to show that a chemical is dangerous, rather than on the manufacturers to demonstrate that they are safe before they are put on the market.

The language of TSCA itself poses another significant problem. TSCA not only requires that the agency prove a substance poses an "unreasonable risk" to health or the environment, but section 6 states that any regulation they enact must be the "least burdensome" to its manufacturers. Rosenthal, Gray, and Graham (1992) argue that the narrative nature of TSCA, which leaves terms such as "unreasonable risk" undefined, "invite EPA to make determinations . . . which will vary from decision to decision based on a discretionary balancing of diverse factors" (Rosenthal et al. 1992, 304). In other words, the necessity of proving "unreasonable risk," in its vagueness, affords EPA administrators significant room for interpretation.[13] It also leaves the agency vulnerable to industry pressure. In practice, the finding of "unreasonable risk" requires a very stringent standard of evidence (Dickson 1994, 20), and mandates that regulators consider economic costs as part of the determination of whether a chemical poses "unreasonable risk." Finally, under section 6, even if EPA determines a substance to pose "unreasonable risk," it is unlikely to remove it entirely from the market. More likely, they would impose "less burdensome" regulatory options such as warning labels or use restrictions.

Often, when EPA does move to ban or heavily restrict a chemical, the manufacturers will take them to court. Such was the case in 1989 when they attempted to ban the use of asbestos. The court overturned the ban on the basis that "the EPA had failed to consider whether regulatory controls other than an outright ban would reduce the level of risk of asbestos to an adequate level" (Dickson 1994, 21). Thus, EPA had violated section 6 of TSCA that requires the least burdensome regulation be imposed.

The Federal Hazardous Substances Act (FHSA), under the jurisdiction of the Consumer Product Safety Commission, is similarly problematic. FHSA permits CPSC to regulate consumer products that "because of toxicity, irritation, sensitization, or other characteristics, may cause substantial personal injury or substantial illness during or as a proximate result of any customary or reasonably foreseeable handling or use" (Dickson 1994, 22). Like TSCA, however, FHSA requires a determination of "unreasonable risk" to human health, a finding that is difficult to achieve since again, regulators must apply a cost-benefit analysis.[14] Although the CPSC has successfully banned a few substances, it too has been thwarted by the legal system and the burden of unreasonable risk. In 1983, the courts overturned its attempted ban of urea-formaldehyde foam insulation on the basis of insufficient evidence of unreasonable risk (Dickson 1994, 22).

Asbestos and formaldehyde have a long history of federal regulatory efforts, and are undoubtedly two of the most well studied hazardous substances. EPA considers both to have significant adverse health effects. They classify formaldehyde as a probable human carcinogen, and have extensively documented its noncancer health effects, especially on the respiratory system. Additionally, EPA scientists have accumulated extensive evidence of asbestos's capacity to cause cancer and other lung diseases. The inability of EPA or CPSC to successfully remove these two substances that they have studied so extensively does not bode well for the future use of TSCA or the FHSA to ban harmful indoor air pollutants. It is thus not surprising that manufacturers lobbying against new indoor air pollution regulation advocated language similar to that of TSCA and FHSA.

Fagin and Lavelle (1996) argue that even the language of TSCA was not accidental. Rather, the "unreasonable risk" and "least burdensome" criteria reflect chemical manufacturers' intense lobbying efforts to ensure that they would be protected from having their products banned. Fagin and Lavelle document how industrial interests pour millions of dollars into congressional campaigns, hire academic researchers to create and exploit scientific uncertainty, and operate intense public relations efforts to persuade legislators and the public that hazardous products are safe (Fagin and Lavelle 1996, xx). Thus, the insufficiencies of TSCA and FHSA have greatly helped manufacturers keep hazardous indoor air polluting substances on the market and in consumer products.

Failed Legislation: The Indoor Air Quality Acts of 1991, 1993, 1994, 1995

In recognition of the inadequacy of existing regulation, Congress considered indoor air pollution legislation in 1991, and then every year between 1993 and 1995. The first incarnation of this legislation appeared as S. 455, the Indoor Air Pollution Act of 1991. The senate passed this bill, but it was never enacted. Subsequent legislation was introduced in both chambers, beginning with H.R. 1930 (Indoor Air Pollution Act of 1993), H.R. 2919 and S. 656 (Indoor Air Pollution Act of 1993/1994), and then H.R. 933 (Indoor Air Pollution Act of 1995). During these years, the text of the legislation changed, as its sponsors "attempted to ease industry concerns and win Republican votes" (Congress and the Nation 1998, 431). Below, I will provide a rough overview of the legislation and industry response. I will focus on S. 656 and H.R. 2919, as Congress held hearings on both of these bills.

The original version of H.R. 2919 allocated resources for indoor air quality research, information dissemination, and voluntary training programs for contractors. However, it also would have directed EPA to compile a list of "common indoor air hazards," and to "issue guidelines as necessary to identify, eliminate, or prevent indoor air hazards" (H.R. 2919, 103rd Cong., 1st Sess. § 2702(a), (b) (1993)). Compliance with guidelines would be voluntary, but this version allowed the administrator to make it mandatory if s/he determined it necessary (Ibid.). This version of the bill also directed EPA to create health advisories in order to increase public awareness "concerning the health risks of, and to encourage action to reduce exposure to, indoor air pollutants" (Ibid., § 2704(a)). As part of these advisories, EPA would set action levels for specific indoor air pollutants (Ibid., §2704 (b)(3)). And finally, section 2712 permitted citizen suits.

Not surprisingly, industrial interests mobilized heavily against this bill. Most of the hearing testimony consisted of speakers from business associations (lobbyists) representing building owners and managers, and manufacturers of chemicals, consumer products, building materials, and furnishings. In their testimonies, they assailed the legislation for creating the potential for mandatory compliance with EPA guidelines, for opening the door generally to regulation of indoor air substances, and for unnecessarily duplicating existing legislation (TSCA, FIFRA, and FHSA).[15] They argued that any regulation (including listing and issuing of advisories) of specific hazardous indoor air substances would negatively impact the market without following proper protocol. They also urged the deletion of the health advisories, citizen suits, and listing of indoor air hazardous on the basis that the legislation permitted regulation based on "loose scientific standards." Above all, they argued that actions other than funding research and disseminating "sound scientific information" to the public were inappropriate market interventions. In short, they disputed the need, legitimacy, and scientific basis for regulation, claiming an information-based, public awareness strategy to be the only appropriate federal approach. Consider the following testimony from the president of the Building Owners and Managers Association (BOMA):

> This issue will not be solved by regulation, and we believe this is where this legislation leads. The solution is more effective research and education . . .
>
> We have three major concerns with the provisions of H.R. 2919. Primarily, while the provisions of this bill are intended as voluntary guidance, the EPA Administrator, at the stroke of a pen, can turn them into regulations. . . . While we welcome practical guidance based on sound

research, we oppose giving the EPA unilateral authority to regulate. . . . BOMA (also) believes that the "pollutant-by-pollutant approach," under which the EPA would establish action levels to reduce exposure to individual contaminants, is ill advised. . . . Clearly this is an area where further study is required, before giving the EPA such an overwhelming and counter-productive task. (George Julin III, President, Building Owners and Managers Association, testimony in hearing on H.R. 2919, 103rd Cong., 1st Sess. (1993), 79–83)

The Business Council on Indoor Air (BCIA) testimony echoes BOMA's:[16]

In light of existing federal authorities and programs, BCIA questions the need for indoor air legislation. . . . With regard to H.R. 2919, BCIA is concerned that the legislation, if passed, would: . . . unconstitutionally delegate authority to EPA to convert its "guidelines" into mandatory requirements, providing no guidance as to the circumstances under which guidelines could become requirements; (and) require EPA to issue market-impacting health advisories, in the absence of a notice-and-comment provision. . . .

BCIA . . . applauds the shift of focus to indoor air hazards rather than pollutants or contaminants. . . .

BCIA's primary concerns with the health advisory section of H.R. 2919, as currently drafted, relate to the scientific standards to which these health advisories would be held and to the circumstances under which they would be developed. . . . Unlike the requirements of existing statutes, H.R. 2919 does not hold EPA to the same minimum standard of scientific evidence that must be satisfied before a health advisory may be issued in the area of controversial scientific theory. The informational intent of health advisories does not justify a lesser degree of scientific scrutiny. (BCIA prepared statement in hearing on H.R. 2919, 103rd Cong., 1st Sess. (1993), 86–91)

Finally, the president of the Chemical Specialties Manufacturers Association (CSMA)[17] expressed similar views:

Section 2704(b)(3) requires EPA to develop at least 12 health advisories for indoor air pollutants within 2 years of enactment. . . . Unfortunately, H.R. 2919's approach to health advisories creates several problems. . . . (T)he health advisories are not required to be based upon sound scientific evidence which has been peer reviewed. The loose threshold of scientific findings necessary to support the health advisories is a departure from other statutes. It is particularly troubling since the advisories will likely have a large impact on the public's choice of products and services which are already regulated under FIFRA and FHSA. Under those statutes, however, a regulatory action of health warning must be supported by sound, verifiable science; and these health advisories should be held to those same standards (99)[. . .]

(The setting of pollutant-specific action levels) . . . is completely inconsistent with a non-regulatory, public awareness approach and can only be regarded as a table-setter for a pollutant-specific command-and-control program. (Ralph Engel, President, Chemical Specialties Manufacturers Association, testimony in hearing on H.R. 2919, 103rd Cong., 1st Sess. (1993), 98–104)

Ten months later, the Committee on Energy and Commerce (to whom Senate referred the bill) reintroduced a highly modified version as the Indoor Air Pollution Act of 1994. The Committee eliminated the sections on health advisories (and action levels) and citizen suits, and changed all guidelines to voluntary. Additionally, they made changes to the language, such as changing the list from "common indoor air hazards" (H.R. 2919, 103rd Cong., 1st Sess. § 2702(a) (1993)) to "common significant indoor air health risks" (H.R. 2919, 103rd Cong., 2nd Sess. § 3(a) (1994)). Although this change may seem subtle, it moves the focus of the legislation away from specific sources of pollution and contaminants to the even murkier realm of "risk." In tandem with the loosening of guidelines, they added language to "toughen" scientific criteria: "It is the intent of Congress that risk assessments conducted under this Act be conducted in accordance with sound, unbiased, and objective scientific practices" (Ibid. § 12(a)). Finally, this new version removed any potential for regulation of indoor air pollutants, and focused instead on information dissemination and research.

While the House debated and modified H.R. 2919, the Senate considered S. 656, also known as the Indoor Air Pollution Act of 1993. This legislation was heavily research focused, but section 8 would have authorized action based on existing statutory authorities (TSCA, FIFRA, FHSA, Clean Air Act, Safe Drinking Water Act, etc.) (S. 656, 103rd Cong., 1st Sess., §8(b) (1993)), and "supporting actings" (Ibid., §8(c)). This section authorized EPA to identify "contaminants or circumstances of contamination for which immediate action to protect public and worker health is necessary," and allowed for the recommendation of legislation, if needed, to address this contamination (Ibid.). Additionally, section 7 authorized a list of contaminants (as opposed to "hazards" or "risks"), and the publishing of health advisories (Ibid., § 7(a),(b)). Overall, this legislation permitted greater regulatory action, and would have provided EPA with the potential to deal with specific indoor air pollutants.

Industry lobbyists testified against S. 656 using much the same rhetoric as they did for H.R. 2919. CSMA testimony, for example, focused on sections 7 and 8:

CSMA could generally support the objective of S. 656, the Indoor Air Quality Act of 1993, specifically: additional research into the causes and effects of indoor air pollution, improvements in building systems, and better public understanding of indoor health hazards. . . .

CSMA has serious problems with the quasi- and preregulatory provisions of the bill, specifically sections 7 and 8. One major concern is with section 7(a) which requires EPA to list all possible indoor contaminants, so broadly defined as to include many substances regardless of frequency or ubiquity of occurrence. We strongly believe that requiring EPA to conduct an exhaustive review of all known substances would be ill-advised. . . . (T)he extensive amount of time necessary to conduct and analyze the necessary studies, coupled with the inevitable legal challenges, make chemical-by-chemical programs unworkable. (CSMA, written statement presented at hearing on S. 656, 103rd Cong., 1st Sess., §8(b) (1993), 139–44)

Despite industry displeasure, the Senate passed S. 656, with some modifications and amendments, in October of 1993. The Senate then requested House concurrence. In October of 1994 (the following congressional session), the House passed S. 656, but only after deleting the entire text and replacing it with the text of the weaker H.R. 2919. This eliminated all possibility for regulatory action. As such, the bill was then sent back to the Senate, which did not take up the amended bill. Thus, no indoor air legislation, even in a much watered-down and industry-friendly version, was ever enacted. In 1995, Joseph Kennedy II (D-MA) reintroduced the bill as H.R. 933, but this too failed—it was referred to the House Commerce Committee, where it died.

This history of failed indoor air legislation shows considerable industry influence. Even though the final legislation did not pass, its later versions removed almost all of the sections to which industrial lobbyists had objected. Today, the EPA indoor air quality strategy looks very similar to what these lobbyists asked for—a research and public awareness approach.

Issue Framing: Indoor Air Is Private Air, Exposures Are Voluntary

The way policy makers frame the problem of indoor air pollution is also an important factor in explaining the adopted approach. An analysis of technical reports on indoor air quality, brochures for the public, and a special issue of the *EPA Journal*[18] reveals that EPA authors frame the problem of indoor air quality as "private," "personal," and individualized. This framing makes the current approach seem completely logical—as a "private" rather than "public" issue caused by voluntary consumer behavior, government regulation in this area seems an inappropriate incursion into citizens' private lives. Instead, informing consumers so that they can make wiser choices about their behaviors within the home seems the most reasonable solution.

EPA scientists and policy makers view air within the home as "private air" that the occupant owns. Put differently, air within the home is private property. Additionally, they frame use of harmful consumer items as "voluntary" "personal activities." For example, cleaning the house with common cleaning chemicals, wearing perfume, or wearing dry cleaned clothes are "personal" activities that expose people to VOCs. Framing IAQ as largely the result of personal activities conducted within private space has serious implications within a U.S. regulatory context. Specifically, it invokes a rhetoric of American individualism and the right to free choice. Seen this way, EPA regulation of IAQ within the home becomes an infringement upon property rights, and the rights of U.S. citizens to make their own choices about how they live their life and what risks they choose to take. Ken Sexton (1993), in the *EPA Journal* special issue summarizes this viewpoint well:

> The role of the government varies according to the 'publicness' of a particular space as well as the nature of air-pollution health risks, either voluntary or non-voluntary . . .
>
> The rationale for government regulation of outdoor air pollution is based in part on a definition of outdoor air as a "public good" and on the realization that those who suffer the effects of such pollution are neither compensated by, nor powerful in influencing, polluters. The situation is quite different for some indoor air environments, especially private residences, for both the costs and the benefits of pollution control are internalized within households . . .
>
> . . . (A)lthough individuals are certainly making decisions about their own air quality, it is not clear that these are 'informed' decisions. Government actions aimed at improving personal decisions about indoor air quality may be preferable to rules and regulations (e.g., simple warning devices, product labeling, or information programs) . . .
>
> Perhaps the most serious impediment to implementing a regulatory approach is public antipathy towards this form of intervention inside the home. (Sexton 1993, 12)

Hansen and Lott (1993) express these same views in their article within the same *EPA Journal* special issue:

> The irony in the current debate over indoor air pollution is that indoor air fits the classic case where economists argue government intervention is most unwelcome. By definition, indoor air is air within a building that someone owns. As long as someone owns the air, he or she obtains both the benefits and the costs from deciding how clean it should be . . .
>
> Cost-benefit calculations done by the government are not a close substitute for private decision making. Individuals' decisions may differ from regulators' because individuals may be inarticulate or uninformed, or perhaps because they may attach different values to their health and length of life than do the regulators.

Cost-benefit analysis goes to great lengths to approximate peoples values for these things, but this is one area where we can simply rely on those affected individuals to reveal this information to themselves. (Hansen and Lott 1993, 30)

And finally, Nichols (1993) echoes the viewpoint:

Increasingly, Americans are realizing that their behavior as consumers has a direct impact on their health and environment, and they are seeking user friendly information to help them act. Governments, in turn, are facing up to the political and financial costs of mandating and enforcing citizen behavior and are searching for nonregulatory tools. (Nichols 1993, 37)

These passages point to some interesting assumptions underlying the way the authors have framed IAQ problems. First, if we look specifically at hazardous consumer products, such as solvents, the banning or restriction of toxic ingredients within the products (in this case methylene chloride) would not constitute intervention within the home. Chemically based products have a complex "life-cycle," from production to eventual usage or disposal in a hazardous waste dump, with many possible stops in-between. For example, methylene chloride may be produced in a chemical plant, then bought by another company and used as an ingredient in paint stripper, then used by a homeowner as part of a remodeling project. Whatever chemical is not used is taken to the dump, where it can become a nonpoint source of water pollution. In these scenarios, people come into contact with methylene chloride in many stages along the way—the workers in the chemical plant where the substance is synthesized and in the paint stripper plant where it is mixed with other chemicals to form the final product, the homeowner and anyone who may live with her when she uses it to remove paint, and finally people who work at and live near the dump. Use within the home is only one possible step in the lifecycle of methylene chloride, and if the EPA or CPSC moved to restrict it, it would be doing much more than simply intervening within the home. Thus, framing IAQ as solely an issue within the home obscures the complexity of the problem, and requires a narrowing of vision. On the other hand, seeing it as only within the home legitimates a hands-off regulatory approach.

It is curious that Nichols puts blame for IAQ problems squarely on the shoulders of people's "behavior as consumers." Also, she views regulation of IAQ sources as "mandating and enforcing citizen behavior" (Nichols 1993). If the EPA banned p-dichlorobenzene from air fresheners, forcing companies to use safer alternatives (many fresheners already on the market do not contain p-DCB), this would not force consumers to change their behavior. Similarly, many manufacturers have voluntarily removed formaldehyde from perfumes and nail polishes, but others have not. If EPA or CPSC banned usage of

formaldehyde in these products, consumers would still be able to wear perfumes and nail polish. *Hence, viewing consumer behavior within the private
space of the home as the site of enforcement as well as the cause of the problem di-
verts responsibility from the corporations that are putting the harmful substances
in the products in the first place. It also takes responsibility off of government regulators to protect consumers from harmful substances.*

Another interesting assumption relates to the rhetorical split between
"public" and "private" spaces, with the space inside the home being the most
"private." In making this distinction, the authors argue that whereas in a "public" space, people have no control over what they breathe, in "private" spaces,
such as the home, people have total control. In order for this claim to be even
partially sustained, one must assume that the person(s) living within the home
are the homeowners. Since many of the most potent VOCs come from building materials, such as particle board walls, floors, or cabinetry, and carpet and
carpet adhesives, the only way a person could have any control over what is
used would be if they owned the house, apartment, or dwelling in question.
Building materials are a key area in which landlords cut costs in order to make
good returns on their investments, and less-toxic materials cost more. Hence,
it cannot be true for everyone that all air within the home is "owned" by its inhabitants. Nor can it be true that those who breathe the air within the home
are always the ones who exercise and bear both the costs and benefits of indoor
air "decisions,"—for renters, it is more likely that they live with the landlord's
cost-benefit decisions, which are unlikely to factor healthy indoor air into the
equation. Even if indoor air were capable of being "owned," it is unwise to assume that the person who owns the air is the person who breathes it. Indeed,
the whole notion of air as something discrete that can be owned is highly
problematic. Air, whether indoor or outdoor, is migratory, and does not recognize borders, boundaries, or economic and political designations as "private"
versus "public." As such, basing policy decisions on these boundaries simply
does not make sense.

Finally, the notion of "voluntary" exposure is questionable, even within the
space of the home and for the most informed individuals. Manufacturers are
not required to list ingredients in most common chemically based consumer
products. Even in the case of household pesticides (bug "bombs" and sprays,
for example) that under FIFRA must list specific "active ingredients," additional toxic chemicals (up to 95 percent by volume) are listed only as generic
"inert ingredients" (Fagin and Lavelle 1996, 135; U.S. EPA and CPSC 1995,
24). This labeling as "inert ingredients" is supposed to protect manufacturers'
trade secrets. When we use these products, or come into contact with them due
to someone else's use of them at home, school, or work, our resulting exposure
is not "voluntary" or "informed." In fact, our exposure to indoor air pollutants
can be just as involuntary and uninformed as exposure to outdoor air pollutants. As Smith (1993), puts it,

(I)t is only partly true that people knowingly decide to bring indoor exposures on themselves. How many members of the public are able to interpret the list of ingredients on a can of household cleaner or pesticide
to decide how much exposure is warranted for them or their families?
How are householders able to judge what chemicals will be released
from a carpet or piece of furniture they buy? What can members of a
single household do to determine what they are being exposed to in the
water piped into their home? (Smith 1993, 8)

Smith points to the deceptiveness of the belief that all exposures to indoor
air pollutants are informed, voluntary decisions. He also highlights the prevailing assumption that all people living within a household are consulted
about every use of household chemicals. Parents routinely make decisions
about what products to use in the home, yet many are not aware that EPA
bases acceptable exposure limits on adult men's bodies. Even if EPA and CPSC
were to mount a massive educational campaign, it is unlikely that most exposures could ever be "informed decisions," considering the sheer number (ca.
70,000) of chemicals available on the market.

Beyond the framework of the home, the notion of voluntary exposure becomes even more problematic, especially in those spaces that fit less neatly into
the already blurry "public/private" split. Take, for example, the common office
building (or nonindustrial workplace). Technically, this would be a "private
space," owned by a business, a nonprofit organization, or the state. Normally
in such buildings, the owners contract janitors (usually choosing those who
offer the cheapest services) to clean the bathrooms, hallways, and other shared
spaces within the complex. The contracting agency determines what cleaning
supplies will be used, mostly on the basis of least cost and maximum effectiveness. The actual members of the janitorial staff are usually not involved in such
decisions, and must use whatever supplies their employer provides. The employees who work within the office rarely have any input into this process either. Thus, it is unlikely that most of the people (janitors and office workers)
who come into contact with the cleaning chemicals or air fresheners are doing
so "voluntarily" or on the basis of "informed decision-making" on their part.
Although it makes sense for employers to make decisions that keep their employees healthy, there are no guarantees that employee health will be safe-
guarded as employers conduct cost-benefit analyses. Employees must rely on
employers' willingness to take account of their welfare.[19]

In sum, the way policy makers frame the issue of indoor air pollution itself
can also be seen as a contributing factor to the discrepancy between risk and
regulation of indoor air pollution. In none of the proposed versions of legislation was a strict regulatory approach truly attempted—the legislation was
never envisioned as such. Furthermore, discussion of regulation of the production and manufacture of indoor air pollutants was completely absent. For

example, consider Senator Chaffee's testimony on S. 656, the toughest of the proposed legislations, which he cosponsored:

> I would like to make it clear that this legislation does not place the Federal Government in the living room of Americans. The bill does not provide authority to regulate indoor air contaminants, but rather takes an informational approach. . . . The best defense we have against an unhealthy indoor environment is an informed consumer. . . . I would like to point out, Mr. President, that this is not the heavy hand of government. This is arming people with information, and allowing them to make decisions about what steps to take. (Senator Chaffee, testimony on S. 656, 103rd Cong., 1st Sess., 139 Cong Rec S 3773, March 25, 1993)

This framing, in addition to the history of failed legislation and inadequacy of existing legislation, make the current strategy seem no surprise. I now turn to an analysis of current IAQ strategy.

EPA Indoor Air Quality Strategy: Informing Target Audiences
Strategy Overview

Wallace (1993) urged EPA policy makers to devote more regulatory attention to the largest sources of human *exposure* to air pollutants (indoor sources), rather than simply the greatest *emission* sources (outdoor sources). As a result of the complex factors presented in the previous section, and in spite of his compelling findings of the harmfulness and prevalence of VOCs indoors, EPA policy has focused primarily on nonregulatory, market-based, and voluntary solutions. In general, these solutions have centered on end-of-the-line strategies. In other words, rather than taking the harmful substances out of the products, EPA efforts have focused on what actors (i.e., "target audiences who can implement our policies and take action to improve indoor air") (Axelrad 1993, 17) can do to lessen the health impacts, once the substances contained by the products reach the home, school, or workplace. Essentially, the goal is to teach "consumers," as well as architects, engineers, and building managers to recognize toxic substances in building materials and consumer products (pressed-wood products, adhesives, cleaning supplies, solvents, air fresheners), and to avoid them by purchasing less-toxic alternatives or lessening the exposure through ventilation. Above all, EPA has centered its IAQ activities on information dissemination.

EPA summarizes its IAQ strategies in *Targeting Air Pollution: EPA's Approach and Progress* (1993). Of the nine stated primary program objectives, five are oriented specifically toward enhancing the information base and public awareness. Only one objective discusses possible regulation of hazardous substances under TSCA or FIFRA (U.S. EPA 1993, np). The information-based objectives are to:

- Establish effective partnerships with organizations representing the range of target audiences for indoor air quality information to communicate specific guidance and information and promote timely action on indoor air quality issues;
- Develop practical guidance on indoor air quality issues utilizing a broad-based consensus approach which includes representatives from industry and public interest groups to ensure that information provided is accurate and practical;
- Design market-based incentives for industries to lower chemical emissions from their products and provide consumers and other decision-makers with information needed to make informed purchasing decisions;
- Identify and fill research gaps in order to provide information to address outstanding indoor air quality issues; and
- Enhance scientific understanding and public awareness of the complex factors affecting indoor air quality. (U.S. EPA 1993, np)

These goals, as well as the sections that follow them on "Information Dissemination" and "Training Key Indoor Air Audiences" make it clear that the EPA approach favors shaping individual decision-making ("informed purchase decisions"), rather than regulatory control (U.S. EPA 1993). In meeting these objectives, EPA has published a number of informational brochures for the public that are available through the IAQ Clearinghouse, a toll-free information service. An analysis of these brochures even further clarifies the EPA approach to indoor air pollutants. Below, I examine two of these brochures.

Brochure 1: The Inside Story, A Guide to Indoor Air Quality

This joint EPA/CPSC brochure is specifically focused on indoor air within the home, and is written for a nontechnical audience. Readers are presented with an overview of common air pollution sources within the home, classified by type (biological, combustion, consumer products, etc.), as well as a chemical-by-chemical profile of the most hazardous home substances. A two-page spread illustrates a typical suburban split-level home complete with attached garage and basement, with sources of pollutants numbered. The introduction explains that the booklet "was prepared . . . to help you decide to take actions that can reduce the level of indoor air pollution in your own home" (U.S. EPA and CPSC 1995, 5).

Although the brochure covers a wide range of types of indoor air pollutants, I focus here on how it discusses VOCs from household products and building materials. Before doing that, however, it is important to note the EPA's "three basic strategies" for improving indoor air quality (as presented in this brochure and others): source control, increased ventilation, and air cleaning devices (U.S. EPA and CPSC 1995, 10).[20] These three methods are sprinkled throughout the text, and (especially the second and third method) typify the EPA's reactive rather than preventative approach to this problem.

After presenting an overview of the potentially hazardous effects associated with the use of household products containing organic chemicals, the authors give advice on ways to reduce exposure. They caution consumers to:

- Follow label instructions carefully.
- Throw away partially full containers of old or unneeded chemicals safely.
- Buy limited quantities.
- Keep exposure to emissions from products containing methylene chloride to a minimum.
- Keep exposure to benzene to a minimum.
- Keep exposure to perchloroethylene emissions from newly dry-cleaned materials to a minimum. (U.S. EPA and CPSC 1995, 17)

Each of these warnings is accompanied by an explanation of why these actions are important, as well as how one can best accomplish them.

The advice the authors give for formaldehyde is similar. First, they provide an overview of health effects, followed by an outline of what types of materials consumers would encounter formaldehyde in. They then recommend the following ways to reduce exposure:

- Use "exterior-grade" pressed wood products (lower-emitting because they contain phenol resin, not urea resins).
- Use air conditioning and dehumidifiers to maintain moderate temperature and reduce humidity levels.
- Increase ventilation, particularly after bringing new sources of formaldehyde into the home.
- Ask about formaldehyde content of pressed wood products, including building materials, cabinetry, and furniture before you purchase them. (U.S. EPA and CPSC 1995, 17, 21)

These excerpts demonstrate that EPA hopes not only to train people to become knowledgeable about a wide range of chemical substances, but also how to avoid them if possible. They further show that they are in fact concerned about the adverse public health effects of these substances.

Brochure 2: Indoor Air Quality and New Carpet: What You Should Know

In addition to its campaign of informing consumers, EPA encourages industry to voluntarily adopt measures to decrease indoor air pollutants. For example, it engaged in what it terms a "dialogue" with the carpet industry and other carpet interest groups in order to develop voluntary installation guidelines.

The Agency recently completed a year long "dialogue" with carpet floor covering industries, unions, public interest groups, and other Federal agencies to explore ways of reducing the emission of VOCs from new carpet and related installation materials, such as carpet cushions and adhesives. As a result of this voluntary process, the carpet industry agreed to test new carpet floor covering materials for total VOC emissions and is exploring ways of lowering emissions of VOCs from carpet products. Most importantly, the industry has undertaken an extensive consumer education program in cooperation with other dialogue participants, designed to provide the public with information on the role that carpet products play in indoor air quality and ways that consumers can make informed purchase decisions. (U.S. EPA 1993)

Basically, through this nonregulatory process of working with industry, EPA hopes manufacturers will provide information to help consumers lessen the impact of harmful consumer products when they reach the home. As a result of the carpet "dialogue," EPA created a dialogue-member[21] reviewed brochure for the public titled *Indoor Air Quality and Carpet: What You Should Know* (U.S. EPA 1992b).

The tone of this brochure is a bit different than that of the *Inside Story.* Beginning with a brief discussion of the importance of indoor air quality and proper ventilation, it explains that while it is good to try to reduce exposure to chemicals, at the same time these products provide benefits "that add to the overall quality of life" (U.S. EPA 1992b, np). It further explains that although new carpet, carpet cushions, and adhesives emit VOCs, "limited research to date has found no link between adverse health effects and the levels emitted by new carpet" (U.S. EPA 1992b, np). Additionally, it states that all odors—"even food and flower odors"—are caused by chemicals, thus we should not necessarily be bothered by chemical odors (U.S. EPA 1992b, np). It then lists "steps to take" to reduce exposure, such as:

- Ask your carpet retailer for information on emissions from carpet.
- Ask for low-emitting adhesives if adhesives are needed.
- Be sure the retailer requires the installer to follow Carpet and Rug Institute installation guidelines
- Be sure the ventilation system is in proper working order before installation begins. (U.S. EPA 1992b, np)

So this brochure, like the *Inside Story,* aims to teach consumers to lessen the impact of VOC emissions through their behavior (ventilation, asking for low emitting adhesives). But one cannot help wondering why it is that consumers (rather than a regulatory agency) must ask installers to follow guidelines and to use low-emitting adhesives. It seems as if the consumer is put in the odd position of enforcer of "voluntary" guidelines. It also seems as if the only people who come into contact with new carpet are those who purchase it themselves (in other words those who "own" it). This raises the question of who, exactly, is empowered to heed this advice, and who is not.

The Assumed Reader—The Middle-Class Suburban Homeowner

These brochures reveal more than simply the EPA's indoor air quality policies. They also bring to light an important problem: although they are supposed to be written for the general public, in fact the assumed reader is a middle-class, suburban homeowner. With the exception of one small (two paragraph) section in the *Inside Story* that is written for people who live in apartments (it advises readers to "encourage building management to follow guidance in EPA and NIOSH's *Building Air Quality: A Guide for Building Owners and Facility Managers*") (U.S. EPA, 7), the strategies recommended in the brochures assume that the reader has the money and time to find and purchase safer products and building materials. It also assumes that all individuals are empowered to make such purchasing decisions.

This assumed reader can also be found in the original TEAM studies themselves, which propose the following "individual actions" for control of emissions:

> . . . (Un)used paint cans, aerosol sprays, cleansers, solvents, etc. may be disposed of or stored in a detached garage or tool shed. Charcoal filters attached to the kitchen and bathroom taps can remove chloroform and other trihalomethanes from water supplies. . . . Discontinuing use of room air fresheners or switching to brands that do not contain p-dichlorobenzene will reduce exposure to that chemical. . . . Dry-cleaned clothes could be aired out for a few hours on a balcony or porch before hanging them in a closet. (Wallace 1987, 8)

Here, the advice to store chemicals "in the garage or tool shed," purchase filters, or hang clothing outside on a porch or balcony assumes a suburban or rural home and the ability to pay for water filters.

This finding is important, for it reveals not only that the brochures are written with middle-class homeowners in mind, but that in fact the entire EPA approach, as currently constituted, can only provide protection for such people. People who do not own homes must rely on the willingness of landlords, building managers, and even other people within the household to follow the EPA's indoor air quality guidelines (such as using low-emission carpet adhesives or pressed wood products with lower formaldehyde content)—they do not have the ability to make such purchasing decisions themselves. Following these guidelines can be costly and time consuming, as alternative products are not only more expensive, they are also not widely available.[22] Even alternative

cleaning products are not carried at most supermarkets and hardware stores—
a trip to a health food or specialty store is usually needed, and again, these
products cost more than comparable, VOC containing products.

Consequences: Environmental Inequality Indoors

We'd all like to see a reduction in CO_2 levels, and clean, sweet, breathable
air for everyone, regardless of their economic condition. That's why we
work so hard to create a future where fossil fuels, petrochemicals, and
the airborne toxins they generate are a relic of the barbarian past. In the
meantime, those of us who are fortunate enough to have the resources to
protect our family's breathing space are foolish not to consider it.
                    —*Real Goods Catalog Spring 1999 (p. 10),*
        text accompanying advertisements for air filtration devices

Although providing unequal protection for people with less financial resources and nonnormative bodies is not the EPA's intent, it is the outcome of
this policy that has centered on training individuals to avoid toxics. In short,
individuals are encouraged to use privilege to secure healthier indoor air for
themselves and their families, while those without privilege remain unprotected. These people without class privilege or household decision-making
power, such as children, women, and the elderly, are doubly hurt by this approach, as not only are they unlikely to be able to implement the EPA recommended avoidance strategies, but the cost of not doing so stands to inflict
greater damage to their more "vulnerable," nonstandard bodies.

The environmental justice/ inequality literature has well established that
environmental burdens are unequally distributed in American society.[23] Beginning with the foundational GAO (U.S. GAO 1983) and United Church of
Christ (CRJ/UCC 1987) reports, these studies have focused primarily on disproportionate group level exposures of poor communities and communities
of color to large, outdoor, stationary sources of pollution from hazardous
waste sites, toxic industries, and dumps. But just as exposure to outdoor environmental hazards is unevenly distributed, the current EPA approach to indoor air pollutants fosters the same kind of disparity in indoor environments.
In short, if protection is provided through consumer avoidance of harmful indoor air pollutants and through the purchasing of more expensive less toxic alternatives, costly filtration devices, or by increased ventilation, only those who
can afford these options can be protected.

Ulrich Beck claims that toxic contamination is "democratic" in that no one
can escape—there is no way one can avoid it, no "safe" place. He further argues
"the class-specific barriers fall before the air we breathe," and "already in the
water supply all the social strata are connected to the same pipe" (Beck 1992,
36). Beck is writing in the German context. In a U.S. context, this work shows
that income does affect the air we breathe, and that although we may all be

attached to the same water system, with the simple addition of a faucet or shower water filter, we do not all share the same exposure to contaminants within it.

Essentially, EPA IAQ policy encourages those who have money, knowledge, and decision-making power to purchase their protection from indoor air pollutants. In 1992, the IAQ Clearinghouse answered 17,000 phone calls and mailed out 130,000 publications (Axelrad 1993, 17). Although this number is impressive, it has hardly put a dent in informing the majority of U.S. residents (how many calls and documents were for the same people?). Water filters run in price from $29.99 for an end-of-the faucet model, $37 for the shower, to as much as $2,000 to $3,000 for a unit which purifies water for the entire house. Air purifiers generally cost between $50 and $400. Alternative cleaning products can cost twice as much as their more toxic counterparts—Real Goods, a popular dealer in "eco-friendly" merchandise, advertises nontoxic kitchen and bathroom cleaning solutions at $10.00 for 32 ounces (Real Goods 2002, website). Alternative building materials are not only more expensive, but difficult to find.

Yet one must ask if the job of the EPA is to bolster the market in goods which help the privileged "privately" avoid toxic contamination,[24] or to protect everyone from environmental health threats. Indoor air pollution emanates from indoor air pollutants; chemical indoor air pollutants are manufactured and then put into consumer products and building materials. Indoor air pollution cannot be pigeonholed as a "private" problem deserving of "private" solutions. People are indoors at home, at school, at work, where they shop . . . and indoor air pollution is experienced in all of these places. Even if EPA were successful in informing every last individual of the hazards of indoor air pollutants (the Office of Air and Radiation notes a "disparity between minority and low-income populations and the population as a whole with respect to indoor air awareness or risk reduction actions" [U.S. EPA 1997, 50]), not everyone could afford to "take action," nor are all in a position of control to do so. The only way to ensure that people will be protected equally is to get the substances out of the water, building materials, or consumer products before they reach the market (or faucet).

Conclusion

My research speaks not only to regulators and policy, but also to broader academic scholarship on environmental inequality. I encourage scholars of environmental inequality to move beyond geography; to look at privilege in order to better understand how inequality is produced; and to pay attention to the embodied nature of environmental burdens. And I call upon policy makers to act as a force for social change, by enacting proactive collective solutions that provide equal protection for all, rather than encouraging reactive private responses for privileged actors.

The story of IAQ policy clearly shows the importance of moving beyond geography and rooted space in trying to understand how environmental burdens (in this case exposure to toxic industrial chemicals) are disproportionately born by disadvantaged groups. Studies of outdoor, geographically specific pollution sources are of critical importance to struggles of community self-determination and power in response to environmental inequality embedded within capitalism. However, as we live in an increasingly more chemicalized world, these outdoor sources become just one of the many ways that hazardous compounds reach disadvantaged bodies.

This situation also exemplifies the need to look at privilege—in this case class, race, gender, and age privilege—to understand how environmental inequality "happens." Just as Laura Pulido (2000) shows the history of white privilege and the processes of suburbanization, as a manifestation of white privilege, allowed whites in Los Angeles to secure cleaner outdoor environments for themselves at the expense of nonwhite Angelenos, so too privilege allows those with affluence, knowledge, and decision-making power to secure cleaner indoor environments for themselves—at the expense of the less privileged who lose potential political allies in the quest for broader regulatory change. The racialized nature of class formation in the United States, along with the gender and age implications of decision-making and power within the home, suggests that multiple types of mutually constituted privileges are likely at work in producing environmental inequality. My work thus leads me to echo Pulido (ibid.) and Szasz and Meuser (1997) in their call to researchers of environmental inequality to shift their focus to the "haves" in addition to the "have-nots."

Finally, the lessons learned from IAQ policy analysis point to the embodied nature of environmental inequality. By assuming a middle class suburban homeowner when formulating regulatory strategy, and a normative, adult male body when analyzing the risks that chemicals pose to human health, policy makers have created a situation where those with nonstandard, more vulnerable bodies are provided unequal protection from environmental burdens. This begs researchers to consider the questions of whose bodies matter, and whose bodies are placed at risk when the raced, classed, gendered, and aged aspects of embodiment are ignored by those producing the scientific knowledge upon which regulatory practices are based.

As for policy, it has been a more than a decade since the TEAM Studies and *Unfinished Business* reported the discrepancy between the threat posed by indoor air pollution and the lack of priority the EPA devotes to it. Since then, the agency has focused its efforts on disseminating information to different sectors of the U.S. public in hopes that with this knowledge, people will be able to avoid or lessen their exposures to toxics in products and building materials. Although indoor air pollution legislation was considered in Congress between 1991 and 1995, none passed, and no version ever considered regulating the *manufacture* of the substances known to pose the greatest threats to human health through indoor air. In a sense, the current policy seems to do more to protect the manufacturers' freedom to market indoor air polluting substances than it does to protect people and vulnerable populations from being exposed to them. Only true regulation of these harmful chemicals can achieve equal protection.

At first glance, the 2001 Senate bill, S. 855, known as "The Children's Environmental Protection Act," appeared to be an exciting new development. This bill contained provisions to start collecting child-specific chemical safety data, and to evaluate existing protective standards to ensure that they adequately protect children and vulnerable populations. But the overall approach remained focused on research and information dissemination, favoring individual action over collective, regulatory responses—for example "(p)rovid(ing) parents with basic information so they can take individual responsibility for protecting their children from environmental health threats in their homes, schools, and communities . . ." (S. 855, 107th Cong., 2d Sess., (2001)). Toothless as it was, S. 855 was referred indefinitely to the Senate Environment and Public Works Committee.

EPA recognizes that environmental burdens (or "risks") are not distributed equally amongst the U.S. populace, and acknowledges that their policies can exacerbate this unequal distribution, as evidenced by the EPA Environmental Equity Workgroup's advice that the "EPA should, where appropriate, selectively assess and consider the distribution of projected risk reduction in major rulemakings and Agency initiatives" (U.S. EPA 1992a). Such an assessment is long overdue on indoor air quality policy. If this policy remains as currently implemented, it can only further environmental inequality in the United States.

Guide to Acronyms

BCIA: The Business Council on Indoor Air
BOMA: Building Owners and Managers Association
CIAQ: Interagency Committee on Indoor Air Quality
CPSC: Consumer Product Safety Commission
CSMA: Chemical Specialties Manufacturers Association
DHHS: Department of Health and Human Services
DOE: Department of Energy
EPA: Environmental Protection Agency
FHSA: Federal Hazardous Substances Act
FIFRA: Federal Insecticide, Fungicide, and Rodenticide Act
GAO: United States General Accounting Office
IAQ: Indoor Air Quality
MTBE: methyl tertiary-butyl ether
NIOSH: National Institute for Occupational Safety and Health

OSHA: Occupational Safety and Health Administration
p-DCB: p-dichlorobenzene
QRA: Quantitative Risk Assessment
TEAM: Total Exposure Assessment Measurement
THMs: trihalomethanes
TSCA: Toxic Substances Control Act
VOCs: volatile organic compounds

3

Chemical Weapons "Dispersal"?

The Mundane Politics of Air Monitoring

MONICA J. CASPER

December, 1998

I am sitting at a long table in a storefront office on Main Street, in Tooele, Utah, with my laptop computer and a notebook open in front of me. It is a sunny, cold day, with a high blue sky and patches of white snow on the ground outside the windows. I am surrounded by files, all of which detail various aspects of the U.S. chemical weapons program, which I am here to research. Aside from the files, the office contains three life-sized mannequins wearing gas masks, and a scale model of the incinerator located 22 miles south of town, in Rush Valley. The synthetic human figures, with their frozen, serious expressions, keep me company while I write.

This is my second day in the Tooele Chemical Stockpile Outreach Office, and my notebook is filling rapidly with information about the arsenal and its destruction. It is fascinating stuff. The office, established by the U.S. Army's Program Manager for Chemical Demilitarization (PMCD) and administered by the public relations firm Booz-Allen Hamilton, contains more data than I ever would have imagined. Not only are myriad government documents present, but so too are reports from the "opposition," including a health survey prepared by local citizens of Tooele and Grantsville and material from citizens' groups across the country opposed to incineration. As I read through hundreds of pages and take notes about the program, I begin piecing together the contours of the controversy surrounding it. My excitement about this project mounts.

But today I am especially eager to be here, as it is Wednesday. This means that at one o'clock in the afternoon, in just about ten minutes, the civil defense sirens will be tested. The Chemical Stockpile Emergency Preparedness Program (CSEPP), funded by the U.S. Army, is a regional system of thirty-seven sirens and emergency broadcasts designed to ensure safe evacuation of residents in the event of a chemical emergency, known as a "hazardous material/ chemical incident." The sirens, with oversight provided by Tooele County Emergency Management, are located in various communities based on their proximity to the Deseret Chemical Depot, where some 13,000 tons of chemical agent are stored.

If and when the sirens erupt, they will be followed by a spoken public broadcast. Such announcements, I am told, range from "Warning, Warning. An emergency condition exists at Tooele Army Depot. Stand by for further instructions," to orders to "shelter in place," to directions for evacuation depending on which way the wind is blowing. Immigrants to the county are given a packet of information, including a description of what is stored at Deseret and a pamphlet entitled *Your Guide When the Siren Rings*. A letter to new residents from the Director of Emergency Management states, "We at Tooele County feel that these sirens give our communities a greater sense of security and a definite 'extra layer' of protection in any type of emergency." I try to imagine what it might be like to move into a new neighborhood and receive material about hazardous, even deadly, materials along with the usual information about schools, libraries, and hospitals.

Since my arrival in Tooele, I have made a point of memorizing the four basic directional routes out of the county, and I always keep the gas tank of my rented SUV at least three-quarters full. I am anxious to witness for myself how effective the alarm system is, having now heard about it from many informants, some of whom sang its praises loudly. So I sit at the table awaiting the *Wah! Wah! Wah!* of the alarm, pen poised above paper, ears sharply attuned. One o'clock comes and goes, and I hear nothing but the sounds to which I am becoming accustomed—traffic passing along Main Street, folks talking on the sidewalk, the dry cough of the office manager, snow crunching underfoot. I wonder if there is a malfunction in the equipment.

Later, I learn that the alarm did indeed go off as planned, just as it does every week at this time. But on this particular Wednesday, I cannot detect the test from within the confines of the very location designed to convince the local public that the chemical weapons program here is safe. I find this immensely ironic, and more than a little disturbing. I do not sleep well that night.

Chemical Weapons in the United States: History and Background

In 1995, a group—or cult, according to some observers—of Japanese terrorists, known as Aum Shinrikyo, released the nerve gas Sarin on a Tokyo subway station platform, injuring thousands of people during the busy morning commute. Subsequent intelligence would reveal that the cult, founded by a meditation center mogul, had $1 billion in assets and access to a cadre of experts capable of manufacturing and procuring chemical and biological weapons. The subway attack shocked the world and called attention to the global community's collective inability to confine weapons of mass destruction to combat situations only.

In the United States, the incident captured the public's attention and sparked some interest in the topic of chemical weapons. The terrorists were, briefly, a favorite target of late-night comedians. But still, Japan was an ocean away, and it was all too easy for many Americans to think of chemical weapons either as relics of past wars, filtered through sepia-toned images of gaunt veterans of a previous generation, or solely as an international concern of interest to the United Nations but not to the average citizen.

But then, on September 11, 2001, tragedy struck closer to home. In the morning hours of that clear summer day, Islamic fundamentalist terrorists hijacked four American planes. One jet, United flight 175, bound from Boston to Los Angeles, was diverted and flown directly into the South Tower of the World Trade Center in New York City. A second jet, American flight 11, also bound for the West Coast, was crashed into the North Tower. A third commandeered jet smashed into one corner of the Pentagon and a fourth plane, diverted by heroic passengers from its intended target the White House, plunged into a Pennsylvania field, killing everyone on board. Shortly after the initial attacks, the World Trade Towers, consumed by fire and chaos, collapsed one right after the other into a mammoth, tangled heap of steel and glass and bodies, forming the hallowed and harrowing site that has come to be known as Ground Zero. More than 3,000 people died that day, and a nation was forever changed.

In the post-traumatic frenzy of media coverage that followed the attacks, as Americans tried to come to terms with their newfound vulnerability and profound grief, chemical and biological weapons (CBW) became a household name. All of a sudden, a topic that had been relegated to the history books seemed all too current. Fear and suspicion pervaded the American consciousness as the populace imagined and tried to protect itself against threats both known and unknown. Every suspicious powdery substance was anthrax, every dark-skinned person a terrorist, no matter that he had been your neighbor for years and loved baseball. Average citizens began stockpiling the antibiotic Cipro, threatening a shortage, while others purchased their very own gas masks.

We also learned about unique threats, such as those to America's chemical weapons stockpile. Chemical weapons stockpile? Yes, indeed. It became chillingly clear to those reading the newspaper or watching the news that the United States has its own supply of nerve gas, stored not far away on some unpronounceable foreign base or in the dank caves of a terrorist cell, but rather in our very own backyards. And these facilities were now considered to be at high risk. The landscape had shifted after 9/11, with consequences not only for the quotidian lives of Americans, but just as surely for the embattled United States chemical weapons program.

The chemical weapons stockpile, contrary to its singular nomenclature, is in actuality spread out across nine different sites. It houses some 30,000 tons of chemical agent, contained in millions of weapons such as rockets and projectiles. Eight stockpiles are located in the continental United States: Anniston, Alabama; Pine Bluff, Arkansas; Pueblo, Colorado; Newport, Indiana; Blue Grass, Kentucky; Aberdeen, Maryland; Umatilla, Oregon; and Tooele, Utah. And one is located on Johnston Atoll in the Pacific, midway between Hawaii and the Marshall Islands. There are also a fairly large number of nonstockpile weapons, dispersed at military bases and in hazardous waste sites across the country. While some stockpiles are quite remote, others are located in towns, near schools, and adjacent to agricultural fields. In short, chemical weapons are right next door.

A chemical weapon is any armament (e.g., bomb, cartridge, projectile, missile, mine, rocket) that contains toxic nerve agent. The United States began researching, producing, and storing chemical weapons during World War I (Price 1997). The most significant agent until the 1940s was mustard gas, but GB/Sarin, VX, BZ, Lewisite and others quickly followed. These agents act on the nervous system and may cause toxicological effects ranging from amnesia to convulsions and death (WHO 1970). Adding these agents to munitions was intended to be a military stroke of genius, making possible the quick death or destruction of an opposing army. In a combat situation, disabled soldiers requiring medical treatment can cause far more trouble for armies than dead bodies, so extreme sickness rather than death is often a preferred goal. However, chemical weapons proved difficult to use in practice—for example, on windy days, they were blown back on the troops that had deployed them—and instead became valued for their symbolic power as a deterrent. Conventional wisdom during this era was that the U.S. would not be attacked with chemical and biological weapons if it had its own arsenal to deploy if needed (Price 1997).

Given this strategic arms control function, the production of chemical weapons increased dramatically in the U.S. during the Cold War, and they began to be stockpiled at the nine different storage facilities managed by the Army. They were also tested on American soldiers and sailors in the 1960s—a legacy only recently disclosed by the Pentagon. Other nations, such as the former Soviet Union, France, Germany, Japan, and China, were also researching and producing chemical weapons, ostensibly as deterrents (Burck and Flowerree 1991). With very few exceptions, none of these weapons were ever used in military combat. One notable, and notorious, case was the use of VX by Iraq against Iran in the 1980s. Iraq has also used chemical weapons against the Kurds.

Despite the historic proliferation of chemical weapons, there has long been a "taboo" (Price 1997) of sorts attached to them, in part stemming from the horror they elicit. This interdiction was first embodied in the 1925 Geneva Convention and more recently in the international Convention on the Prohibition of the Development, Production, Stockpiling and Use of Chemical Weapons and on their Destruction (CWC). The CWC was opened for signature in 1993 and accompanied by a flurry of positive media coverage (Smithson 1993). This global treaty requires all signatory countries, of which there were 169 as of 1998, to destroy their current chemical weapons stockpiles and to refrain from developing more. It is the first international treaty designed not only to prohibit use of weapons of mass destruction, but also to prevent further manufacture and to eradicate existing stockpiles. Signatory countries are charged with disposing of their chemical arsenals in a safe and environmentally friendly manner. Implementation of the treaty falls under the jurisdiction of the Organisation for the Prohibition of Chemical Weapons (OPCW), based in The Hague, which provides weapons inspection among other functions.[1]

Prior to the CWC, there was growing awareness that aging stockpiles may be ecological hazards, and some nations, especially those with small stockpiles, had already begun to demilitarize their weapons. In the United States, which has one of the largest stockpiles, second only to Russia, production of most chemical weapons had ceased by 1968. Then, the Army began disposing of its outmoded stockpile by deep ocean dumping, land burial, and open-pit burning (Bernauer 1993). Increased environmental awareness led to restrictions on these methods (they are now specifically forbidden by the CWC), and the Army began researching other strategies for destroying the weapons (Zakin 1987). Although neutralization using biologic agents was considered an option in the 1970s, the Army decided in 1982 to adopt incineration as its baseline technology. At the time, incineration was believed to be easier, faster, and cheaper than any other method. It has turned out to meet none of these criteria, although the Army still portrays it in glossy PMCD promotional materials as "a safe, proven disposal process."

The first incinerator was constructed on Johnston Atoll—"miles from nowhere," as one informant told me—as a prototype for subsequent continental sites and is known as the Johnston Atoll Chemical Agent Disposal System (JA-CADS).[2] Burning of the stockpile there, about 6 percent of the total U.S. chemical arsenal, was completed in 2001 and clean-up activities are underway. In 1995, a second incinerator known as Tooele Chemical Agent Disposal Facility (TOCDF), similar to the first but with some modifications, was constructed in rural Utah, and others are in various stages of planning or construction. The incinerators in Umatilla, Oregon, and Anniston, Alabama, were recently completed but are not yet on-line. In Alabama, this is due largely to poor results on emissions tests, opposition from the Governor, and ongoing public concern (Bragg 2002).

Focused on its mission to rid the nation of leaking and potentially dangerous chemical weapons, the Army pursued incineration with very little input from local citizens at or near the sites targeted for the construction of burn facilities. Subsequent political activism has affected, and in some cases impeded, disposal plans at some of these sites, causing the Army to add public relations to its list of chemical weapons related activities. Two sites, in Maryland and Indiana, are using alternative technologies, primarily because those stockpiles contain limited types of weapons. The Aberdeen facility houses only mustard agent, while Newport houses VX contained in ton containers rather than in munitions.

Incineration may seem like an odd choice. As environmental activists have argued for years and scientific evidence is increasingly documenting, incineration and its by-products pose a number of health problems (WHO 1970;

Zakin 1987; Crone 1992; Szasz 1994). These problems may be amplified when the materials being incinerated are themselves toxic. In addition to nerve agents, which are deadly, other materials of concern in chemical weapons incineration include dioxins and furans, and at least forty-eight other organic substances including original chemical agents and chemicals produced from incomplete combustion (Crone 1986; Chemical Weapons Working Group 1997). These chemicals include a variety of substances with both known and unknown risks to human and ecosystem health (Carson 1962; Ahlborg et al. 1995). During incineration, these agents may be released into the air through either *direct exposure pathways*, which are direct releases out of the furnace smokestacks, or through *indirect exposure pathways*, in which materials are deposited onto the ground and travel through different media (water, soil, food). Once introduced into the human body, the endocrine system and other bodily functions may be severely disrupted (Colborn, Dumanoski, and Myers 1996; Environmental Protection Agency 1997).[3]

To incinerate chemical weapons at these expensive, state-of-the-art facilities, the Army and defense contractors must manually transport munitions from storage areas. This is one of the most dangerous parts of the operation, as workers are directly handling and moving the deadly agent. Once at the incinerator, workers disassemble munitions, separating explosives from liquid chemical agents, and then initiate the automated process by which chemical agents and bulk containers are burned. The facilities must manage waste materials (atmospheric releases and solid waste) after incineration. Four separate furnace systems are required to carry out these activities. Both TOCDF and JACADS have been beset with numerous technical problems, on several occasions resulting in accidental releases of toxic waste into the atmosphere (Raloff 1994; Crawford-Browne 1996; Harrison 1996; Webster 1996). TOCDF has also garnered its share of whistle-blower cases requiring Federal judicial intervention.

In addition, burning of chemical weapons has generated millions of pounds of toxic waste (Kentucky Environmental Foundation 1998). For every pound of chemical agent destroyed, 15 pounds of waste are produced; after just a year and a half of operations, TOCDF produced over 45 million pounds of waste. This waste includes decontamination solutions and contaminated brine, ash, and dunnage, which is transported across the country and oceans to be burned, landfilled, or otherwise disposed of. A massive quantity of solid waste from the JACADS operation, for example, was barged from the South Pacific to California in 2000, while hazardous liquid waste was simply placed in barrels and restocked in bunkers, awaiting future disposal.

The process of incineration, with its multiple potential by-products, has led skeptical observers to categorize the program as chemical weapons *dispersal* rather than disposal (Chemical Weapons Working Group 1998). Indeed, incineration may not meet the basic obligations of the CWC which requires safe and environmentally sound disposal practices. The terminology of chemical weapons "destruction" seems to imply that the weapons completely vanish in a *poof!* of smoke. But it is impossible to obtain complete destruction with zero production of residues, due to the law of conservation of matter as Hugh Crone defines the problem. He writes, "[W]hat goes in at the front end comes out in equal mass but different chemical form at the other end. Thus destruction is conversion to different chemical form: Nothing is lost or disappears; the substance merely changes" (1992, 95). For many critics of the U.S. chemical weapons program, this form of destruction is simply not adequate for protecting ecological and human health.

It seems, then, that destroying chemical weapons poses many of the same technical difficulties as using them did (SIPRI 1980; Crone 1992). The Army can move forward only when it convinces regulators and the public that its practices are safe—and so far, the public is not convinced (Morrison 1991; Satchell 1993; Brown and Johnson 1994). There are several ways that program managers attempt to build safety into the operation. Risk assessments, for example, are ubiquitous, although tremendous differences in interpretation exist among proponents and opponents of the chemical weapons program. Other strategies include technical solutions, such as air monitoring systems designed to ensure environmental quality.

The Strategic Significance of Air Monitoring

The importance of air monitoring cannot be overestimated, both in ecological and political terms. For all practical purposes, a clean, chemical-free environment—broadly or narrowly defined—is linked to healthy bodies, whether of workers or citizens. Two methods of verification are used by the OPCW in determining whether signatory countries are abiding by the terms of the treaty: the continuous on-site presence of trained inspectors, and the use of on-site monitoring equipment. Carefully engineered filtering and monitoring technologies are designed both to keep the environment as clean as possible *and* to convince the public that it is being protected. Yet, as we shall see, air monitoring systems are suspect in the highly contested arena of chemical weapons "dispersal."

Each chemical weapons incinerator is equipped with two types of monitoring systems. The most significant is the Automatic Continuous Air Monitoring System (ACAMS), which is finely calibrated to rapidly detect an agent leak or spill anywhere in the facility. The second system is the Depot Area Air Monitoring System (DAAMS), which does not have the same capabilities as the ACAMS. Instead of catching leaks on the spot, the DAAMS system collects air samples over a longer period of time, usually 12 or 24 hours. This system is used to verify ACAMS results and to provide a more sustained record of air quality in a given area.

Monitoring conforms closely to standards determined by the United States Public Health Service (PHS), based on toxicology studies done prior to the

Occupational Health and Safety Act (OSHA) of 1970. Additionally, in 1988, a working group convened to investigate the health effects of long-term exposure to low doses of chemical agent, reexamining standards for GB, VX, and HD. The group's updated recommendations were accepted by the PHS, which determined maximum permissible exposures for workers and for the general population. These standards are used throughout the chemical weapons program to interpret and act on data from the air monitoring systems.

For example, the Airborne Exposure Limit (AEL), also known as the Time Weighted Average (TWA), is the concentration that unmasked workers putting in a full eight-hour day for five days per week may be exposed to without suffering any ill health effects. In practice, the AEL is used as an alarm threshold; if the agent is detected at amounts above the established AEL, protective masks must be immediately used. The General Population Limit (GPL) is the amount of agent that the general public may be exposed to indefinitely (24 hours per day, seven days per week) without adverse effects. Inside chemical processing areas, the Army adheres to a more stringent standard known as the Immediately Dangerous to Life and Health (IDLH) limits. Toxicologically speaking, this is the maximum concentration from which a worker, unmasked or with failing equipment, could escape within 30 minutes and still live. Chemical facilities also must comply with an Allowable Stack Concentration (ASC), a standard based not on health effects but rather on concrete emission quantities.

These standards are subject to extensive review and analysis, suggesting that they are scientific and objective, and thus adequate. Moreover, the Army's chemical weapons program is subject to oversight by a host of Federal and local agencies. The Centers for Disease Control and Prevention (CDC) works closely with the Army on all aspects of air monitoring. For example, the CDC offers assistance on locating and operating monitoring devices, on quality control issues, and on the establishment of exposure levels for all chemical agents. The CDC also reviews Army monitoring data every two weeks to affirm that data quality objectives are met. These objectives include whether monitoring devices are performing adequately, and also whether agent is being detected at the lowest level of health concern.

In addition to the CDC, the chemical weapons program is monitored by Congress, which maintains legislative oversight of the entire chemical demilitarization program; the National Academy of Sciences, which provides scientific and technical advice; OSHA, which provides safety oversight for employees of the program and enforces safety regulations; the Office of the Secretary of Defense, which reviews all disposal site plans and safety requirements and confirms that all DOD and Army safety regulations are being met; and state and local agencies, which enforce EPA and state regulations, oversee disposal operations, and enact state laws to protect public health, safety, and the environment. All of this monitoring, both technical and organizational, lends credence to the idea that air monitoring standards are sufficiently tough and appropriately managed.

However, even proponents of incineration, echoing scientist Hugh Crone, acknowledge that it is impossible to completely annihilate burned material. While they claim that the amounts emergent from the stacks are at *low enough* levels as to produce no threat to human health, they do admit that errors might occur. (And many errors have occurred, with accidental releases reported at both JACADS and TOCDF.) The PMCD asserts, somewhat disingenuously, that "although there is no indication of low levels of agent being released from the stacks, there are limits to the levels that the instruments can measure."[4] The agency also acknowledges that "the absence of 'any' agent is difficult to quantify. Detection must occur at a discrete, measurable level."[5]

Yet it is precisely these "unmeasurables" that local citizens and activists are concerned about. Such gaps in expert knowledge and exceptions to the mundane reliance on technology speak to some of the doubts held by opponents of incineration. Outside of the carefully constructed "fact sheets" outlining the parameters of the chemical weapons program, and inside the communities and homes of the people most likely to be affected, it becomes quite clear that not everyone agrees with the Army's assessment of the thoroughness and safety of current air monitoring practices. This contention matters significantly in terms of the ultimate success of an embattled public program.

In what follows, I describe chemical weapons activities in Tooele, Utah, and suggest that there are varied, competing perspectives on environmental quality in this region. Air monitoring, I suggest, means different things to different stakeholders. While it may be a perfectly adequate technical solution for the OPCW, the U.S. Army, public health regulators, and defense contractors, it is not sufficient for the residents who fear for their health and lives, and the activists who claim to speak for them. The politics of air monitoring embody concerns about how toxic chemicals migrate, and with whom they come into contact.

Chemical Weapons in the West Desert

Tooele County is about thirty miles southwest of Salt Lake City and due south of the Great Salt Lake. It contains Tooele, Rush, and Skull Valleys as well as the Oquirrh and Stansbury Mountains. By many in the Salt Lake area and elsewhere, Tooele County is considered an outdoor paradise, a sportsman's haven. Maps of Tooele show numerous campsites, ski runs, hiking trails, and fishing holes, and the area is also known for motorized recreation on the Bonneville Salt Flats. Ironically, despite the natural beauty of the place, Tooele County is also home to the West Desert Hazardous Industrial Area and a number of military installations. The industrial corridor contains two commercial hazardous waste incinerators, one commercial hazardous waste landfill and treatment facility, and one low-level radioactive material repository. Magnesium Corporation of America, known as MagCorp, is located there and is considered one of the nation's top polluters (Ward 1999).

The military installations, clustered relatively near each other in the starkly beautiful and wide open West Desert valley, include Dugway Proving Ground, Tooele Army Depot, Deseret Chemical Depot, and CAMDS. Dugway has been historically a site for testing of nuclear, biological, and chemical weapons, and Deseret houses just under 40 percent of the nation's chemical weapons stockpile, the largest of any of the nine sites. CAMDS, adjacent to the chemical depot, was an original hub for research into alternatives to incineration of chemical weapons. The area is a local portrait, in desert hues, of the military-industrial complex.

There are about 40,000 residents in the 7,000 square mile county. Many are Mormon, mirroring the population of the rest of the state. In spite of the toxic load in Tooele County, its major towns—Tooele (the county seat) and Grantsville—are rapidly booming bedroom communities for Salt Lake City. Cheaper housing, natural beauty, small town life, and job opportunities draw new residents. The major employers in town in the public sector are Dugway, the Army Depot, the Chemical Depot, and CAMDS, and in the private sector, EG&G Defense Industries (which runs the chemical depot), MagCorp, and Detroit Diesel. The military has been around the longest, and has employed hundreds of people since the 1930s at Dugway Proving Ground.

Many of the people I spoke to work at one of the military facilities or have relatives and friends who work there. In many ways, the military is a more integrated part of the community than the private facilities and is thus somewhat more accepted. For example, there is almost uniform disgust with MagCorp, which routinely spews chlorine into the air around Tooele County. Although residents to some degree distrust the military, and "government" in general, the Army is also seen as a rather benevolent employer. This despite the fact that, as some residents mentioned, from the 1950s through the 1970s almost 500,000 pounds of nerve gas were released into the air at Dugway. Also during these years, some 1,200 open-air test firings of munitions filled with nerve gas were conducted (Marshall 1996). In addition, in March 1968, nerve agent was sprayed from an F-4 Phantom jet, resulting in the death by exposure of 6,000 sheep in the aptly named Skull Valley. Everyone I spoke to commented on the sheep incident, but with very little open malice toward the Army.

TOCDF, the 22 acre chemical weapons facility designed to eradicate the stockpile, was completed in 1995 and fired up for its first burn in 1996. It is difficult to convey the surprise of finding a modern incinerator in the middle of the majestic high desert. When I visited the site, I came around a bend in my 4×4 and all of a sudden, there was the smokestack rising from the valley floor, silhouetted against the craggy, snow-covered mountains in the background.

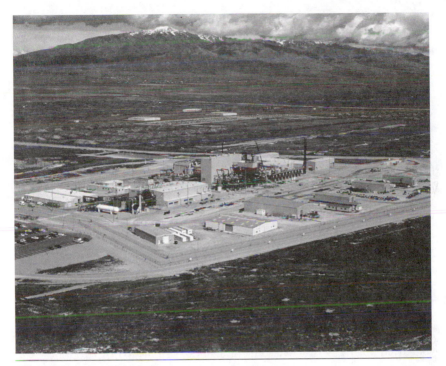

Official U.S. Army photograph.

With 840 miles of electrical wire, 33 miles of pipes, 16,000 valves and instruments, and 2,000 pieces of automated equipment (Grossman and Shulman 1993), TOCDF looks like some sort of Rube Goldberg creation done in teal, black, and red. It operates around the clock and is staffed by some 600 people. To visit TOCDF, I had to first watch two safety videos and be fitted for a gas mask. Once my mask was declared safe, I had to carry it with me in an Army-issue canvas bag along with three syringes of Atropine, a nerve agent antidote. In the event of an emergency, I had to be prepared to use both the mask and the syringes. (Although "incidents" requiring gas mask usage are quite common, nobody has ever had to use the syringes at TOCDF, according to informants.) I also had to wear a hard hat at all times and, in some areas, ear plugs. TOCDF is extremely noisy, like many industrial sites.

TOCDF ran at half-capacity for almost two years until the end of 1998, when it received approval from the Utah State Division of Hazardous Waste to run a full-scale operation. The project is managed by EG&G Defense Industries, whose employees far outnumber the military personnel on-site. (In fact, during my visit I saw only one person in uniform; everybody else appeared to be civilians.) Since its inception, TOCDF has concentrated almost exclusively on M-55 rockets. Manufactured during the 1960s, the M-55s contain GB (sarin) and are particularly prone to leakage. The chemical agent interacts with the aluminum in the warhead, creating a "leaker," as they are known. GB is one of the nerve agents that acts almost instantly, "clenching the body's muscles and heart in an unyielding death grip" (Grossman and Shulman 1993). Despite its emphasis on M-55s and Sarin, the Desert Chemical Depot contains every other kind of chemical agent—and TOCDF is slated to destroy them all.

Whose Environment? Competing Perspectives on Air Quality

Mabel Thomas is 84 years old, a Mormon widow with 36 grandchildren, 37 great grandchildren, and 7 great-great grandchildren. She has survived cancer, asthma, and her husband, a coal miner who died of black lung disease. We spoke on a cold, dark evening about her family, her health, and her views on chemical weapons disposal. One of the most striking things about our conversation was her lack of faith in the Army's ability to protect the public, which had prompted her to become involved in some community activities against incineration.

A few weeks prior to our interview, she told me she had experienced what was most likely a severe respiratory attack after exposure to chlorine gas. To my mind, the obvious culprit was MagCorp; chlorine is a byproduct of magnesium production, and I had already heard numerous stories about harmful chlorine exposure. Yet chlorine has also been used as a weapon. Mabel was convinced that her ordeal had something to do with the Army. This is how she described it:

> I had this terrible cough . . . I got to coughing so hard that I was throwing up. . . . I smelled this horrible chlorine gas coming in the window. . . . It came from out at one of these plants out here, north of us here. And I didn't know anything about it until afterwards, and then it came out in the paper, you know, that there had been a leak. . . . And I thought maybe it was something from the base because once in a while when I'd go outside, you know, when we have these little leaks, and I know they say it doesn't come out in the atmosphere, but I don't know. But anyway, I don't go out too much when I know there's anything like that because then I start breathing and having problems.

Mabel told me that when she first moved to Tooele from Montana, the air "was so clear and it was so nice." Now, "you can come out from Salt Lake City and look out over this way, we've got nothing but a blue haze over here." I asked her about the origins of the blue haze, probing specifically to see if she would target MagCorp or the other industries in the area. Instead, she again pointed her finger at the Army:

> It is scary, it's real scary. We talk among ourselves a lot about it, you know, and how concerned we are over what could happen. . . . The thing I don't understand with the base, when they always come out with the

deal of, you know, no harm to the public and all this kind of stuff. . . . But when you see that stuff coming out of that stack there, you still know there's something going into the atmosphere. And I don't know how they're trying to fool us or why they're trying to fool us, because I mean, we're not that dumb, I don't think, that we don't know something's coming out of that stack there.

When I asked her to be more specific about what might be coming out of the stack or what could happen because of the emissions, she remarked:

If it's something that's in the air, it could hurt our minds, you know, I mean we could start having trouble that way with memory. . . . And then the little youngsters that is growing up, what's going to happen there, too? I hope that it doesn't cause any deformities. . . . We don't know what kind of chemicals they are because we're in the dark. And this is something that I dislike very much. I think we should be told what kind of chemicals they are, what they can do to the body and what they can do to the nervous system and so forth.

She talked at some length about "the government," and her concerns reflect a lifetime spent in the shadow of twentieth-century military activities in the American West:

They're wrong in keeping everything back the way they do. . . . You almost feel like a guinea pig, you really do. . . . They're going to do what they're going to do, and you're the little man over here, so they're not worried about you. . . . It's the wrong way to think about a human being, really. . . . And I think about what they've done down in southern Utah, those people down there. . . . the A-bomb, you know, when they exploded, and all the cancer those people are suffering with down there. . . . And then look at Dugway over here with the sheep, when they had that deal over there, and they kept saying no, that had nothing to do with it.

I asked Mabel if and how the community could take care of itself in the event of a hazardous incident. She replied:

You know, one thing, who's got a mask here? Who's got the equipment here that you could help yourself? They give you a little kit and bring it around for you to hang on your door, but all that is material to read on what to do. Like I said, I'll get in my car and head west, if I can get out of here . . . and every Wednesday afternoon that siren goes off. You know, we can't hear it down here. And I've gone out on the porch and I thought, well, maybe it's me. So I've asked the neighbors to go out and see if they can listen for it too. They can't hear it either. So I know it isn't me. . . . You know, I've got a grandson that works out there, and of course, I'm always saying to him, "What if anything happens?"

Toward the end of our interview, I asked Mabel what she thought the community could do to help change the situation in Tooele. She sighed and told me,

> There's nothing we can do, like I tell you, our hands are tied. There's nothing we can do. You can talk all you want, you can tell people all you want about things. Nobody listens. . . . Look at darned WWI, how some of our people were even gassed with some of the things that was used. WWII, look at how our men were used during that war. So why don't we think that we could be used that same way here? And it's horrible to think that way about your government, it really is. But that's the way I feel.

Blake Robeson is a local activist, committed to making the Tooele-Grantsville area cleaner and safer for residents. An articulate, intelligent, married father of two, he has longstanding ties to the community. But he admits that he did not know quite what his family was getting into when they moved to the area, which he described as "a hazardous waste zone out in the west desert." He finds incineration of chemical weapons by the Army to be troubling:

> This is an agency of the government that's handling an incredibly toxic substance, they're using a very controversial way of getting rid of it, it's an agency of the government that has a shameless record of disregard for public health and safety, especially here in Utah. And you know, you add that all together, you've got a program that's in trouble. . . . And of course, the worst case scenario is you have a leak that sends gas downwind. People don't die, but they're exposed. They don't even know they're exposed. They cover it up, and then they go on.

He expressed considerable concern about the handling of the program, including technical issues:

> I couldn't figure out why this program was so troubled. [A whistleblower from the plant] said, "Well, it's systemic." The intent of Congress made sense, you know, for anything, whether you were using incineration or whatever. Build a prototype, test it out; build a pilot, test it out; redesign, move on full-scale. Start, better, best. But they never tested one out before they went on to the design of the next. So all the flaws were passed along. . . . Our first week was very instructive. At JACADS they always had this problem with a leak on this one wall in their filter bag, so when they built this thing . . . they added a vestibule of wooden sheds with insulation and monitoring equipment in it. Seventy-two hours after they fired it up, the thing leaked, they detected it, caught it, and said, "Hey, no

problem, it didn't migrate off the base." Well, it didn't, but it was caught in a big wooden bandage. I mean, that's *not* state of the art.

I asked Blake about political activism and what could be accomplished in the community:

> People here are remarkably—I don't know if the right term is numb—or whether they're in denial. I think it has more to do with the fact that in this level culture, risk is just background. . . . MagCorp is a hellish environment. . . . We have a friend whose face was burned off out there. If you work at the smelter, that's not safe; underground mining, which is what people did for years, that's dangerous. If you worked at the depot, you were handling munitions. I mean, the attitude is sort of like, well, I go to work, I risk my life. What's the deal?

He later remarked, sadly, that "sometimes you feel like you're dealing with addicted, traumatized amnesiacs. They have somehow forgotten a lot of elemental things." I was not sure if he was referring to the residents or the Army officials.

Another activist, Eric Stevenson, with roots in the more widely known and controversial group Downwinders, shed some light on this phenomenon of routinization, in which urgency seems to take a backseat to mundane concerns:

> When it became clear that it was too late to stop the plant from being built . . . it became a question of how do you best monitor this situation, make sure that the Army was constantly aware that people were all over their backside so that they wouldn't become complacent? It's easy when you're operating a plant seven days a week, 24 hours a day for ten years, or whatever it takes, that workers get into a routine and there's a complacency sets in, and that's when mistakes happen, when people are not on their toes. . . . We felt it was important to keep that kind of scrutiny, and intensely enough that their own internal controls were also augmented by community snooping and oversight.

This is certainly a different notion of oversight than that articulated by the PMCD. The remainder of my interview with Eric reflected his extreme concern about the direction the program was taking and about the lack of public input into the process.

I also spoke with public health officials in Tooele County, first with a health department official and then with a group of regulators from the Division of Solid and Hazardous Waste (DSHW) in the Utah State Department of Environmental Quality. Both interviews were instructive, differing as they did from my conversations with activists. Health officials were far more likely to speak in the technical language of the PMCD.

Marvin Baxter, a county official, provided some background on monitoring activities in the region:

We started an air monitoring program back in the county when all these industries started up. It's really the State Department of Environmental Quality's responsibility. After we'd started doing our air quality monitoring program, then they set up their own shop, and that allowed us to back off of doing our own. It seemed like we had to initiate the state in order to do that. Although levels that they found are very low, it's still something we thought they should have taken an active role before we had to.

I asked Marvin about risk and he answered me in fairly technical terms:

Try to look at risk as far as from a scientific standpoint. What we try to do is we try to, from a Health Department standpoint, we try to look at all the different cancers in the area over the last twenty-three years. We've tried to look at birth defects, we've tried to look at other types of multiple sclerosis, those types of things. . . . True risks are hard to look at. . . . The risks that concern me in a lot of places is how close people might be working with the jobs and what's going on with their health. . . . I think the citizens are more worried about an environmental hazard and the risks need to be evaluated and looked at, even though they might live 50 miles away from the source, there still is a potential for concern.

The Health Department's interaction with the chemical weapons facility, according to Marvin, is largely tied to "what if" scenarios:

The only time we get called in is if we go through scenarios. If there is release, then we get called in and we decide when something is clean. . . . We do a lot of role playing here, trying to prepare for if there ever was an accident. Our main role would be . . . to go back and say, okay, this area is clean enough to go back in or not. So we would probably spend a lot of time in mediation.

Echoing Blake Robeson's comments about the local citizenry and politics, Marvin remarked,

As a general rule, I see people more apathetic. We do have a smaller group of people who are very concerned about the environment, and trying to make sure things are okay. A lot of people think everything's okay.

My interview with Marvin also provided one of the most humorous moments of my stay in Tooele. After we had finished talking and I was outside scraping ice off the rental's windows, Marvin came running out in his shirtsleeves to tell me a story, firmly implicating the Army (with tongue in cheek) in local social problems:

> Well, Tooele County has one of the highest, if not *the* highest, teen pregnancy rates. We had a meeting about it, a public town hall meeting. Lots of people came and offered ideas and solutions. One older gentleman, he raised his hand and said, "I'll tell you what's causing the teen pregnancy rates to go up; it's that damned nerve gas!" I'm not sure if he meant to be funny or not, but he did get a laugh. I thought you would appreciate that bit of news about health in our county.

I also spoke with three state regulators, much less witty, who discussed at length the DSHW's monitoring activities. This includes an office at TOCDF adjacent to the control room, from which environmental engineers can monitor air quality, provide oversight of the facility's own measurements, and assure adherence to Federal and state toxicology standards. All three men felt that monitoring was adequate and that emissions were at low enough levels as to avoid human health hazards. But what they described was a reactive organizational structure rather than a proactive one, despite public perceptions that they do take an activist role. In the words of Dan Martin,

> The industry side, in this case the Army, often feels like we're being too stringent, you know, we're putting too many controls on them. The other side, that is in opposition to the facility, feels like we're caving in to them and we're giving away the farm, and we're not being stringent enough. And so our job, and I think this is an important point, is not to decide for the Army what the best technology is to dispose of these weapons. Our job is to take whatever technology the Army chooses, as long as it fits within the legal requirements, and make sure that if they're going to operate it, they do so safely.

What is striking in this passage is the DSHW official's assumption that it is neither state regulators *nor* the public that should select a baseline technology, but rather the Army. For this environmental engineer, monitoring was defined as something technical (and thus perhaps apolitical), relevant only after a disposal method has been chosen and implemented.

Finally, I spoke with Fred Hart, one of the managers of EG&G, the defense contractor running the incinerator. A proponent of incineration and a businessman first and foremost, Fred's answers were unemotional and clipped. He did not allow that there might be room for error in the standard-setting process, but he did speak to the political nature of the chemical weapons program. His remarks contained considerable faith in the scientific basis of monitoring as described above:

The interesting controversy that's going on right now is what is the toxic level of agent when you expose it to a newborn or whatever. And if you go to the people who are fundamentally against it, they have a great distrust in the people who set the standards for what is and is not safe. And these are people like the CDC, DHHS. . . . It's interesting to watch those interactions and see, you know, is it 0.00002 mg per cubic meter or is it 0.00001? I don't care. As long as we're in order of magnitude below that, we're fine. So they can argue about the one-two as long as I'm ten away from it.

Despite his rationalist bent regarding monitoring, Fred exhibited some passion when talking about the value of his work. He firmly believes that his company is doing a good thing by ridding the planet of chemical weapons. He remarked,

I find these weapons very distasteful and an insult to humanity and they need to be gone, period. We should find ways to never do this kind of stuff again. . . . Chemical weapons are not designed, they're not useful to kill military folks. They're not a military advantage. They're used against civilian populations. That's all they're good for. They're terrorist weapons. You can't stop an army with them, but you can sure kill a city. Terrific, huh?

Contested Environments, Invisible Bodies, and the Future of Chemical Weapons

So what are we to make of these different perspectives on environmental quality in the chemical weapons program? Clearly, for people like Mabel Thomas, Blake Robeson, and Eric Stevenson, air monitoring standards are not sufficient to allay their profound concerns. This can be explained in part by a lack of trust in the Federal government, as represented by an Army that has not always told the truth to the American public. It can also be linked to deep-seated and entirely justified fears of the noxious chemical agents being incinerated in these people's backyards.

I would like to suggest that something else is happening here, too. Different stakeholders in this arena have various, often competing, notions of what the environment is. For incinerator proponents and regulators, the environment seems to refer simply to air quality; if standardized technologies are in place and found to be functioning, then the environment—that is, the local environment in and around the incinerator—is being protected. Environment is understood here in technical terms of parts per million of possible contaminants. And unless sirens erupt or monitoring systems are activated, the assumption is that what emerges from the smokestack should not be a problem for anyone.

However, local citizens and activists have a very different notion of environment, one that is not merely spatial and/or technical. I want to suggest that theirs is a more embodied sense of environment, one that recognizes that "parts per million" matters not just to cubic volumes of air, but to the beings that inhabit that space. Air quality is understood in terms of who will be affected by contaminants in the environment—whether it is Mabel Thomas coughing up blood after being poisoned through her bedroom window, or the children of Blake Robeson walking home from school with their friends. Rather than being "irrational," as some incinerator proponents describe citizens and activists, this seems to be a quite sensible assessment of the proximity of workers, neighborhoods, schools, and whole towns to some of the deadliest chemicals known to humanity.

Consider the following passage from my interview with Blake Robeson, which we might view as the foundation for an embodied notion of environment: "The odd thing is that everything I learned while I was living in the wilderness was the lens that I used when I came out here, and that's one of the reasons I'm involved in all this. Because it's never about the topic; it's about people reconnecting. It's amazing that people don't know where their own damn bodies come from. Over and over, I try to say, you know, your bodies are passed through. *These decisions are translated into flesh and blood*" (italics mine). What these citizens and activists make clear is that bodies are present and should be made visible in public policy about chemical weapons.

What are some implications of this for the future of the disposal program? Obviously, despite a costly public relations campaign, the public in Utah and other communities with stockpiles is far from convinced that incineration is safe. Nor is it likely to be so, given that the Army is instituting public relations *after the fact* of choosing and implementing incineration. As Blake Robeson put it, "[the Army] plays by different rules or no rules or their own rules, and the decisions are always made and then the people are asked to comment on them." Citizens are also likely to not be convinced as long as decisions are made in exclusively technical terms that refuse to make room for the flesh and blood consequences of those decisions. It is ironic that President Bush has publicly stated that chemical weapons in the U.S. are not a great threat, despite the events of 9/11. His administration is more concerned with Iraq and North Korea, which seems to suggest that chemical munitions are an international, but not a domestic, issue.

What might an alternative approach be? Again, Blake Robeson: "[Democracy] means that people get a real say in what the criteria are for the decision, and if there are alternatives, looking at them before you get to the point where we were with chemical weapons, where they are all so heavily invested in their careers and reputations and contracts that nobody could get off the train." It also means incorporating diverse perspectives into decision-making, including those that might be at odds with the party line. Where differences exist regarding definitions of the environment, policy makers and program managers would do well to err on the side of precaution. For citizens frightened of toxic chemicals, technical solutions are simply not enough.

And finally, an alternative approach means making bodies visible, rescuing them conceptually and practically from the mundane politics of air monitoring. For it is human bodies that will be marked—perhaps fatally, certainly tragically—by the presence of chemical hazards in communities. Ridding the planet of lethal munitions is a worthy goal, and the United States is absolutely correct to be attempting to meet the terms of the global CWC. But implementation of the treaty should emphasize disposal and not dispersal, and citizens' fears of chemical pollutants need to be taken seriously for the program to succeed. Surely the Army, defense contractors, and policy makers will want to guarantee that the planet's inhabitants are not destroyed along with chemical weapons, in a haze of malignant smoke.

PART II

BODIES

4

Chemical Politics and the Hazards of Modern Warfare
Agent Orange

DIANE NIBLACK FOX

As an issue that has persisted for more than forty years despite various attempts to define and resolve it through science and politics, Agent Orange links local to global and bodies to nations across divides of class, gender, ethnicity and nationality, with meanings that change from person to person and from context to context, and referents that range from the technical to the metaphoric. These few pages do not pretend to fully enumerate, let alone to settle, the controversies that surround this chemical; rather, they explore what might be added to those discussions by people as yet little heard from, people the Red Cross designated in 2001 as "the disabled poor, including those thought to be affected by Agent Orange."[1]

This chapter is derived from a longer study that seeks to bring into dialogue public and private discourses about Agent Orange: discourses of science and politics with those of individual and community experience; discourses of nation-building and national security with the words of people whose bodies suffer the consequences of those processes. The first part of the chapter considers varied uses of the term. The second describes Agent Orange as a chemical. Next comes an introduction to some of the political controversies, public outcries, and scientific inquiries engendered in the United States by its use and the aftermath of that use. The last part treats Agent Orange as an experience, in the language of people in Vietnam who believe they may be bearing the consequences of that use.

An Excess of Meaning

Since the late 1960s, and especially since the mid 1970s, emotionally charged controversy has surrounded the topic of Agent Orange. But what is Agent Orange? At times, it is a code name for a chemical, at times, a metonym for TCDD dioxin, or a generic term for all the chemicals used during the war in Vietnam, or a synecdoche for all the environmental damage that lingers from that war, or even more globally, for the consequences of war. At other times, it is the name of an illness: "My uncle's daughter is suffering from Agent Orange"; or, "I know a man who can cure Agent Orange." In some popular uses it seems to serve as a synonym for "birth defect." The disabilities associated with it are sometimes taken as a sign of the workings of the law of karma, or of the hand of fate (*Vietnam Courier* 1998). To the extent that illness in Vietnam can be described as a matter of balance and integration of the personal and the natural worlds (Marr 1987, 167), 'Agent Orange' may be read as a metaphor for a world out of balance, dis-integrated.

In America, Agent Orange has been called "a symbol of deceit and betrayal" (*Vietnam: A Television History* 1983); ". . . a metaphor for everything that was wrong about the most unpopular war in American history" (MacPherson 1984, 601); and a marker for "a sea change in the way Americans think," for the deep embedding in American thought of a "profound suspicion of science, government, and technology" (Burkett and Whitely 1998, 551). A Pulitzer Prize–winning journalist who has covered science, medicine, and the environment for some thirty years calls it "technology gone bad, Frankenstein, the best and the brightest, civilization turned dark," adding: "The opposite side of the coin is romanticism gone paranoid and luddite." It is also, he continues, "a cover word for damages due, for the reparations no one can give as reparations, . . . [a] cover that allows us to proceed without looking too closely at what happened and confronting where we are in history. . . " (Franklin 2000).

Some call Agent Orange a diversion. One American physician, Marshall Goldberg, could barely contain his frustration: "You have a war that has destroyed the health system, destroyed the infrastructure and created problems of pollution, hunger, malnutrition and their associated diseases—and you are going to sit around arguing over one small part of the total damage, pouring millions of dollars into research rather than helping people?" An American scientist who has long worked on the effects of dioxin raises another caution about Agent Orange's potential as a diversion: "If we assume certain health consequences are from Agent Orange when they are not, we may not be focusing on causes we can prevent in the future" (Schecter 2002). We should recognize long-term effects but be careful not to overgeneralize.

In March 2002, when representatives from the U.S. and Vietnam met in Hanoi for their first bilaterally government-sponsored conference on the consequences of Agent Orange in Viet Nam,[2] the American ambassador called Agent Orange "the one significant ghost" remaining from the war, while the Vietnamese vice-minister for Science, Technology, and the Environment called it "chemical warfare."

Agent Orange is not only a marker of ghostly silences, silencings, and hauntings[3] however, but also a vehicle that opens dialogue, expanding the "moral community" (Morris 1997), as American veterans, seeing the similarities between the illnesses that mark their own lives and those that mark the lives of Vietnamese thought to be affected by Agent Orange, call on the U.S. government and the chemical firms that sold it Agent Orange to fulfill their "moral duty" by compensating Vietnamese as well as Americans (Brunnstrom 2002). For some people in both Vietnam and the United States, Agent Orange has become a possible way of understanding the complex of forces that have shaped their experience of life and suffering, a way that links personal lives to societal problems.[4]

Agent Orange as Chemical

Strictly speaking, however, 'Agent Orange' was a nickname for one of the 16 main chemicals used tactically by U.S. and Saigon forces from 1961–1971,[5] during the war in Vietnam. It was one of a group of six chemicals rather euphemistically referred to as defoliants and herbicides, one of three that was contaminated by dioxin. Approximately 90 percent of these chemicals were used for defoliation, and 10 percent for crop destruction.

The term "Herbicide Orange" was the U.S. Defense Department code name given to a reddish-brown to tan liquid formulated to contain a 50:50 mixture of the n-butyl esters of 2,4-dichloro-phenoxyacetic acid (2,4-D) and 2,4,5-trichloro-phenoxyacetic acid (2,4,5-T). It got its name from the orange stripe painted around the 55 gallon barrels in which it was stored, and its nickname Agent Orange from the media. Agent Orange (and Agent Orange II) made up roughly 61 percent (44,953,560 liters) of the 72,740,400 liters of herbicides and defoliants deployed from 1961 to 1971.[6] It was used in roughly 66 percent of the missions for forest defoliation, and 40 percent of those for crop destruction (Lewy 1978, 257; Westing 1984, 4, 7).

One part of the toxicity of Agent Orange comes from its 2,4,5-T, which the U.S. officially recognized as potentially teratogenic (causing malformations) in 1969, contributing to the April 1970 order to suspend its use in the war, and to restrict its domestic use in herbicides (Lewy 1978, 263). Another part of the toxicity of Agent Orange and the three other defoliants that contained 2,4,5-T (Agents Purple, Pink, and Green) was TCDD dioxin, an unwanted by-product generated during the manufacturing process. TCDD is both very persistent and exceptionally toxic, often being referred to as the most toxic man-made chemical (Young and Reggiani 1988, 11; Le Cao Dai 2000, 35–39). Discussion of Agent Orange today is frequently more exactly a discussion of dioxin.

While Agent Orange and five of the other chemicals (Agents Purple, Pink, Green, White, and Blue) were generally referred to as herbicides and defoliants, they were used in concentrations and dosages higher than those recommended by their manufacturers. How much higher? Accounts vary. Ensign (144) says concentrations were 13 times higher, Westing (1984, 5) says dosages were 20 to 40 times higher, and a document prepared by the chairman of the Agent Orange/Dioxin Committee of the Vietnam Veterans of America puts the strength at 6 to 25 times those used for civilian purposes (Sutton 2002, 3–4; see also Cecil 1986, 225). Given the thousands of individual sorties involved in the spraying (see Cecil 1986), it seems reasonable to assume that concentrations and dosages varied, as did the number of sprayings applied in a given area.

Though Agents Purple, Pink, and Green were the first chemicals used in the war, Agents Orange, White, and Blue were the main chemicals used during the peak years of herbicide spraying, from 1967–1969. Agents Orange and White (a 1:4 mixture of picloram and 2,4-D) killed plants by mimicking their hormones to interfere with normal metabolism and were generally used for forest destruction. Agent Blue (active ingredient, cacodylic acid, an arsenic compound) was a desiccant that killed by preventing plants from retaining moisture, and was primarily used for crop destruction (Cecil 1986, 225; Westing 1984, 5).

While the image most often used to portray the defoliation is that of the low flying C-123 transport planes of the "Ranch Hand Project"[7] aerial spraying, the chemicals were also sprayed from riverboats, from trucks and other vehicles, and, around the perimeters of bases, by hand-held canisters.

Accounts of the extent of upland forests, saltwater forests and croplands that were sprayed vary somewhat and are at times incommensurable, though the total number of acres defoliated is frequently given in round figures as 5 million, with another 500,000 acres of crop destruction [cf. Harnly 1988, vii]. More precisely, according to Lewy (1978, 258), who bases his account on figures from MACV Command History, 4,747,587 acres were defoliated, and 481,897 acres of crops destroyed. He gives the proportion of cropland sprayed as 3.2 percent,[8] while the Committee of Concerned Asian Scholars quotes Air Force statistics that report nearly 10 percent of all arable land had been sprayed by 1969 [1970, 113]. Work to check and complete the accuracy of these statistics continues to this date.[9]

The official U.S. Air Force history estimates that 20 percent of the jungles of the south were sprayed (Buckingham 1982, iii). Harnly records 20 percent of the saltwater mangroves as having been destroyed, the Air Force history puts the figure at 36 percent, while the American Association for the Advancement of Science reported 20–50 percent of the mangrove forests "utterly destroyed" (Neilands et al. 1972, 274).

Lewy claims 46.4 percent of the total forested area was sprayed more than once; Harnly gives a figure of 32 percent for repeated spraying of upland forests. Vo Quy, internationally respected director of the University of Hanoi's Centre for Natural Resources Management, adds napalm, saturation bombing (25 million bomb craters in an area roughly the size of New Mexico), and bulldozing to the effects of spraying, coming up with a figure of 22,000 square miles of forest and farmland, mostly in the south, destroyed by thirty years of warfare (Vo Quy 1992, 13–16).

The long-term ecological impact of the spraying is still being studied. The effects in a given location varied with the kinds of vegetation sprayed, and the number of applications: according to one source, trees over seven years old were generally able to recover from a single spraying, but younger trees, certain mangroves, and other susceptible plants were not (Cecil 1986, 226). While great efforts at reforestation have reclaimed some areas, others remain covered in a tough, economically useless tall *imperator* grass that has been nicknamed "American grass," or by forests of low-grade bamboo (Vo Quy 1992, 14).

Lewy (1978, 258) gives the proportion of the population living in sprayed areas as something under 4 percent; Stellman (2000) estimates that 1 million people lived in heavily exposed areas. Given the great population movements during the war—of soldiers, evacuees, and some 2 million internal refugees in the south—it should be asked whether these figures include the number of people who later lived in or passed through these regions. The effect of spray drift and contaminated water and soil movements also complicate the compilation of accurate statistics.

Vietnamese estimates of people affected are sometimes given as 30,000, sometimes 70,000, and sometimes 1 or 2 million. This range can be partially understood as a result of the difficulty of developing statistics when there is no commonly accepted set standard for conditions that are linked to Agent Orange exposure, coupled to factors such as the unknown number of people thought to have already died, and the number who continue to be born with what may be second or third generation effects. Statistics are further complicated by new exposure that continues in a limited number of specific locations where spills occurred, storage containers leaked, or a plane was shot down with a full load of chemicals, or in locations that were repeatedly and intensively sprayed at close range, such as the perimeter of bases (cf. Dwernychuk et al. 2002; and Schecter et al. 2001).

Agent Orange As Controversy

The use of chemicals was controversial from the beginning, in both military and civilian circles. A full, balanced account of the histories of those controversies has yet to be written; here I can raise only a few points.[10] When experiments at a joint American-South Vietnamese Combat Development Test Center led, in November or December of 1961,[11] to requests that chemicals be used for a "crop warfare program," the U.S. at first declined, concerned about adverse political affects on the South Vietnamese, and about charges of chemical warfare that might be brought by the communists. In January of 1962, however, President Kennedy authorized the first use of defoliants. The first crop destruction mission followed on November 21 of that year.[12]

Arguments within the military and the administration that the use of herbicides and defoliants was banned by the Geneva Protocol and that their use would expose the U.S. to charges of barbarism were countered by arguments that the concept of chemical warfare applied to people and animals, not plants (Buckingham 1982, iii; Cecil 1986, 155). Cecil recalls arguments that killing plants instead of people would blunt guerrilla activity without inflicting direct injury on enemy, ally, or innocent (179). Another argument was that herbicides were "an economical and efficient means of stripping the Viet Cong of their jungle cover and food" (Buckingham 1982, iii).

It was not the use of herbicides and defoliants, however, that first caused public alarm over the use of chemicals in Vietnam. The use of various nauseating and asphyxiating gases, including apparently limited trials of the potentially lethal arsenic-containing DM (Neilands et al. 1972, 30–32, 47), drew a strong outcry at home and abroad in early 1965, before the beginning of the most intensive use of herbicides and defoliants. While President Johnson's press secretary called the materials used 'standard-type riot control' agents, a foreign doctor in Vietnam chronicled the casualties and fatalities he treated as a result of those gases (Neilands et al. 1972, 102–13), and the *New York Times* editorialized "... ordinary people everywhere—have a strong psychological revulsion, if not horror, at the idea of any kind of poisonous gas...." (Lewy 1978, 102–13).

Once the herbicides and defoliants were in full use, assessments of their effectiveness varied, particularly for the part of the program aimed at crop destruction. In 1967, for example, the Air Force noted success in achieving one of the objectives of the program, "to separate the VC from the people by forcing refugee movements into GVN [Government of Vietnam—a reference to the Saigon-based government] controlled areas."[13] A Rand Corporation study that same year concluded that the program was probably counterproductive. Estimating that 325,000 villagers had been affected by spraying operations that destroyed their crops and produced food shortages, the Rand study found 80 percent of the villagers they interviewed blamed the US/GVN for the destruction of their crops, with 74 percent expressing "outright hatred" (Lewy 1978, 260).

Scientists Raise the Alarm

Scientists were among the first to publicly question the use of chemicals. A March 1964 statement of the Federation of American Scientists read in part: " ... we are concerned with reports of the field use of chemical weapons in Vietnam. Allegations relating to the use of anti-crop agents under American supervision have been officially denied. However, reports that defoliating agents have been used to destroy protective cover have been confirmed by representatives of the Department of Defense. These charges give rise to the broader implication that the U.S. is using the Vietnamese battlefield as a proving ground for chemical and biological warfare. We ... feel that such experimentation involving citizens of other countries compounds the moral liability of such actions." The Pacific Division of the American Association for the Advancement of Science (AAAS) echoed these concerns in a June 1966 resolution, noting that the biological effect of the agents being used was not known, and that scientists had a special responsibility to be fully informed, since the products were the result of scientific research (Neilands et al. 1972, 118). Two of the first scientists to rally their colleagues to research were the liver specialist Professor Ton That Tung in Vietnam, and Harvard Professor Matthew Messelson, who was head of the Herbicide Assessment Commission of the American Association for the Advancement of Science.

In February 1967, 5,000 independent scientists, including 17 Nobel Prize winners and 129 members of the National Academy of Sciences petitioned President Johnson to order a stop to the use of herbicides and recommended a review of U.S. policy towards chemical and biological weapons. The Pentagon ordered a review of all published and unclassified literature "related to the ecological consequences of repeated or extended use of herbicides," which was carried out by the Midwest Research Institute and reviewed by the National Academy of Sciences (NAS). The results spoke of the destruction of vegetation, the unlikelihood of human or animal fatality, and the inconclusiveness of data "with respect to chronic toxicity and many other issues." In transmitting the results to the Pentagon, the NAS president cautioned that the study was only a "first step in investigating further the ecological consequences of the intensive use of herbicides" (Young and Reggiani 1988, 36–37; Neilands et al. 1972, 118; Uhl and Ensign 1980, 142–47).

Inconclusiveness of the data is a theme that runs through early studies of the effects of these chemicals on human health, as well. Wartime conditions were cited, along with inadequate health statistics. In 1969, E. W. Pfeiffer, a zoologist at the University of Montana, and Gordon H. Orians, a zoologist at the University of Washington, came home from a two-week field trip to Vietnam speaking of great environmental destruction, but unable to confirm reports of human and animal abnormalities (Orians and Pfeiffer 1970). The 1970 AAAS study, while finding "no definite evidence" of adverse health effects, did however find flaws in an earlier Army study that showed a downward trend for stillbirths, placental tumors, and malformations coincident with the peak of spraying.[14] A study begun in 1970 by the National Academy of Science at the request of Congress and the Secretary of Defense, concluded in 1974 that "no evidence substantiating the occurrence of herbicide-induced defects was obtained. However, "the potentially most definitive aspect of this examination has not yet been completed" (Young and Reggiani 1988, 35).

In the summer of 1969, a Bionetics Laboratory study that as early as 1965 had linked 2,4,5-T to malformations in test animals resurfaced, leading to further study and the order to suspend the use of the chemical in Vietnam and at home, pending yet further study (Lewy 1978, 263).[15] After several military units illegally continued using some of the 2.25 million gallons of Agent Orange stored in Vietnam, Cecil reports, the remaining barrels were shipped to Johnston Island in the Pacific in April 1972. In the summer of 1977, they were taken out to sea by the Dutch ship *Vulcanus* and incinerated, along with 860,000 gallons from storage at the Naval Construction Battalion Center at

Gulfport, Mississippi (Cecil 1986, 165). In the interval, over 250,000 pounds of Agent Orange had leaked into the soil of the island (Casper 2002, 17–19).

U.S. Veterans

In 1978 and 1979, a class of over 2.4 million U.S. veterans, their wives, and off-spring brought suit against seven chemical companies for injuries they alleged they suffered as the result of exposure to Agent Orange. The case was settled out of court, with the companies agreeing to pay $180 million, the largest award ever made to that date (cf. Young and Reggiani 1988; Cecil 1986; Shuck 1986). A lawyer who works with ongoing veterans' claims describes these early suits as "premature," given what was then known about the effects of dioxin (Smoger 2002). It was not understood at the time, for instance, how dioxin could affect the workings of the body; the mechanism by which dioxin affects multiple cell functions, its binding to the Ah receptor, was only discovered in the 1990s. Once again, this is a story that deserves a full telling, but can only be mentioned in passing here, to mark the importance of the veterans' role in bringing the issue before the public and motivating scientific study. (Another major part of the story that exceeds the limits of this chapter but deserves full and careful study also surfaces in these few lines: the role of the chemical companies, and the profit motive, both in the development and production of these chemicals, and in the handling of knowledge about their toxicity. More research is needed on this issue.)

By 1988, ten major epidemiological studies of Vietnam veterans, Agent Orange, and TCDD exposure had been completed under various auspices: the U.S. Air Force, the Veterans Administration, the Centers for Disease Control, the National Institute for Occupational Safety and Health, and the National Cancer Institute. Five further "health surveillance" projects were ongoing: three by the Veterans Administration Agent Orange Projects Office, one with the cooperation of that office and the Environmental Protection Agency, and the fifth by the Armed Forces Institute of Pathology (Young and Reggiani 1988, 59–61). Cecil mentions thirty-two studies underway by 1982, and another twelve being planned (1986, 171).

Controversies, questions, and denials beset these early studies. Those who believed that Agent Orange had no harmful consequences apart from chloracne, a serious skin condition generally accepted as caused by exposure to dioxin, blamed the media for overblowing the evidence in response to veterans' anger and their search for meaning in their lives and ailments (cf. Young and Reggiani 1988, 300–304). Those who believed it had greater effects than some of the studies showed, claimed a too-limited sample size (Cecil 1986, 170), bias, or falsification of evidence (see AP for one example). The senior counsel assisting in the Australian Royal Commission study that found "no connection between unfavourable outcome and exposure to Agent Orange" writes about the clarity of the scientific evidence (Young and Reggiani 1988,

304–305) with conviction equal to that of a member of the U.S. Agent Orange Scientific Task Force that determined there was enough scientific evidence of a link to grant compensation to veterans (Webster and Commoner, in Schecter 1994, 19), to give but one example of the difference of opinion resultant from exhaustive examination of the evidence.

Accumulating Evidence

Amidst controversy and debate, however, the list has been growing of diseases and conditions for which the U.S. gives compensation due to their possible link to exposure to Agent Orange. Although there is as yet no internationally accepted definition of diseases and conditions related to Agent Orange, since 1996 the U.S. Institute of Medicine has listed ten diseases—five cancers, two nervous disorders, two skin conditions, and one birth defect—as having "sufficient" or "limited" evidence of a link to exposure to Agent Orange (IOM: 7).[16] Dr. Dai, long-time researcher and head of the Agent Orange Victims' Fund of the Vietnamese Red Cross, believed there was enough evidence to add these conditions to the list as well: primary liver cancers, metabolic disorders (cerebro-arterial and coronary-arterial disorders); "unusual" births (spontaneous abortions, premature births, stillbirths, molar pregnancy, chorio-carcinoma), and a variety of birth defects affecting the first and second generations (Le Cao Dai, 2000 157–58).

Vietnamese research, though long hampered by wartime and postwar conditions and a lack of sophisticated equipment, has amassed a body of what Dr. Dai calls "suggestive" evidence. A Harvard researcher calls it "anecdotal," adding that such evidence, "when there is enough of it, becomes quite persuasive" (Constable 2002). Dr. Dai spoke of research he had conducted in a district of Ha Bac province in the north that suggested that veterans who fought in the south had more children with birth defects than those who fought in the unsprayed north, and that the longer they stayed south, the more likely they were to have such children. He spoke as well of ongoing cooperative research near a former U.S. base in Bien Hoa where chemicals were both stored and dumped, showing dioxin in the blood of patients at many times the acceptable level set by the World Health Organization (Schecter et al. 2001, 435).[17]

Yet again, a comprehensive study would be useful: a compilation of major Vietnamese research to date, translated into English, including the volumes of surveys and other research conducted by the National Committee to Investigate the Results of Chemical Warfare in Vietnam (known as the 10–80 Committee), as well as other research that has focused on reproductive issues and pregnancy outcomes, neural disorders, digestive illnesses, skin diseases, cancers, and immune disorders (Le Cao Dai 2000, 138–54). Such a translation must be done meticulously, with a goal of contributing to knowledge and clearing up misunderstanding, to prevent the distrust and disrespect that occur when words are used in a highly charged context in slightly different ways without recognition of their shifting nuances.

At the public health level, doctors at the Vietnamese Committee for Protection and Care of Children (CPCC) and the Red Cross have several answers in response to questions about why they think certain diseases may be linked to Agent Orange. The head of a provincial branch of the CPCC spoke of starting to suspect Agent Orange when he and a doctor from the Red Cross were looking for common factors in a certain clustering of unusual birth defects found in his province; they noticed that these children had at least one parent who had fought in sprayed areas in the south (Pham). A doctor working for the Agent Orange Victims Fund of the Vietnamese Red Cross gave as suggestive evidence the experiences of men who fathered children with birth defects with one wife, and then divorced that wife and remarried, only to again father children with birth defects; he also spoke of men who fathered healthy children before they went to war, whose children born after the war suffered a variety of conditions. In addition, he pointed to the unusual distribution of the children born with these birth defects: normally, he explained, only one child in a family suffers birth defects, but in these cases, many children—sometimes all—were affected.

Recent international research seems to support some of the observations made earlier by Vietnamese scientists.[18] In 1997 the International Agency for Research on Cancer (IARC) designated the form of dioxin found in Agent Orange (2,3,7,8-tetrachlorodibenzo-p-dioxin, known as TCDD) as a known human carcinogen, as did the U.S. Public Health Service's National Toxicology Program in 1999, and the U.S. Environmental Protection Agency (EPA) in its more than three thousand page report, released in 2000 after ten years of work. At the conference on "The Ecological and Health Effects of the Vietnam War," held at Yale University in September 2002, the director of the experimental toxicology division of the EPA named the following as findings of dioxin's effects on humans: "cardiovascular disease, diabetes, cancer, porphyria, endometriosis, decreased testosterone, chloracne," along with developmental effects on the "thyroid status, immune status, neurobehavior, cognition, dentition, [and an] altered sex ratio" (Birnbaum 2002).

Today ongoing scientific debates are carried on in terms that include: the possibility of developing valid exposure assessments; dioxin levels in soil, human tissue (fat tissue, blood, and breast milk), and animal tissue samples;[19] the possibility of male-mediated birth defects that occur years after exposure (Erickson 1984; Young and Reggiani 1988, 304); the possibility for valid epidemiological study given the passage of time and the absence of baseline data; whether TCDD is an initiator or promoter of damage, or a complete carcinogen; whether there is a threshold level (the shape of the dose-response curve); and what should be the role of scientific uncertainty in regulatory policy ("proof of harm," "acceptable risk," or "precautionary principle") (Webster and Commoner, in Schecter 1994, 15–16).

Though the research on Agent Orange and its contaminant dioxin is ongoing, the work that has been done is suggestive enough, and the political pressures have been strong enough,[20] that the U.S., Australian, South Korean, New Zealand, and Vietnamese governments have all established plans to compensate veterans who were exposed to the chemical. For the purposes of this paper it is important to recognize, however, that this is a topic that takes us to the limits of what is currently known by science. Such recognition can help us raise questions that may lead to a better understanding of appropriate roles for science: both what it can do, and what it cannot. Recognizing that a consideration of Agent Orange exceeds the discipline of science opens the possibility of investigating the chemical as an intersection, a "dense site where history and subjectivity make social life" (Gordon 1997, 8). Or, in this case, history, technology, and subjectivity.

This section has attempted to provide a brief introduction to some of the ways Agent Orange is spoken of as a subject of political controversy and an object of scientific study. The next section attempts to introduce some ways it is spoken of by people in Vietnam for whom it has become a way of making sense of the suffering they and their families and communities have experienced.

Agent Orange as Experience[21]

As a first step towards understanding how people in Vietnam treat the question of Agent Orange,[22] I visited Dr. Nguyen Viet Nhan, a professor in the physiology department of Hue Medical School.[23] Hue, a city of great beauty and great tragedy situated in the center of Vietnam, was not directly sprayed itself, but lies just south of Quang Tri province, and downstream from the mountains traversed by the Ho Chi Minh Trail—two of the most heavily sprayed regions during the war.

"Before . . ." Dr. Nhan tells me, "I spent all my time reading and teaching. I didn't know anything. . . ." We are in his office at Hue Medical School, where he has spent the last several hours patiently explaining his research, a three-site study of the links between Agent Orange and birth defects. Dr. Nhan began the study as his doctoral thesis, working on the hypothesis that Agent Orange would have had an effect on the germ cell, causing mutations, and that the occurrence of disabled children would serve as an indicator. Working with local health workers in three areas (the city of Hue, the mountainous district of A Luoi, and the village of Cam Lo in Quang Tri province), he selected 600 children with disabilities out of an original pool of 10,000 children who were "normal and not," as he puts it. When we spoke, he had not yet finished analyzing his data.

"It is hard to measure the results," he tells me. "We don't have enough modern equipment to evaluate the presence of dioxin in the soil, water, leaves, etc.;

we lack specialists in epidemiology; we don't have enough money to organize a large investigation; and the length of time is a problem. Twenty-five years ago [as I write, it is now thirty]—that's too long to evaluate accurately.

"But truly," he continues, "we don't need to know about the past. The war is behind us. We know a lot about dioxin already. What we need now is knowledge to help these children and their families."

He concludes our conversation with an invitation. "This morning we have talked a lot," he says, "but you will never understand anything if you just sit here with me. So this afternoon I plan to take you to visit some of the families."

That day we paid visits. Three years later, with the help of the Committee for the Protection and Care of Children (CPCC) in Thai Binh, and the following year with the help of the Red Cross in Ha Nam, Thua Thien Hue, and Dong Nai, I conducted the interviews from which the following stories are drawn.[24]

Following Dr. Nhan's formulation of how we may come to "know something," this section begins with stories of families the CPCC and the Red Cross have designated as "thought to have been affected by Agent Orange." One story will be told in detail, to provide some understanding of the context. Fragments of a few other stories will be excerpted.

The first story is from an interview conducted with a family in a northern province of Vietnam in the spring of 2000, where I was led by Tran Thi Lang, a friend who had worked for many years on malnutrition and maternal health issues. As a native of the province, her sympathy for those who suffered the consequences of Agent Orange there had been aroused both through her personal experience and through a collection of vignettes titled *Di Hoa Chien Tranh* [The Disastrous Consequences of War] (Minh Chuyen 1997).

Interview in a Rice-Farming Village

When we arrived at Mrs. Ha's home,[25] she was cooking lunch over an open fire in the detached kitchen. They had expected us earlier, but we were late, so the family had gone back to work, thinking our plans had changed. Mrs. Ha's husband, Mr. Binh, had gone to the communal warehouse to get wine to sell in the village, and Mrs. Ha wanted to wait for his return to begin the interview. As we hesitated a moment in the courtyard, family and neighbors began to gather. An old man, giving me a sideways glance, tested my Vietnamese. "What is this in Vietnamese?" he asked. "*Mot ngoi nha*—A house," I answered. He nodded vigorously, and walked up the steps into the new cement house.

It turned out "house" was indeed a significant word, symbolizing the care given by the extended family. Mrs. Ha's older brother pointed to a mud-walled, thatched-roofed house on a low-lying piece of land across the way. "You see, that house over there was their house. The relatives got together to loan them money to buy this house." It is a loan the relatives know cannot be repaid.[26]

"My sister and her husband are far too miserable," the brother continues. "I mean, in a year—in roughly 12 months—they had to go to the hospital thirty times, and each time there is only us to count on." I think of what it would take to get a sick person to the hospital from there: down the village lanes to the dike; a kilometer or so along the top of the dike to the small country road; through neighboring villages to the main provincial road, and then an hour or so by car to the provincial capital. But they would not go by car. Would they go by motorbike? I have only seen bicycles in the village. I think of the children left behind, the house to look after, and the crops to tend.

We went into the house and sat on plastic stools around a low table, where Mrs. Ha's brother poured us cups of tea. While we were waiting, Mrs. Ha spoke of her husband's many illnesses, recalling: "There was a time when the doctors at the hospital in town said 'That's all we can do; let him go home and wait for death. If he craves anything, let him have it.' His stomach was swollen like this, and his skin was completely swollen, and he couldn't go to the bathroom. Neighbors, and then other women, and then organizations gave a bit of rice, a few potatoes, and some kernels of corn, and then I had to beg for each nickel and dime.

"Then I had a dream about going into the forest to get medicine for my husband, so I 'dove through the mud' to get to the forest—all the way to Sa Pa—and there was the medicine to give my husband, folk medicine, and he took it and got better, and did not die."

Lang turned the conversation to strains these illnesses have put on the marriage. "Do you ever get angry or think of leaving?" she asks. "Sometimes I refrain from speaking," Mrs. Ha replies, "and sometimes I argue a sentence or two. Then I reflect, and pity him, and cry, not knowing what to do. He is so thin, his skin is so dark. He is now reaching the time of old age and weakness. His life is like the wind."

She turns to speak to the family and neighbors who fill the house, listening to our interview. "When you are happy, do you think you can stay that way forever? We can't be miserable forever, uncles and aunts, grandfathers—can we? That's right—I have to encourage my husband."

When Mr. Binh comes in, he tells us that in 1972, before the Paris Agreements, he was a special forces soldier in reconnaissance in Tay Ninh, a heavily sprayed region in the south. Where he was stationed the trees were denuded of leaves; he lived in tunnels, "bareheaded, barefooted, barechested"—"camouflaged by spreading mud on his body," interjects another man. "We saw 200 liter barrels with yellow stripes," Mr. Binh tells me, "they had three yellow stripes. We had only been through high school, so we could only read the word 'Dio xin,' or 'zio xin,' or something like that. At that time, we thought whoever died, died at once, and whoever lived, lived whole."[27] Mr. Binh came home with many diseases: diseases of the skin, of the nervous system, of the circulatory system, of the digestive system.

"The very regrettable aftereffects of that war you see in the first fetus my wife gave birth to," he tells us. "*My* wife, right here. It was like a monster, a monster in a fairy tale. You know, it didn't have a human shape. And a few minutes after it was born, it died. Very, very hard. And my very own wife has many illnesses, most of them women's illnesses. Women also bear the consequences of this war."

The couple's second child was slow-witted. He "doesn't know anything," they explain; he just turns from side to side. Their third child, a daughter, was born epileptic and blind, with no pupils. Their fourth child was sixteen at the time of the interview, and enrolled in school.

After her daughter was born, Mrs. Ha said to herself, "Enough!" She didn't know if it was because of the war or because of fate, she says, but she went to be sterilized. The procedure, which involved inserting medicine into the fallopian tubes, led to many complications, much loss of blood, and repeated operations. As we spoke she was in pain, with one half of her stomach swollen.

"I only believe in science," she explains. "As for the traditional village healer, I don't dare believe, because my child's brain and eye are very very important. Therefore, I totally and completely only believe in science. Science says she can't be cured. Then we must bear it, helplessly. What can we do? We can't do a thing.

"This all started from giving birth to children like this, and voluntarily going to be sterilized. Then I was unlucky and the consequence of sterilization was much illness. That made us spend a lot of money, money that a poor family doesn't have . . . very hard, very desperate. But it's all for my husband, all for my children, so I try to overcome the difficulties. Such a hard situation, but I still have to look after my husband, after my children. I know that my life is deeply entwined with his. I link my whole life with my husband and with my children, to 'carry the rivers and the mountains' to my last breath, and only because of war."

Mrs. Ha's brother says he wants to ask me just one more question. "In your country," he begins, "are there children like this?" He gestures around the room. I do not understand his implication, and cannot answer. "Children this strong, this tall, this big—or smaller?" One of the women sitting on the bed laughs and says "I've seen on TV—they are big. Vietnamese are the smallest." Mrs. Ha's brother continues: "Our life here should be like that of our international friends. But because the war lasted far too long—all our lives—we lost the chance to study, because at eighteen we left school and took up the gun. When the enemy was gone, we came back . . . back to feed our children, but there was not enough, so they are sickly and puny like this. You see?"

"These are the consequences of war," Mr. Binh explains. "What he is saying is that the consequences of war are very great. . . ."

Earlier Mrs. Ha has thanked me, and the American government, for paying attention to them and trying to help. When Mr. Binh again thanks me as a representative of the American government, I explain that I do not represent the government, that I do not know if the government will help, but that I believe ordinary people will. Mrs. Ha's brother replies, "Because everything comes from the people, doesn't it?" When he sees I am again not fully following his meaning, he explains: "Because if the people have sincere hearts and make demands on their government, most governments must execute those policies, because the government is for the people, isn't it?"

Mr. Binh has a request: "I want to ask you to say this to the American people. An unavoidable war broke out between our two countries. In reality, nobody wanted it. Now both sides understand each other, and the two countries are friends, and trade business. Close the past and open the future. The two countries circulate goods. They've exchanged ambassadors already. But what happened before—that is, the consequences of the bombs and bullets, and of the chemicals, outrages the Vietnamese people. Yes, because the result is not to kill a person at once, but the result waits for the children, and for the grandchildren.

"So I really hope the American people, together with the Vietnamese people, will demand that the American government not produce those chemicals any longer. Don't take them to make war with any other country. What is banned by international law should not be used. So stop using them. Yes . . . not just I myself in particular, or just the Vietnamese people in particular, but the whole world in general opposes these chemicals."

After saying good-bye to the family, we walk back along the dike. A stony silence I dare not break separates me from my friend. In the car, the man I take to be from security softly marvels, "That place was truly 'far away and remote.' "[28]

A year later, when I come across Gordon's words, the image of this family comes to mind. She writes: ". . . those who live in the most dire circumstances possess a complex and oftentimes contradictory humanity and subjectivity that is never adequately glimpsed by viewing them as victims or, on the other hand, as superhuman agents" (1997, 4).

*****

The stories told by Mrs. Ha and Mr. Binh are not meant as representative, but as samples. As a colleague from the local Red Cross in another province observed, with a shake of his head and a sigh at the end of our eleventh interview there: "Every family—its own set of circumstances."

Science, Politics, and Moral Responsiblity

If politics asks these families for patience until the scientific verdict is in, and science asks them for samples of blood, breast milk, and fatty tissue, what do these families ask of science and politics?

"Responsibility," as one interviewee put it. "The word in Vietnamese is responsibility."

One question is how these families' illnesses are related to Agent Orange. To that question, neither the families nor the scientists can reply with absolute certainty. A pharmacist with two severely paralyzed sons put it this way: "I am the only one in my family with this problem, and the only one who was a soldier. I supplied medicines—also insecticides—but friends who worked with me weren't affected. Professors expert in this field must research more—I can only say this much. Quite a few friends in my same unit also have similar problems—continual miscarriages, for example."

Like many of the people I spoke with, the pharmacist muses about the link between fate and Agent Orange as he searches to make sense of his life. "That is my situation," he says. "I see the fate of the Vietnamese people. Why is my fate so unjust, so severe? When I review my own life, I see that there are no faults worth mentioning—from childhood to now, I've generally lived compassionately with my friends, behaved carefully and properly, kindly . . . didn't fight, or play rough. I was naughty, but I never fought anyone. When I went into the army I was lucky—I didn't have to carry a gun to fight anyone directly. My duty was to take care of the medical supplies for the soldiers."

Other people spoke of making offerings, praying, and visiting fortune-tellers, physiognomists, and geomancers, looking in vain for an explanation. "I was told there was nothing wrong with the graves,"[29] said a woman who had fought in the south, "and nothing wrong with the way my family lived. Our parents on both sides were very gentle, good people . . . three generations were landless laborers, five generations were revolutionaries." What she would like, she said, is recognition, official recognition that she and her family had made a contribution to the nation, so that people would know that their suffering was not because they were bad people. As an afterthought she added that 100,000 Dong ($7) would be useful.

These families ask questions about morality, questions of meaning, and questions of ultimate significance, questions science and politics cannot answer. Taken together with critiques raised by medical anthropology, various environmental sciences, and science and technology studies, these questions draw attention to the ways, as Keyes (2002) puts it, "modern societies organized around secular institutions, science, and rationalized action have not only failed to provide people with adequate means to address [. . .] suffering, but [. . .] have also generated new forms of social suffering."

Looking at Agent Orange as both an artifact of the chemical age and as a marker of social suffering expands the conversation to include the multiple layers of meaning distilled into the term, enabling us to take its moral dimensions seriously, and to ask accountability of the social, economic, and political forces that led to the creation and wartime use of chemicals. Such a treatment brings together questions that have been "sealed off into incommensurable problems," to use Latour's phrasing, ". . . questions that cannot be solved separately but rather must be tackled all at once" (1999, 310). These questions entail a careful look not only at the relationships between knowledge, politics, economics, and ethics, but also at where we have come as a nation, at whether we intend to be here, and at how we might redirect our energies towards creating a world that is safer and healthier for us all.

"We know we sprayed Agent Orange," mused a toxicologist at a preparatory meeting for the first official talks between U.S. and Vietnamese scientists. "We know Agent Orange contains dioxin," he continued, "and we know a lot about the effects of dioxin already. What is it that we need to know?"

How do we know when we know enough? And in the meantime, in the midst of our uncertainty, how do we respond to human suffering? The question, then, is only partly who these families are in relation to Agent Orange; equally important are questions of who we are in relation to our own humanity, and of how we may dispel the ghosts of the past that still haunt our relations with the world.

5

From Metallic to Sickly

*Chemical Waste,
Environmental Discourse,
and the National Body
in Post-Socialist Hungary*

ZSUZSA GILLE

The environmental problems of the former socialist countries of Eastern Europe and the former Soviet Union have been often identified as being among the worst, if not the worst, in the world. The environmental problem of state socialism has been constructed in both scholarly and journalistic accounts as the result of inefficiency and backward technology. The main culprits were large, out-of-date, uncompetitive enterprises in heavy industry, primarily metallurgy and the coal-based energy sector, that were shielded from the world market and thus produced inefficiently. Inefficiency, in the language of neo-liberal economics, is not only the greatest sin but also the main cause of environmental problems. This representation of state socialist environmental problems, however, ignores some more recent, but no less significant, sources of environmental harm, such as the electronics industry, the nuclear energy sector, and the chemical industry.

Many countries under state socialism could boast a modern, competitive chemical industry, often relying on Western technology and know-how, that cultivated strong ties with the world market and produced quite efficiently. While the environmental and public health burdens of chemical production are very serious, and it is a well-documented fact that hazardous wastes are produced overwhelmingly by the chemical industry, its pollution has never been treated as somehow "representative" of state socialism.

Blaming environmental degradation entirely on the dinosaurs of coal-based heavy industries gives the illusion that if only these factories went out of business or were modernized, the problem would be solved. This, of course, effectively disarms present efforts to politicize the environmental problems produced by the nascent economic order, and by nonparadigmatic polluters in particular.

Ignoring the chemical industry in representations of state socialism however also leaves a series of institutions, a certain material culture, and a particular ideology that emerged under state socialism hidden from view or explained away. I show that the chemical industry played an important role not only in the material and economic foundations of socialism but also in self-representations of the socialist nation. These roles changed over time as the relationship between society and materiality/nature and that between the state and citizens went through transformations. I argue that such historical processes have tangible consequences for environmental policies in the present. To provide a sharp and empirically grounded argument, I use the case of chemical wastes in Hungary as a lens through which we can understand this history.

Body and Nation during Stalinism

The 1950s in Hungary was a time of high modernity, at least as it concerns Stalinist industrialization and urbanization based on centrally defined over-ambitious production targets. The voluntarism of economic planning relied on an extreme "social constructivist" notion of human and nonhuman nature. According to this position, socialism was the society that could overcome the obstacles to production posed by the social contradictions of capitalism, most notably the separation and conflict between use value and exchange value.[1] In socialism, workers supposedly had an objective interest in the development of the means of production, including technology and their own productive capacity, and thus gave their best to plan fulfillment and the building of communism. To entice them just a little more, the Stalinist party-state organized work competitions, in which workers of a plant or district challenged their counterparts elsewhere to fulfill the plan faster or to overfulfill it to a greater extent by the end of a certain period. The best known of these "production-helping," consciousness-raising campaigns was the Stakhanovite movement, in which workers competed with each other in breaking the norms ascertained for a certain work task. This voluntarist attitude, the idea that simply by making an effort, more can be produced from the same amount of resources and by the same number of workers, presupposed and ultimately forced an extreme flexibility both on human and nonhuman nature.

The conquest of nonhuman nature was hailed, and the aesthetics of socialist realism openly celebrated the transformation of idle nature into useful, productive nature with the industrial landscape advertised as the right natural environment for the Socialist Man. Morning or night, winter or summer, the industrial plants of Stalinism permeated the natural environment, creating what we might call socialism's second nature.

> The sky is clear. It was dawn not long ago, and now the summer sunshine is peeking into the wide yard of the morning. The factory however knows neither night, nor dawn, nor morning. It only knows shifts following one another. The factory rules the entire landscape. (Vészi 1952, 11)[2]

It was a beautiful summer night. The noise of the millworks almost belonged to the sound of nature around here. (Vészi 1952, 45)

Similarly it went with human nature. Workers' bodies were construed as flexible enough to work not eight but twelve to fourteen hours a day if necessary and to break the records of the already backbreaking norms. What supposedly made this voluntary and painless for the workers was their identification with the productionist goals of the regime and the rigorous disciplining of their bodies. "Today, in contrast,"—argued a contemporary propaganda brochure—"things are different: the country is ours, we are its stewards. We know that we are working for ourselves, for the benefit of our country" (Iron Workers' Union 1951, 4).

Representing workers' bodies as such was elevated to a new kind of aesthetics and ethics that materialized in paintings, sculptures, and literature that quickly filled public spaces and the shelves of libraries,[3] a fleet of loud monuments to the rule of mind over body and the rule of society over nature.[4]

This rule seemed to be most complete in the metallurgical industries of the 1950s. As the primary task was to modernize the nation to build communism, metallurgy and the heavy industries in general took on a central role. Metallurgy and engineering were not only strategically important, but also the symbolically most relevant industries of state socialism. The Soviet economic and political model that by then had been operating for three decades also suggested that a true socialist economy must be based on the central role, if not the idolization, of metals, not just in the economic sense but in the political sense as well. Communists considered metallurgical and metal workers the most trustworthy stratum of the working class, because of their skills and activist past. Metallurgy and engineering quickly became an ideological metaphor for communism. Metal and mechanical symbolism grew strong initially in the early Soviet era in the futurist works of artists and poets such as Mayakovsky, but there were numerous other less well-known worker-poets, such as Aleksei Gastev, who used iron and steel as a metaphor for the workers' hard and hardworking bodies and the metallurgical production process as a metaphor for the individual worker's identification with his tools and work task and his dissolution into the collective (Hellebust 1997, 505).

> Flywheels in motion.
> A hundred thousand workers to the task.
> We go fearlessly into the iron.
> We give it our hearts.
> (Gastev, *The bridge*, 1918, quoted in Hellebust 1997, 515)

Soviet leaders were also fond of assuming metallic names: Molotov from *molot* (hammer) and Stalin from steel (Hellebust 1997, 501).

The economic and geopolitical pressures coupled with the cultural-aesthetic regime of Soviet state socialism led to a modernization project that prioritized heavy industry and particularly metallurgy and engineering. As a result, the training of cadres emphasized the same industries, and the prevailing mental image of production became that of metal manufacturing, a production process relying on discrete production tasks (rather than "continuous production processes"),[5] mechanical (rather than chemical) transformation, and on individualizable ("Taylorizable") performance. Metallurgy not only became overemphasized as the foundation of society, it was held up as the model for planned production for the rest of the economy.

The prevalent waste discourse of Stalinism could not escape this imposition either. This discourse conceptualized waste as primarily metal scrap, as entries under waste in Hungarian dictionaries published in early state socialism testify. Definitions offered for waste are not abstract at all, rather they amount to no more than a collection of examples from metallurgical and engineering waste practices. The 1962 edition of the *New Hungarian Lexicon,* for example, explained the concept of waste this way:

> The remainder of the processed material left after tailoring or working to a given size (e.g. metal shavings, waste sheets, etc.). The reduction of waste is an important economic interest, which can be achieved by, for example, precision casting and the appropriate composition of pattern designs. Depending on their quality and size, wastes can in many cases be utilized (e.g. re-smelting) and this has great economic importance.

As if the metallic examples were not enough, the lexicon refers the reader to the heading "Metal wastes," while making no mention of other types of waste.

Besides the mentioned priority given to the metallurgical and engineering industries in the 1950s, there were two other factors that contributed to this rather limited view of waste. With the onset of the Cold War, Western countries placed an embargo on metal exports to socialist countries, which for a country poor in metal ores, such as Hungary, potentially spelled disaster. In addition, the steel manufacturing technologies of the time—primarily the Siemens-Martin technology—relied heavily on iron-scrap for the efficiency of combustion. In sum, cultural, political, economic, and technological reasons all contributed to the exclusivity of a metallic waste model in policies dealing with wastes.

Beyond the explicit identification of waste with metal scrap, production waste tended to be visualized as metal waste, or at least the characteristics of metal scrap—its solid state, its finality, its tangibility, its discrete nature—were readily assumed to be universal for all production wastes. Liquid or gaseous wastes, or wastes that were produced continuously rather than discretely were ignored. As a result, the primary methods of waste reduction and reuse could be applied only to discrete and solid materials. This new approach, unlike recycling, gave priority to reusing waste materials in their original quality and function without chemical or substantial mechanical transformation. As Géza Gazda, the "hero" of the Stalinist material conservation campaigns put it,

> The correct interpretation of material conservation is to transform all those lay-away materials, that are found in iron scrap, for example, used axle materials, tracks and other steel materials, into useful materials *by by-passing the Martin furnaces, and occasionally even the rolling mills,* in the production process. (Minutes. Document Number 33. Box 5. 1951. Central Council of Hungarian Trade Unions. Department of Economics, 3—my emphasis)

He himself attracted the attention of the party with his innovation that made steel scrap immediately reusable without melting it down: he built a series of rollers that flattened out the pieces of scrap cold (!) into sheets which could then be used as if they were made of new materials. Reusing waste without chemical transformation strikes us today in the West as a rather progressive approach. After all, it not only encourages material conservation and a preventative attitude to environmental problems, but it prioritizes reuse over recycling, which is the more efficient of the two. This model worked quite well in industries that turned out discrete products, such as leather, paper, textile and wood. However, it turned out to be inapplicable in the chemical industry.

The Chemical Industry as a Class Alien in Stalinism

If metallurgy and metalworking industries were strategic and constituted an indispensable representational role in state socialism, other industries, primarily the chemical industry, were considered to be an alien territory for state socialism. Let us review the causes of this ideological hierarchy.

The kind of production processes that characterize the chemical industry did not lend themselves easily to the organization of central planning and the disciplinary organization of production. In order for certain social and political elements of what Burawoy (1985) calls the factory regime to work, it has to dovetail with the human-material connection in a given production process. This has to do with the nature of the human-material connection in the chemical industries in general. First of all, chemical production is a continuous process, as Robert Blauner summarizes:

> chemical processes cannot be subdivided to the extent that the mechanical operations in assembly can be. Chemicals are not discrete units upon which a number of operations can be performed very quickly, but liquids and gases that flow continuously through a series of automatic operations, each of which takes a considerable amount of time. (1967, 163)

In the chemical industry, products and semi-finished products are produced in large batches, then the production line is reorganized, and another product or semi-finished product is created. Since one batch may take several weeks, no single finished product is turned out for weeks or months. For this reason, work competitions based on monthly targets did not succeed very well. As a trade union report explained,

> This method [breaking up quarterly quotas into monthly ones] is especially incorrect in chemical industries, where the monthly production program within the quarterly one changes frequently. In case of a change in the program, it may happen that the worker works on an entirely different task than s/he made a pledge for. As a result, the competition only exists on paper. (Report on the Situation of Socialist Work Competitions, January 16, 1953. Department of Wage, Production, and Economics of the Central Council of Hungarian Trade Unions. Box 12/90, 2)

It was not only the temporal breakdown of plans that caused problems but also the breakdown of plans into quotas for individuals. In the chemical industry, as Blauner argues, work tasks are less individualized. Workers mostly add or drain materials, check meters and weigh materials and provide a control over the otherwise quite automatic chemical processes. Here work cannot be as standardized as in the mechanical process or assembly line industries, because a lot depends on the chemical or biological givens of each unique production process. For the individual worker, this means that s/he has less control over her/his individual performance. Speeding up, looting, or slacking off are difficult. As a result, the socialist work competitions that urged the break-down of plans into individual workers' quotas and a rivalry among individual employees had poor prospects for implementation.

> The detailed breakdown of the plans met with serious obstacles, because they only broke down the plans to shifts. Since in the great majority of the chemical plants the product of each shop goes through various labor processes, it is necessary to break down the plan in such a way that would determine for the individual worker the task per shift so that the individual final results of each worker in the shop add up to the targeted goal. (Report on the Socialist Work Competitions of Chemical Plants—second quarter of 1952 and beginning of first quarter of 1953. Department of Wage, Production, and Economics of the Central Council of Hungarian Trade Unions. Box 12/90. February 2, 1953, 2)

The idea that production is an aggregated total of tasks performed by individual plants, shops and workers is a characteristic logic of central planning predicated upon a schematic understanding of mechanical or metallic production models. Chemical industries rely on a different set of relationships between the human and the material aspects of production. High-level party and trade union officials, however, rejected this essentialist view of materiality and nature, and their unwillingness to "make exceptions" for the chemical industry aggravated technical managers.

> The breakdown of plans in such a way met with a serious resistance by the technical employees, what's more the enterprise triangle [a body consisting of the management, the party and the trade union officials] in the Budapest Sulfuric Acid Factory could only be persuaded after a several hour-long debate. (Report on the Socialist Work Competitions of Chemical Plants—second quarter of 1952 and beginning of first quarter of 1953. Department of Wage, Production, and Economics of the Central Council of Hungarian Trade Unions. Box 12/90. February 2, 1953, 2)

Indeed, reports indicated that chemical plants were lagging behind in the socialist work competitions. When explaining the poor records of chemical plants in these competitions, party officials often referred to the "special situation" of the industry.

> The chemical industry differs from other industries to the extent that in it work not skilled workers [i.e. with special learned skills] but well-trained workers with long experience. The labor processes are not mechanically visible [sic] processes but chemical processes that take place in a closed system. For this reason, the rationalization of work is more difficult than in those industries which have mechanical processes. (Report. October 30. No document number. Fonds 276. Group 116. Preservation unit 40, 138)

As a solution, the report suggested organizing the Stakhanovite movement not by individuals but by teams, brigades, and plants; and instead of the criteria of production volume, it considered innovations and material conservation. Nevertheless, a later decree strongly pushed for individual quotas and as a result, a 1954 report still found that "on the terrain of the chemical industry, the organized direction and control of the work competition is not sufficiently held in hand and, as a result, there are not enough efforts made to correct mistakes" (Report on the Work Competition of the Chemical Industry, October 30, 1954. Department of Wage, Production, and Economics of the Central Council of Hungarian Trade Unions. Box 174).

In terms of the planning of material use, chemical plants were also in an ambiguous position. On the one hand, as a contemporary evaluation suggested,

> [b]ecause the use of auxiliary materials cannot be deduced from the chemical equations of the technological process, and their "wear and tear" depends on a lot of different factors, the calculation of material norms requires an even more careful pioneering work that can transplant experiences onto a scientific foundation. (Jávor 1954, 11)

On the other hand, it was also claimed that "[o]n the terrain of raw materials what makes our [the chemical industry's] situation easier and helps us to recognize our mistakes is the fact that in the chemical industry one can establish what the theoretically necessary amount of raw materials is needed for the production process." (Report on the Situation of Material Conservation in the Chemical Industry. June 6, 1956. Department of Economics of the Central Council of Hungarian Trade Unions. Box 8, 2)

But this was a double-edged sword: the precision of chemical laws could not only help determine more easily what constitutes a wasteful use of materials (although not the use of auxiliary materials), it could also pose definite limits to thrifty material use and was probably seen as too strict to allow spectacular achievements in material conservation.

One of the plants in the Chinoin pharmaceutical company also invoked such biological and chemical givens as reasons for a lack of plan or pledge fulfillment.

> The Penicillin plant pledged to fulfill its July and August plans by August 20. Unfortunately we could not fulfill this partly for technical reasons, partly for reasons that have to do with work discipline, and partly for reasons of the nature of production. We have overcome the technical obstacles, and there seems to be a definite improvement on the terrain of work discipline. *We know that the biological process influences our production to some extent, but not entirely.* We will strive to manage production in such a way that these factors don't hamper our production. (Minutes at the party meeting on August 29, 1951. Chinoin. Fonds 176/2. Group 184. Preservation Unit 2, 15—my emphasis)

In the eyes of the authors of some of these reports, however, this technological uniqueness did not absolve the Hungária Chemical Works and the Chinoin pharmaceutical factory from their poor record in the Stakhanovite movement. The general reasons for such bad performance might be technological but the specific causes had to be political. The report claimed that in these factories "there were a lot of fascists and social democrats among the lower-level technical cadres" (Report. State Economy Department of MDP. October 30, 1951. No document number. Fonds 276. Group 116. Preservation unit 40, 138). Another article not only excluded such technological arguments but identified those as suspect when it alleged that "in the organic and inorganic chemical industry they are avoiding the question under the pretext of various special situations" (Document numbers 12227 and 30581. Fonds 276. Group 95. Box 46).

This mistrust was partially the result of the mentioned uniqueness of the industry and especially its strong reliance on high-level technical and scientific knowledge, and thus of a certain sense of insecurity in the economic and ideological leaders. Put yourselves in the shoes of these party apparatchiks and trade union representatives whose level of education was rather low. "Fifty percent of the cadres in the statistics did not complete the eight-year elementary school," recounted an internal survey report, which then suggested to increase the proportion of the technical intelligentsia (Report by the Department of Party and Mass Organizations of the Political Committee of the Budapest Party Committee on the 1952 cadre statistics. Fonds 95/2. Preservation Unit 282). A 1954 report, however, still found only 5.7 percent of party cadres to be intelligentsia, and even within this group the proportion of the technical intelligentsia represented only 2.8 percent. At the same time 69.2 percent of the paid party activists were workers employed in factories. It is quite reasonable to expect that such officials felt intimidated by the kind and level of knowledge that the management of chemical plants required. For them, such production processes remained inscrutable, and thus dangerously out of their reach of control. Suspicion must have been their natural reaction.

This suspicion probably also had a lot to do with a severe mistrust of the class basis of the chemical industry employees, and of engineers and professionals in general. A memorandum by the Chemical Workers' Union from 1952 warned that "we still have functionaries who loathe the technical employees and, generalizing, identify everybody with the technical employees of capitalism" (Memorandum by the Trade Union of Chemical Industrial Workers, to the Wage and Production Department of the Central Council of Hungarian Trade Unions. Box 127, 4).

From the foregoing discussion and pieces of evidence, the chemical industry emerges as an alien territory for the building of communism. The metallic production culture imported from the Soviet Union and the political suspicion towards the chemical industry led to an exclusionary representation of waste as metal, or metallike, often explicitly as steel scrap. This resulted in a waste model that was based on a metonymy in Gudeman's (1986) sense: the schema planners in early state socialism applied to the economy was steel manufacturing, which was to stand in for the entire economy, turning metal waste into the icon of all wastes. Once the idea that wastes are raw materials that could help fulfill plans faster took root, it was easily applied to all other branches of industry. I discuss the consequences of this model in the next section.

The Problem of Chemical Wastes

The imposition of the metallic waste model on a widely diverse set of industries led to some counterproductive outcomes.

The kind of built-in recycling that characterizes many chemical production processes was not the kind that the party could show off as new, and the achievements of chemical wastes were thus not as spectacular. In fact, a trade union representative suggested that there is a confusion about what workers can pass off as new. "The widening of the Gazda movement in the chemical industry creates a problem, because there are a lot of materials that the plants reused before, and they wonder whether this [practice] is a part of the Gazda movement" (Report on the Gazda movement. December 5, 1951. Department of Wage, Production, and Economics of the Central Council of Hungarian Trade Unions. Box 5/34, 1).

To the extent that the point the party tried to drive home was that wastes are always useful, the propagandistic value of the kinds of products made out of chemical by-products was lower than of those manufactured out of metal, textile, or wood. Consider the following quote from Gazda: "What can you use a thousand tons of [scrap] reinforcing iron for? For the ferro-concrete ceilings of 750 two-room apartments, or for covering the iron needs of three buildings as big as the Sport Stadium of Csepel, or, . . . 50,000 bicycles or 64,000 sewing machines, or 160 large, radial drills, or boiler tubes for 300 engines" (Gazda 1951, 1). What would be the rhetorical impact of this claim if we were to replace the recognizably useful goods produced out of metal wastes with products such as acetic acid anhydride, brenzkatechin, or papaverin—compounds suggested to be made out of chemical wastes by industry representatives in the early 1950s?

The dominant discourse on waste constructed it as something useful, and therefore the Hungarian state's task was to make sure that appropriate use values were given to waste. Wastes were not to be thrown out but to be kept in production and be circulated in the economy as long as possible. If technical conditions for the reuse of certain wastes were missing this was viewed as a temporary problem that rapid technological development and the genius of socialist workers would solve shortly.

There was only one decree, the No. 2500–21/1954 decree of the head of the Central Planning Office on the collection and utilization of wastes, that indicated what was to be done with wastes for which no uses have been found yet. It ordered waste generators to

> bring the attention of their superordinate authorities, the Ministry of Light Industry, or other competent organs (such as research institutes) to so-far unutilized wastes, to ask for their advice and opinion and, if a utilization opportunity is available, to organize the collection, utilization or sale. If the experiments to find uses for certain wastes in the local industry has been successful, the supply boards of the ministries are obliged—at the request of the Minister of the Light Industry—to have the waste generators complete their plan for reusing the wastes in question.

However, the decree still did not give any instructions as to what should happen if the experiments for reuse were not successful, and what other institutes/organizations could conduct experiments and what practical steps those results entitled them to take. Ultimately, it left the burden of determining utility and economic feasibility, but most importantly, the task of dealing with unusable wastes, on the shoulders of managers.

A key area in which such nonrecyclable wastes piled up was the chemical industry. The chemical industry turns out nondiscrete products, which make the applicability of Gazda's model difficult. Gazda noted this difference in his talk at a discussion group on the achievements of his movement.

> I must note that in one respect, the workers of the chemical industry are in a more difficult situation than, for example, those in the steel or timber industries. The wastes whose reuse possibilities we ponder in the steel industry are more tangible than in the chemical industry. Waste in the chemical industry leaves in a gaseous state, which is intangible. (Minutes. Document Number 33. Box 5. 1951. Central Council of Hungarian Trade Unions. Department of Economics, 8)

For Gazda, however, the problem of chemical wastes resided in the technical difficulties of reusing and recycling wastes and not in the pollution such wastes might cause: "It hadn't occurred even to me when leaving the factory and passing by the gas plant, where we always have to walk carefully to avoid the constantly leaking tar water, how much money must be poured in the Danube annually" (Minutes. Document Number 33. Box 5. 1951. Central Council of Hungarian Trade Unions. Department of Economics, 8). In his eyes, what was poured into the Danube was not polluting materials but money that could have been saved by reusing these materials. What kept Gazda awake at night was not public health that might be endangered by dumping wastes in the main river of the country but rather that materials this way became lost forever from the circle of resources available for the party-state to use for designated production goals and ultimately for the building of communism.

Another problem created by chemical wastes, as an industry report pointed out, was that the uniqueness of each production process places limits on its wider applicability: "The chemical industry is in a unique situation in this regard, because it is difficult to find methods that could be applied in other plants due to the fact that the production processes markedly differ from each other. This is so even within individual branches of the industry" (Report on the Situation of Material Conservation in the Chemical Industry. Central Council of Hungarian Trade Unions. Department of Economics. Box 8. June 6, 1956, 5).

In the chemical industry, waste reuse in most cases was, for technical reasons, restricted to recycling, that is the reuse of materials altered by some kind of chemical transformation. Gazda's notion that wastes are 100 percent recyclable was not adaptable to the chemical industry. Metal wastes, in general, could indeed be reused over and over again, and even if they were left to rust they did not constitute a significant source of air or water pollution. To deal with chemical wastes, whose reuse or even recycling was a technically much more thorny problem, and whose accumulation in storage *was* an environmental threat, would have required a more flexible attitude. Problems created by such wastes called for a much more rigorous focus on source reduction, and especially facilities for safe waste treatment and dumping. Source reduction was not prioritized because the metallic waste model suggested endless reusability, which belief was manifest in waste quotas that enterprises had to fulfill. Requests for disposal, on the other hand, were denied because dumping would have meant renouncing a secondary raw material. This emphasis on reuse and recycling is a progressive direction in environmental policies that, in the West, have until relatively recently dealt with wastes through end-of-pipe technologies—dealing with pollution by dumping and incineration rather than preventing it, thus not only wasting resources but also polluting air and water. However, applied as it has been in Hungary, without any consideration for wastes that cannot be unproblematically reused or recycled, it produces unintended consequences and another set of environmental problems. To wit, not only was the idea of useless wastes precluded, but so was the idea that wastes might be harmful. One area where this created many problems was again the chemical industry.

First of all, the by-products of the chemical industry tended to be dangerous to health; second, due to the rapid growth of the chemical industry, such by-products were now created at an unprecedented rate. The significance of chemical investments grew due to the increase of hydrocarbons among energy and raw material sources and due to the industrialization of agriculture. Between 1960 and 1970 the chemical industry was the fastest-growing branch of the economy. The annual average rate of growth was 13.3 percent, double the average industrial growth rate (Pető and Szakács 1985, 553). As the supply of the population with consumer goods received greater political and economic priority after Kádár took over in the wake of the 1956 Revolution, the provision of agricultural chemicals became a key area of expansion, actually suppressing growth in other areas of chemical production.[6]

Despite this fast growth, socialist countries, including Hungary, still needed to import pesticides from capitalist countries, a reliance on the enemy that was unacceptable. In 1970 the share of domestic production of all pesticides was 39 percent, the share of imports from socialist countries 13 percent, and the share of capitalist imports 48 percent (Vegyiművek, March 1, 1971, 1), pushing Hungary to keep increasing pesticide production and chemical production in general. The slogan "we'll be a country of iron and steel" was replaced with the slogan "Let's chemicalize!" and within a decade nonreusable and untreated chemical wastes piled up on factory yards all across the country to such an extent that they created not only bottlenecks in production but also environmental hazards. Local government officials started complaining about illegal dumps appearing both next to dumps managed by councils (local governments) and on the territory of filled dumps where the land had already been put back into cultivation. In 1967, the Executive Committee of the Council of

Table 5.1 The average annual rate of growth in chemical production (1960–1970) (percentages)

Area of production	1960–1965	1965–1970	1960–1970
Fertilizers	21.2	14.3	17.7
Pesticides	35.0	−1.5	15.3
Plastics	22.4	15.0	18.7
Synthetic fibers	8.4	8.6	8.5
Petroleum processing	8.8	11.7	10.3
Pharmaceuticals	26.1	12.2	19.0
Rubber and plastics processing	15.4	7.5	11.4
Chemical Industry Total	14.9	11.8	13.3

Source: Pető and Szakács 1985, p. 557.

Budapest was forced to admit the void in the regulation of industrial waste disposal. Yet the Hungarian state did not accept dumping and incineration as appropriate for dealing with waste until the 1980s.

Body and Nation in Late State Socialism

Starting in the 1970s, the chemical industries gained more importance in state socialism as well, following worldwide trends. Subsequently, by the mid-1980s, a new waste model became dominant in public discourse and policy making: the chemical waste model. The ascendance of the chemical model to hegemony was rooted primarily in the increasing professionalization of economic management and the significance of knowledge-based industries in keeping the economy afloat.

As the professional intelligentsia increased its importance in economic management, its cry for a way to deal with nonrecyclable and nonreusable wastes became louder and less suppressed. At a conference in 1981 on the liquidation of hazardous wastes, a high-ranking official of the Ministry of Industry, a chemical engineer himself, posed the question, "why is it that the Budapest chemical plants and the world-famous Hungarian pharmaceutical industry still do not have a modern incinerator that could guarantee legal air quality standards?" (Szász 1981, 6). In his narrative, the chemical and especially the pharmaceutical industry appear as pioneers that strove to establish safe incineration practices already in the 1970s, but whose requests for permits for a safe incinerator in Budapest were repeatedly turned down by one authority or another. The reasons usually had to do with the councils' interest in a conflicting path of development for the proposed location. The quoted high-ranking official, and this was a theme repeated in my interviews, criticized the

1981 hazardous waste decree for only punishing the enterprises but not establishing the technical conditions to comply with the law. This way, the blame for illegal dumping was pushed back on to the Hungarian state:

> One thing is certain: as long as the chemical plants and plants applying chemical technologies have no possibility to incinerate or have their wastes incinerated in modern facilities, the danger will always remain that they will choose the undesirable path of making materials disappear. (Szász 1981, 6)

From the perspective of the chemical industry, waste reuse, recycling or source reduction through modernization were insufficient. These are all partial solutions, mostly because the processes on which chemical production is based are irreversible, and usually only a small amount of the products and byproducts can be regained or reused. In the chemical model, production is not a closed cycle in the sense that all materials produced can be recirculated into production. The reduction of by-products also meets greater difficulties than in other industries due to the mentioned precision required for successful chemical processes. Finally, dealing with these mostly hazardous substances requires immediate and safe handling. In the chemical waste model, propagated with increasing loudness and success by industry representatives, wastes appear as negative and harmful, and they are best kept away from production and people. They are to be liquidated by end-of-pipe technologies, primarily by dumping and incineration.

Ultimately, the chemical waste model relies on a radically different notion of human body and agency from that of the metallic waste model. In the metallic waste model the key human agency brought to bear upon the production process was that of the worker. This worker had such control over his or her body that substantial tampering with nature and material processes was possible. The same voluntarism that characterized and fueled production pervaded the Stalinist waste reuse campaigns based on the metallic waste model: "Need to melt down metal scrap before reuse? Who says? Nonsense! That's the capitalist way of doing things. In socialism there are no more fetters on progress and on the free development of humans. So let's just roll out the metal scraps cold."

In the chemical industry, as demonstrated above, the precision required for controlled chemical reactions and the time of chemical and biological processes imposed strict limits on how much human ingenuity and stronger, more metallic, bodies could improve on the efficiency or speed of production. Most importantly, however, the type of body present in the background of the chemical model is not a working body but rather a consuming body—a body that consumes, willingly or unwillingly, the products and by-products of the chemical industry.[7] The key concern is not so much with controlling production but with controlling the consumption of products and by-products.

The acknowledgment of the seemingly obvious fact that bodies do not just produce but also consume literally revolutionized environmental discourse. In the slowly lifting fog of omnipresent censorship, effects of decades of illegal dumping of chemical wastes came to light, Western pieces of ecological and public health information crept through the iron curtain, and details of the Chernobyl nuclear power plant were revealed piece by piece. In the representation of these cases, bodies lost their metallic strength and their immunity to natural laws and were rather portrayed as frail, vulnerable, and sickly. The public became sufficiently "primed" for a different way of dealing with wastes, one that emphasized protection from and thus the safe disposal of harmful wastes—not their collection and reuse.

As the chemical model achieved dominance by the mid-1980s, previous measures to encourage waste reduction and reuse were weakened and incineration became an increasingly accepted option. Subsidies and preferences were stopped: initially 20–25 Forints (Fts.) preferences (exemption from import duties and accumulation tax) were provided for each 100 Fts. of an investment, in 1985 the amount was only 7–8 Fts. By 1986, analysts noted the sudden reduction in waste reusing and waste reduction investments, describing the 1981 Waste and Secondary Raw Material Management Program as a campaign "out of breath" (KSH 1988).

The Hungarian state now shifted its efforts to assist in the siting of waste treatment facilities. In 1985, the party daily broke the news about the construction in Dorog of the country's first modern hazardous waste incinerator, and the news of the siting of other incinerators and dumps sited followed. In 1986 a new hazardous waste dump was opened in Eger; in 1987 Rudabánya found itself assigned as the location of a new incinerator; a new temporary hazardous waste storage with a capacity of ten thousand tons was sited in Hernádkércs (Borsod county), to be operated by the local agricultural cooperative; still the same year plans were announced to build a hazardous waste storage site in Szöreg (Csongrád county). In 1988, the Lábatlan cement kiln announced plans to incinerate pharmaceutical wastes; the same year Szolnok, Békés, Csongrád, and Bács-Kiskun counties cooperated to establish a storage site in Kétpó, which was later developed into a complex waste treatment and disposal site; and the state assigned Ófalu (Baranya county) as the country's first nuclear waste dump site.

Most of these sitings—those of the incinerators in Dorog and Lábatlan, and those of the dumps in Szöreg, Ófalu, and Aszód—met with the resistance of the local population; and this time their resistance was not silenced in the media. These cases indicate a radical transformation in the relation between state and civil society, and are in stark contrast to similar cases that emerged fifteen years earlier in which citizens failed to defend themselves from unwanted dumps, as in the infamous case of Garé.[8]

In 1985 the first public protests against waste imports from the West occurred. In 1985 the news also broke that the Austrian city of Graz was planning to store municipal wastes in western Hungary without the knowledge of environmental authorities (B.Sz. 1985; Ferenczi 1985). In 1986, however, these authorities stopped a similar scheme in which Vienna, the capital of Austria, began delivering contaminated soil to Hungary, containing hazardous waste from the construction of its subway, in order to dump it (Mélykúti 1986).

The emergence of the chemical model was thus initially a positive development to the extent that it forced the Hungarian state to acknowledge environmental claims for what they were, rather than viewing them as simply impediments to production, and to the extent that it facilitated a cautious opening of the state to environmental claims makers. The issue of waste distribution was no longer a taboo; not only were dumping and incineration acceptable ways to deal with wastes, it also became increasingly possible to question the siting of dumps and incinerators. The successes of the fledgling civil society in environmental politics made the few years between 1985 and 1990 appear as the years of hope—namely, a hope for a transition to a society based on freedom and democracy while also working towards an environmentally sane economic future. The curious elective affinity between privatization and democratization on the one hand and the chemical waste model on the other, however, turned these hopes ephemeral.

The Contradictions of the Chemical Waste Model in Postsocialism

Representatives of the chemical industry raised the legitimate claim that society needs protection from chemical by-products in the form of safe dumps and incinerators. But why was it in the interest of the chemical industry to add to public panic by emphasizing the dangers of its wastes? Initially, at the beginning of the 1980s, these interests resided simply in establishing a standardized legal and technological routine to dispose of hazardous wastes as a protection from the state's fines and from the anger of the public. Many Western corporations in the chemical industry in fact did not wait for their respective states or other industries to come up with a solution. Around that time, in the early 1980s, an increasing number of chemical companies started to design, construct, and operate their own disposal and incineration facilities in Western countries. Such chemical companies metamorphosed from troublemakers into problem solvers, even though dumps and incinerators are known to cause serious environmental problems.[9]

The collapse of state socialism, however, added a new motivation for propagating end-of-pipe solutions to wastes—one that turned out to be rather consequential for the direction of postsocialist environmental policies. Privatization opened up the possibility of operating waste dumps and incinerators as privately owned, profit-oriented facilities rather than as public utility companies. That is, rather than hiding their wastes from view as evidence of some shameful incident, chemical plants could now turn them into a "raw material" for a profitable venture. Many chemical companies started to dump, treat, or burn other plants' wastes for money—a lot of money.[10] To the extent that in the case of privatized and profit-oriented incineration operation at the fullest possible capacity is more of an imperative than in the case of state-owned facilities that are run as public utility companies, the choice of entrepreneurial solutions is likely to have significant environmental impacts. The pressure to run an incinerator at maximum capacity not only increases pollution but also has the effect of expanding the circle of "wastes to be liquidated by incineration." The increase in end-of-pipe capacities and the market pressures to run these at the fullest possible capacity, make preventative waste policies, such as reduction, reuse and recycling, appear increasingly less cost-effective and more irrational. As corporations reach for this cheaper way of dealing with their wastes, they will also increase pressure on state agencies to give up their reuse and recycling demand for a certain circle of wastes or for a certain portion of their wastes—a trend that has clearly begun in Hungary. Thus the chemical model of waste coupled with privatization does not so much eliminate wastes as much as it produces them in an endless cycle. This, however, is not the only shortcoming of the prevalence of the chemical waste model.

Simultaneously with privatization, Hungary also saw the collapse of the dictatorial, one-party structure and started enjoying the spread of democratic institutions. Environmental policy also came to be "democratized." As mentioned, the chemical model, relying on an image of a consuming body, initially opened up channels between civil society and the state to negotiate the siting of dumps and incinerators. After 1989, the parameters of these channels became solidified in the framework of environmental public hearings. The procedure of these hearings rests on the obligation of companies to prepare and make public the environmental impact assessments of the proposed facility. Affected residents have a certain amount of time (usually about two months) at their disposal to access these documents and make up their minds as to the desirability of the proposed facility. Then residents can voice their opinion in a public hearing organized by the local environmental authority. It is this authority that decides whether to grant the permission, to deny it, or to withhold it until further conditions are met. While this is a huge step forward from the practice under state socialism in which localities had no say whatsoever in the siting of a hazardous facility, we must also recognize the limits of this "democratic practice."

First, in the case of public hearings about dumps and incinerators, by focusing the debate solely on a particular facility, the question of whether the country should establish more of such facilities does not even emerge. To the extent that environmental impact assessments and public hearings must concentrate on one concrete investment, extralocal impacts, such as the effect of an increased incinerator capacity on the country's waste practices, are necessarily ignored. Second, since the system of obligatory and publicly available environmental impact assessments and public hearings is put in motion by the investor, and since, as such, they are limited to the discussion of one concrete solution, these seemingly democratic institutions cannot present actual choices to the residents whose opinions they are meant to solicit and respect. The only choice residents have is to agree or disagree with the proposed facility. Because of this limited choice, even citizens or groups otherwise open to some aspects of the proposal have no other choice than to vote against it. No wonder that in the majority of such public hearings, affected residents will, "just to be safe," vote against the proposed incinerator or facility. Then, it is easy to ridicule them as irrational, ignorant country people who are afraid of modern technology, a rhetorical practice I found repeatedly in Hungary. It is also quite understandable why industry representatives quickly find themselves calling for limiting "democracy." During my research on a siting conflict over a hazardous waste incinerator proposed for Garé, informants repeatedly cited a quote from Edward Teller: "democracy is dangerous because in democracy, a few clever individuals have to convince a lot of stupid ones."

Are these procedures truly representative of democracy, however? Public hearings certainly appear democratic in form, but are they democratic in content? Not only do public hearings concentrate on one facility and exclude nonlocals from participating, public discourse in general is limited to issues of waste distribution. Issues of waste production—that is, the questions of whether to manufacture something with by-products the safe treatment and disposal of which is difficult to solve technologically or is uneconomical, or whether to explore reusing or recycling options—do not even emerge. The chemical waste model instituted in the context of a privatized economy limits public discourse to issues of waste distribution, and thus communities find all their energies funneled into passing around environmental hazards as hot potatoes. The hegemony of the chemical waste model thus produces not only waste but also spaces to be cleaned up in an endless cycle. The presently dominating chemical waste discourse views environmental politics as a zero-sum game: "we don't care where the waste goes, as long as it is not here." It is easy to see how this model of democracy fails to promote solidarity among communities and how this process is doomed to repeat itself ad nauseum in a Sisyphusian effort of society to protect itself.

Conclusion: Which Nation, Which Body?

I described the nature of early socialist ways of dealing with wastes in Hungary, and captured their logic in what I termed the metallic waste model. This approach, based on practices in metallurgy, prioritized waste reuse and recycling over dumping and incineration—a seemingly progressive policy. Unfortunately, the methods of implementation, and especially the imposition of this preventative approach on industries, such as the chemical industry, where reuse and recycling were not technically or economically feasible led to unintended environmental consequences, such as illegal dumping and incineration practices. Environmental and public health grievances resulting from such practices played an important role in revitalizing civil society in Hungary in the 1980s and they created a favorable atmosphere for replacing the prevalent preventative waste policies with what I termed the chemical model. The chemical model operates on the assumption that bodies are not primarily producing bodies—as with the metallic model—but they are consuming bodies, ingesting and absorbing pollutants and toxins. The chemical model thus prioritizes safe disposal and incineration over recycling. Unfortunately, the economic conditions in which this discursive shift was made from preventative to remedial policies at the end of the 1980s, such as privatization and the general retreat of the state from the economy, discredited any preventative approach as too much state intervention and dismantled the otherwise well-functioning infrastructure for waste collection, reuse, and recycling. The role of public control now shifts from control over production to the limited control over distribution, in which people can only have a say in where to dump and incinerate and not in what to do with wastes or whether to even engage in production with unrecycleable by-products.

The state, corporations, and civil society are all locked in the vicious circle of producing waste that needs to be dumped or incinerated, regulating these technologies but not finding willing communities to live with waste elimination facilities. However, since such decisions are made based on science, democratic legislation, and public hearings, the entire regime of waste production and dealing with wastes appears perfectly rational and democratic. Consequently, this hegemonic discourse makes alternative solutions appear irrational and undemocratic. No wonder that after 1989 the Green movement in postsocialist countries, especially its segment critical of end-of-pipe technologies, lost its credibility despite its prominent role in bringing state socialism down.

Furthermore, some environmentally concerned activists have become attracted to self-consciously irrational and undemocratic politics. One of the first Green parties, the Party of Hungarian Greens, went as far as making the historic connection between environmental pollution and the health of the nation. By 1992, this culminated in an agenda in which declining health and growing sterility were primarily interpreted as a problem of national survival, and in which concerns with the cleanliness of the body and nature quickly led to calls for racial purity.[11]

Fortunately, Hungarians do not find this party attractive, although in 1994 preelection polls gave it 10 percent of voter support. By comparison, no Green party in Hungary has yet reached the 5 percent threshold necessary to get into Parliament. It must be realized that this chauvinist wing of the Greens is further discrediting the environmental movement.

It is also clear that the conservative parties in government have established a hegemony by appealing to citizens' patriotism and their feelings of vulnerability as a nation. Environmentalists in Hungary will have to learn how to constructively engage with concerns about the survival of the nation without slipping into extreme nationalist, xenophobic ideology. One place to start would be to analyze how the presumption of consuming—and thus sickly— Hungarian bodies in the presently dominant waste and environmental discourse toe the line of an industrial lobby vehemently opposed to democratic public control over waste production.

6

When a Child Has Cancer

Protecting Children from a Toxic World

VIRGINIA ADAMS O'CONNELL

We live in a toxic world, full of offending chemicals and radiation. We generally accept living in a toxic environment in exchange for a life filled with abundant food and modern conveniences. We may believe that we are slowly poisoning our bodies and our environment, but we are willing to do so in order to live a desired way of life. We understand that in our old age, we may suffer from cancer, cardiac disease, and other respiratory ailments, conditions related to the behaviors we adopted during our lives, but we resign ourselves and say, "We all have to go sometime from something." We live our lives today with some hope that by the time we fall victim to a disease, the doctors will have found a cure, or a treatment that will offset our suffering. We have hope that tomorrow's technology will solve the problems created by the technologies we employ today (Palmlund 1992, 218).

But what happens when that trade-off we make has a devastating and untoward effect? When the price paid for a way of life is paid by someone who is not old and has not enjoyed a rich and satisfying life? These are the issues I address in this chapter as we examine the experiences of seven families whose children were diagnosed as having pediatric cancer. The parents of these cancer patients formed their own theories of etiology to help explain the event of cancer in their child's life. Their theories addressed all three points of the health constellation: the environment, the microbe (or offending substance), and the vulnerability of the individual. All of these families believed that they live in a hazardous world. They saw their environments as full of toxic materials. But they also recognized that we chose to live in this noxious environment in exchange for a desired way of life. When their children developed cancer, however, the price paid for that lifestyle suddenly was too costly since the parents believed that exposure to toxic chemicals, radiation and other environmental carcinogens caused their children's cancer. The cancer laid bare the contradictions they faced as parents and as members of a wider society. They were challenged to protect their children in a world that was basically unsafe. They did not, however, blame big government or big business for their children's exposure. Rather, they blamed themselves for failing to take some necessary precautions to protect their children when the children were in a particularly vulnerable state. Their theories and the amount of responsibility the parents accepted for their children's exposure greatly influenced their cancer experience, especially when the children returned home after treatment. Their experiences help demonstrate that people live with contradictions and opposing demands on their lives. It also shows us that we believe, falsely or not, that we can impose order where there is chaos, even in the face of scientific uncertainty. And because we believe that we can impose order on our local environment, we are less likely to challenge the disorder we see in the wider environment.

Before we review the experiences of these families, I want to briefly discuss the different values Americans place on health, risk, and development in our society.

Competing Values: Health, Risk, and Development

Few would argue with the statement that people generally value good health. We all need a certain level of health and functioning to fulfill our everyday roles and obligations. In order to participate in our world and interact with others we need a certain level of physical fitness, the requirements of which can vary greatly depending on our roles and obligations. The professional athlete needs a different level of fitness than the desk clerk to fulfill his or her occupational duties, but both can be brought down by a bout of the flu.

Not only as individuals, but also as a society, Americans value good health. Our value is demonstrated in part by our continued investment of huge amounts of our collective resources in the pursuit of conquering sickness and disease (Weitz 1996). In this quest for domination over disease, we as a nation spend more than any other developed nation (OECD Health Data 2002). The media celebrates each new advancement in the search for cures. The public is fascinated with attempts to master our physical bodies and all their processes. Life and death events hold a fascination for us all as they most dramatically represent the never-ending human drama, our movement in and out of the social world.

But health is not the only thing we value, as individuals or as a society. In fact, the life lived in pursuit of health alone would be considered by most a dull life indeed. Whether for entertainment, in the pursuit of knowledge and greater understanding, or for the benefit of others, we purposefully place our lives and safety at risk even though these actions seem to contradict our stated value of health. We find physical release from the stresses and strains of our human existence in the pleasures of smoking, drinking, and other drug consumption even though we know without a doubt that these activities are "bad for our health." Many people find the experiences of downhill skiing, car racing, skydiving, and numerous other sport activities exhilarating even though these activities carry their own risks of injury and harm. We believe that human progress and greater understanding comes from pushing the borders of human understanding and knowledge and going "where no man has gone before" even though that unknown chasm may be full of danger and peril. Development is seen as rising from the brave human spirit that drove men and women to go beyond the known and take a risk in search of knowledge. And what of the most profound form of altruism, whereby one person risks his or her life for another person—this is the very epitome of human compassion and sacrifice. We live every day with the contradiction that we value both health and the pursuit of knowledge, daring, bravery, justice, altruism, and sacrifice (Whipple 1992, 351).

As discussed above, we do not put ourselves at risk just for the sheer sake of putting ourselves at risk but in exchange for some "offsetting advantage" (Viscusi 1983, 37). What is defined as "an advantage" for one person may be different for another (Renn 1992, 95). The advantages may be physical, economic, psychological, and/or spiritual. The risk of drinking alcoholic beverages may bring physical relief. Certain risky occupations may bring economic rewards. Certain altruistic endeavors may bring great psychological and spiritual rewards. There are many reasons why we chose to risk our health and safety in order to meet the needs of the many different components of our beings: our bodies, our minds, and our spirits.

One of the advantages from human development and technology is a certain quality of life that Americans have come to cherish. We like the convenience and advantage that new products, procedures, and processes offer us. We are happy that life is no longer brutish and short, that we have cars to drive, plentiful food, medicines, cheap electricity, and so on. We are pleased with these developments even though we recognize that some of these technologies and our subsequent way of life may actually harm our health. The pollution from cars is deemed worth the convenience in travel. The pesticides lingering on our food and collecting in our bodies is the trade-off for an abundant harvest. Medicines help keep us alive even though some may damage our livers. And we exchange the risk of radiation exposure for inexpensive nuclear power. What is implicit is that we are exchanging short-term benefits for long-term consequences. It is this "gamble now and pay the devil later" nature of the exchange that also informs the kind of solutions we implement for the problems created by new technologies.

The medical profession has been greatly criticized by social scientists in many fields for ignoring environmental health over individual health. Cures are developed to fix what is wrong after it is broken. Few medical practitioners try to fix the environment or change the behavior that causes illness in the first place. The reasons why the medical profession's focus is on the individual rather than on the wider societal context are numerous and have been addressed by many authors (for examples, see McKinlay 2001). I argue, however, that *both* the medical profession *and* the public generally prefer the quick fix to revamping of the social order. We want to smoke, drive fast cars, and skydive with the hope that should we fall ill, someone will be there to put us back together. We want to engage in spontaneous sexual activity without worrying about pregnancy or sexually transmitted diseases. We basically want to "have our cake and eat it too," and we keep alive the hope that if we throw enough money and brainpower at the problem, the fix will be found. In fact, we are surprised when we face a problem that has no easy solution. I have often overheard at cancer support groups the unbelieving phrase, "They can put a man on the moon but they haven't found a way to cure me yet!"

But how do individuals and their families cope when faced with the daunting realization that at least in some cases, you cannot have it all? How do people react when the accepted trade-offs affect their bodies in unforeseen and terrible ways? How do parents react when the price for living in a toxic environment is paid by a young body riddled with cancer? By looking at the experiences of the following seven families, we will see that many of them felt trapped. According to these families, since there is "no safe place" to run to (since the whole world is polluted and toxic), they had to do the best they could in the context of their lives to make the world as safe as possible for them and their children. How they managed to accomplish this demonstrates a basic human need to feel some sort of mastery over the world, and the realization that, statistics aside, we are all convinced that we have personal control over the magnitude of the risk we face despite the calculated odds (Renn 1992, 65). This personal conviction may be based on falsehoods and misconceptions, but it helps to motivate our lives, to take action in an uncertain world. It may also, unfortunately, lead us to take action ONLY in our own backyards rather than to take on the wider toxic world. If we believe that the fix comes from controlling our own immediate environments, then there is no need to address the larger social context.

Method and Sample

I conducted interviews with the families of seven children who had been treated at a children's hospital in the Mid-Atlantic region between 1976 and 1988. Two of the survivors were first treated in 1976 and 1977, while the other five were first seen between 1983 and 1988. All of the initial interviews were conducted in the spring of 1989. I was then in periodic contact with the families over the next four years. This chapter, originally written as my master's thesis, was updated and re-worked for inclusion in this book.

Pediatric oncologists today still do not know what causes childhood cancers (National Cancer Institute Cancer Facts 2002), so little has changed since the 1980s and 1990s. Parents facing a diagnosis of childhood cancer today face the same uncertainties regarding the cause of their child's cancer that the families cited here faced.

Two of the children had been diagnosed as having ALL (acute lymphocyctic leukemia), the most common pediatric cancer, while the other cancers represented in my sample were neuroblastoma (2), medulloblastoma (1), optiglioma (1), and Burkitt's lymphoma (1). The age at first diagnosis was between ten months and six years, and the length of treatment lasted between two and five years. All patients were in post-treatment remission and had been at this stage of their cancer experience for a period of a few months to ten years. The ages of the former pediatric cancer patients were between four and seventeen.

Parents' occupations included (in no particular order): factory worker, high school teacher, secretary, college professor, restaurateur, housewife, dairy farmer, engineer, mechanic, and maintenance worker. The educational background of half the parents was "some college" or "college degree"; six had high school diplomas and one had "some high school."

I conducted seven separate interviews with the families in their homes. In all but two cases, the children joined the interview. Although the responses were primarily provided by the parents, the children often added impressions of their own or corrected their parents. The parents, however, felt better equipped to tell the story of their cancer experience since many of the children were quite young when the cancer was first diagnosed.

Each interview lasted between two and six hours. During the interview, the parents were asked to narrate their cancer experience starting with the first appearance of symptoms. They discussed the process of diagnosis and treatment, and the patient's current posttreatment status. I also asked them to discuss their interpretation of the cause of their child's illness, and of the survivor's risk of recurrence or secondary occurrence. After defining the broad issues I wanted discussed, I left my participants to create their accounts and only interrupted to clarify points or to follow up on an interesting aspect of their experience. This particular format gave the families a chance to tell quite varied stories. Even though there were five different forms of pediatric cancer represented in my sample of families, however, there were more similarities than differences in their accounts.

Lay Theories of Etiology

When illness strikes, those affected by the illness try to make sense out of the event that has introduced chaos into their lives. In the medical sociology literature, much has been written about the patient's identification of the cause of the illness, or his/her "lay theory of etiology" (Dingwall 1973; Locker 1981; Schneider and Conrad 1983; Williams 1984). In his work, Locker found that people had to find "answers to at least two questions" (Locker 1981, 49) before order could be reestablished after the appearance of an illness. The first is, "What is wrong?" which is often answered by a medical diagnosis. The second is, "Why has this happened?" or more specifically, "Why has this happened to me at this time?" Both of these questions are addressed in the patient's theory of etiology and it is this going beyond the medical diagnosis that primarily distinguishes between the medical and lay perspectives. Much of the literature has focused on how these lay theories help the ill individual and his or her family gain some sense of control over their illness by helping them to discover ways to manage the illness and/or avoid future episodes. The theory both cites a diagnosis and identifies the event or series of events that prompted the development of the illness.

This second component, however, goes beyond the mere citing of the event(s). The event(s) is also evaluated for its social and metaphysical significance. The question, "Why?" is also answered by evaluating the values, goals, and desires that motivated the individual's participation in the event(s). These values, goals, and desires that ordered and informed the individual's decisions and actions for some time, but have now resulted in an unfortunate illness. This information of the most personal kind, the identity of personal motivations, helps the individual make sense of the current dilemma by setting the event within a personal biography, rendering it a part of his/her total life experience and worldview (Schneider and Conrad 1983, 127; Williams 1984). It is also argued that this process helps to empower the individual since it presumes that by understanding how the unfortunate illness was contracted, the individual can modify some of his or her behavior, and the motivations that inform that behavior, in order to avoid future episodes. Schneider and Conrad refer to this phenomenon as gaining a "prospective" (Schneider and Conrad 1983, 127) understanding of the illness experience, and Dingwall suggests that this kind of insight helps patients "act upon" (Dingwall 1973, 130) and gain some sense of control over their current dilemma. Palmlund also states that since "human action [is] always producing a future and present from a past, we have to deal with all three of these dimensions" in our analysis of human behavior (1992, 211)

There are, however, limits to this process. Individuals who suffer from poorly understood illnesses may find it extremely difficult to compose a coherent theory. The information that could help make sense of their situation just does not exist. In other cases, there may be information available, but none of the information helps these individuals gain some sense of control. Two examples of this situation exist for patients of some genetic disorders and for victims of some types of environmental contamination. The information these patients receive about their conditions often leave them feeling like little more than victims of random biological or environmental mishaps over which they have no control (Brown and Mikkelsen 1990; Bosk 1992).

In most cases, however, the patients find themselves on some middle ground. They find that some of what is known about their condition can help them to understand the illness and take action against it, while other bits of information and lingering unknowns about the illness may challenge their efforts to achieve and maintain a comfortable level of control. How their personal theories are composed can either exacerbate or alleviate some of the uncertainty.

The Families' Theories

As noted earlier, oncologists still do not know for certain what causes the various forms of pediatric cancer. A list of possible causes includes genetic predisposition, contact with certain viruses, exposure to magnetic fields, and exposure to certain environmental carcinogens (National Cancer Institute Cancer Facts 2002; Kinlen and Balkwill 2001; UK Childhood Cancer Study Investigators 1999). Poor diet and unhealthy personal habits, estimated to contribute to between 60 to 70 percent of all adult cancers (AICR 2002), do not appear on this list. Even mothers who may have engaged in unhealthy behaviors during pregnancy are usually reassured by doctors that nothing they did during pregnancy could have caused their child's cancer even if these behaviors had other untoward effects on the child's development. Most pediatric cancers are diagnosed at such an early age (an average age of three) that it is considered improbable by the medical profession that substances such as fatty foods, cigarette smoke, and/or alcohol could be considered contributing factors since only repeated and long-term exposure to these substances are believed to cause cancer.

When asked to cite the cause of their child's cancer during the interview, five of the seven sets of parents said that their child's cancer was caused by his/her in utero exposure to a carcinogen. As a hospital maintenance worker, one mother worked with cleaning products, which she described as "strong chemicals," all through her pregnancy; another mother claimed that spending time in a cigarette smoke filled room while she was pregnant, and her exposure to smoke detectors that were leaking low doses of radiation, caused her daughter's cancer; one father worked in a wood-treatment plant and believed that he brought home remnants of very powerful chemicals on his skin and clothes while his wife was pregnant;[1] a fourth mother talked about her regret for having gone to visit her sister who lives near the Three Mile Island nuclear power plant in Pennsylvania the very day of the nuclear accident while in her second trimester; and the fifth mother believed that a fateful drive through the industrial area of northern New Jersey, "just off the Turnpike, where you always have to hold your nose," affected her unborn son.

Another child, who had been adopted, was described by his parents as a very "fragile" baby because he had been born prematurely. The parents felt that his initial fragility, coupled with living in a cancer belt, accounted for his cancer. The seventh cause was also attributed to exposure to carcinogens. According to the parents, the child had been repeatedly exposed both to the "winds from Harrisburg, from the Three-Mile-Island nuclear power plant" and to insecticides that were sprayed on the family's dairy farm.

The parents drew their list of probable carcinogens from the well of general popular knowledge about cancer. As the parents remarked, "everyone knows" that industrial pollutants, leakages from nuclear power plants, and even secondary cigarette smoke are likely causes of cancer. As Nelkin and Brown point out in the opening of *Workers At Risk*, we choose to live with carcinogens everyday when we "clean our ovens, paint our houses, spray our gardens and polish our boots" (Nelkin and Brown 1984, xiv). As expressed by these families:

> You know, so many things are called carcinogens—the stuff we use everyday to clean our homes and all the waste from the industrial plants that gets in our air and water. We're all surrounded.

> You can't pick up a newspaper or magazine without seeing some article on cigarettes and cancer. Or radiation and cancer. We saw lots of those articles about the dangers [of radiation] right after the accident at Three Mile Island.

This list of possible carcinogens did not come from the oncologists who treated their children or from other medical staff. The medical personnel repeatedly contended that the cause was just not known. Thwarted in their attempts to get information from the doctors, the parents got their information from other sources. They stated that most of their information came from a variety of articles they had read about the link between the carcinogens they identify in their theories of etiology and cancer in general. They encountered these articles both in scientific journals at the hospital and in newspapers and popular magazines like *Good Housekeeping*.[2] However, none of the parents could cite a particular article that they had read. Rather, they regarded the information as "common knowledge."

Two of the families believed that just a brief exposure to a powerful cancer-causing agent(s) (a brief ride through northern New Jersey and central Pennsylvania) rather than "repeated or long-term contact" (DHHS 1987), was sufficient to produce cancer in their children. And all of these families believed that industrial pollutants and leakages from nuclear power plants account for many of the cancer statistics in cancer belts. According to reports from the American Institute for Cancer Research, industrial pollution and occupational exposure are estimated to account for only about 6 percent of all cancer deaths in America. There is quite a discrepancy between the "official" statistics and the beliefs of the families I studied.

Whether or not the doctors believed that exposure to these particular carcinogens could account for their child's cancer did not really concern the parents. The parents regarded them as plausible explanations because of all of the evidence cited in general media sources that linked these carcinogens with various forms of cancer. The articles that the parents had read or heard about clearly demonstrated to them a cause and effect relationship. Although the parents reported that their doctors thought their deductions were faulty, as

Blaxter, and Schneider and Conrad found in their studies, they were "not in principle unscientific," but drew on acceptable scientific thought processes for their development (Blaxter 1983; Schneider and Conrad 1983, 132). The parents' theories identified a known carcinogen(s), identified a period or moment of exposure to the carcinogen(s), and deduced that the exposure caused the cancer. The parents identified a biological process that is akin to the "germ theory" but that is used in varying degrees to explain the occurrence of some forms of cancer.

These explanations helped the parents set the event of the cancer in the family's personal biography. They answered the question, "What is wrong?," and also identified the event or series of events that led to the development of the cancer. The event(s) identified the moment when exposure to the carcinogen occurred, but the parents still needed to answer the question, "Why did the event(s) occur?"

A diagnosis of pediatric cancer is a rare event. Only about 8,600 new cases of pediatric cancer are diagnosed each year in the United States compared to 1.3 million cases of adult cancer (National Cancer Institute Cancer Facts 2002). Other researchers have found that individuals with rare medical conditions often express feelings of being singled out for suffering. As Davis (1963) found in his research on polio, people diagnosed with rare conditions often feel marginalized. Cancer patients have also been known to interpret their suffering as a form of religious retribution. Throughout history, people generally believed that such a dreadful disease could only be inflicted on the sinful (Patterson 1989, 161). This view is not unique, however, to cancer patients. Bosk recently found couples in genetic counseling invoking religious explanations to make sense out of their predicament (Bosk 1992, 50).

Coming into my research with this background information, I suspected that the families I interviewed would both express feelings of being singled out for suffering and incorporate some religious explanations when addressing the question, "Why me (us)?" I was surprised, therefore, that none of the families expressed either of these sentiments. Instead of feeling singled out, the parents repeatedly referred to many other current or former cancer patients in their neighborhood and immediate vicinity, describing a common bond between them and many of their neighbors. This reference to the prevalence of cancer in their area, however, did not mean that their child's cancer was unavoidable. Instead, they stated that everyone who lived in the area was at risk of contracting some form of the disease.

The difference between their experiences and their neighbors' was that they had battled pediatric cancer while their neighbors had been or were currently patients with various forms of adult cancer. The environment was basically functioning as expected until the occurrence of pediatric cancer. The common perception was that cancer was a disease of old age that "people get after living in the area for many years." Cancer was an unavoidable consequence of "life in these parts." The disease was an unfortunate part of the "fabric of our society." The parents did not blame the government or big corporations for polluting their environment and putting them at risk. Cancer was considered the price we pay for the kind of lives we want to live (cf. Edelstein 1988, 141; Krimsky and Golding, 1992, 14). We are caught up in a chemical society (Nelkin and Brown 1984, 174). People want cheap electricity from nuclear power, abundant milk from the use of hormones, antibiotics and pesticides, and homes that stand up to the weather because the wood has been treated:

> I'm a farmer, I use pesticides. I have to use pesticides if I want to make a living.

> I work in the wood treatment plant down the road. The stuff we use to treat the wood is nasty stuff, but the wood holds up for years after it's been treated.

We want to eat what we want to eat, drink what we what to drink, and engage in whatever activities make us happy:

> Sure, our eighty-year old neighbor has lung cancer, but she's smoked over a pack a day her whole life. It's just the price she's paying for enjoying those cigarettes for all those years.

Others have echoed these same sentiments. For example, in Nelkin and Brown (1984) we hear Ken, an electrician at a chemical plant say:

> A lot of things that are good for me and give me enjoyment come out of all this technology, things I wouldn't want to give up. It's nice to return to the basics, but I don't know if I would want to live on a farm and cut my own wood. I know that things that give me pleasure are also bad for me or somebody else . . . (p. 174)

The price of a particular lifestyle, however, is only supposed to be paid by an older person who has already lived a comfortable life (Patterson 1989, 203, 268, 289). As expressed by the popular author, Erma Bombeck, cancer represents a "period of uncertainty and pain usually inflicted on the elderly who *had lived rich long lives*" (Bombeck 1989, intro—emphasis added).

The parents, therefore, did not view their children's cancer as an inevitable event. It was a risk they faced because of where they lived (Brown and Mikkelsen 1990, 61), but it was an event that the parents believe they could have avoided had they made different decisions. Very strong feelings of having made the wrong decision were expressed most clearly by four of the mothers who believed that exposure to the culprit carcinogens occurred while their child was in utero:

I know now that I should have stayed away from those cleaning fluids, being pregnant and all, but I knew we needed the money, especially with the baby coming, so I just kept on working right up until my due date.

As soon as we walked into the party and there was all that smoke in the room, I said to myself that we should leave because of the baby, but it was a case where it would have been very uncomfortable to leave. When I first learned that she had cancer I thought of that party and all that smoke.

I should have never gone to see my sister that day, but I hadn't seen her in such a long time and she wasn't feeling well, so even though I was pregnant and I didn't have much energy myself, it was one of the few free afternoons that I had, so I went, and have regretted it ever since. (drive near Three Mile Island)

We were moving from Brooklyn down to Philadelphia . . . my husband was starting up his new business. . . . It was a bad day the day the kids and I made the drive and I remember how polluted Northern New Jersey was. . . . I should have never gone that day but my husband was already down in Philadelphia and I wanted us all to be together.

These excerpts identify what the women came to see as conflicting desires. Although all recognized the importance of taking very good care of themselves during their pregnancy (the value of health), they felt that they could not always do that sufficiently and fulfill some of their other responsibilities. A desire for financial security motivated one mother to keep working; a desire for maintaining social relations motivated one mother to stay at a party; a desire to see a beloved sibling led to a car drive near Three Mile Island; and a desire for family unity led to a car ride through northern New Jersey. The mothers all felt that their intentions had been good, but their actions had put their unborn babies at risk. When they made what they later deemed the wrong choice, they failed to protect their child against a risk that they had accepted as part of their environment (Crawford 1981).

Even the dairy farmers blamed themselves, not for using the pesticides (which they felt they clearly had to do in order to succeed in their business), but for spraying them too close to the home. And the father who works in the wood treatment plant regretted not having washed off better before he came home. Although all the parents were reassured by their doctors that nothing they did or did not do caused their child's cancer, the doctors could not relieve the parents' feelings of guilt since they felt as though they had failed to prevent a putative cause (Comaroff and Maguire 1981, 15B:115–23). They had thus failed at one of the most fundamental tasks of parenting: protecting their child from harm.

But why did so many of the families believe that the child was exposed in utero and not after birth? As many authors have documented, since the nineteenth century it has been a common belief that the fetus is especially impressionable in utero, and that the mother's physical and emotional states directly affect the fetus' development (Christensen and Casper 2000; Rapp 1999; Casper 1998; Petchesky 1990; Rosenberg 1976). Partially in response to the abortion debate and to the rash of malpractice suits that have been brought against obstetricians in the last few decades, there has been a renewed focus in America today on the fragility of the fetus. Alcoholic beverages carry warning labels addressed to pregnant women, news reports show us heart-wrenching pictures of drug-addicted babies born to mothers using crack, and newly pregnant mothers are warned that taking even a simple over-the-counter drug like aspirin might harm a fetus. As the authors cited above note, we consider the fetus particularly vulnerable to the adverse effects of a variety of poisonous or harmful substances.

Additionally, the average age at diagnosis for pediatric cancer patients is three. Since the parents are aware that many cancers tend to develop slowly, most contend that the child must have been born with the disease. In fact, some of the families in this study were told that this was probably the case by their doctors.

And finally, the in utero explanation helps account for the fact that it is almost always true for families who have had a child with cancer, that only one child in the family ever has the disease. The in utero explanation describes the child's exposure as occurring during a time when ONLY he or she was highly vulnerable. Focusing only on environmental causes, or on possible genetic predisposition, would not account for the absence of disease in the other siblings who share both the survivor's environment and his/her parents' genetic background.

In summary, the parents in my sample stated that their children's cancer was caused by exposure to a carcinogen(s) when the child was in a highly impressionable physical state. The children were exposed because the parents acted against their better judgment and allowed certain unfortunate events to take place. Although in hindsight the parents believed that they demonstrated poor judgment, they were in fact trying to fulfill other social obligations by participating in the unfortunate event.

Protecting Priceless Children

Why is the occurrence of cancer in a child seen as costly, tragic, and unacceptable, while adult cancer is accepted as part of our society? In her seminal book, *Pricing the Priceless Child*, Viviana Zelizer (1985) tracks the changing attitudes about the value of children from the late nineteenth to twentieth century. Whereas in the nineteenth century children were valued to a large extent based on their economic value, by the early twentieth century, children had become priceless. Their value was measured in term of the endless and unmeasurable emotional joy they provided. Children's lives became uniquely sacred and children's illness and death became singularly tragic (Ibid., 32). The worth we as a society place on the sacredness of childhood comes into direct conflict with our willingness to exchange a toxic environment for a way of life when a child appears to be hurt by that environment. The damaged child not only forfeits an idyllic childhood, but pays a price without reward: the pediatric cancer patient has not lived a "rich long life." That is why these families both accepted living in an environment full of risks while also seeing the occurrence of their child's cancer as something unacceptable and tragic.

As noted before, relatively few cases of childhood cancer are diagnosed each year compared to the total number of adult cancers. But even if one child is potentially harmed by exposure to environmental toxins, why do we not make a greater effort to clean up the environment? We already have examples of implementing safety measures that in essence only protect a very small number of children. Consider as an example fire-retardant sleepwear. Each year, about 1,000 children die in residential fires (American Academy of Pediatrics 2000). There are currently approximately 58 million children in the United States under the age of 15. Only 0.000172 percent of these children (1000/58 million) are at risk of dying in a residential fire, and yet parents are encouraged by pediatricians and makers of children's clothing to dress ALL children only in fire-retardant sleepwear. Fire-retardant sleepwear is a safety measure we have adopted for the majority of children when in practice only a very, very small percent of children are at risk. Likewise, we have mandatory infant and child car seats, and countless product recalls for toys and devices that may prove to be only minimally dangerous to a very few children. We buckle and pad our children in the name of safety when only a small percentage of these children may be at risk for injury or death. One accidental death of a child is considered one death too many.[3]

So why are we not doing more to protect the 8,600 children who will be diagnosed with cancer this coming year? I suggest that the answer to that questions lies in part on the visibility or invisibility of causal links. While it is clear to see the effect a car crash has on an unbuckled child, or our own reactions to the heart-wrenching sight of a child's burned body, it is much harder to see the immediate and direct effects of the "winds from Three Mile Island" on a handful of children scattered across central Pennsylvania. While the wrangled body of the young car crash victim can quickly move legislation on car seats through bureaucratic hurdles, and the picture of the young cancer victim can raise a lot of money for finding a cure, it will do less to raise the call for a moratorium on nuclear energy. Who is to say that the "winds" really caused that child's cancer? Could it have been pesticides, some genetic defect that only he/she has, a virus, or a number of elements uniquely and tragically combined? The route of transmission and occurrence is neither clear nor proven. The possible dangers posed by the "winds" are invisible and therefore easier to ignore by the wider public.

Toxic Treatments

All the previous pediatric cancer patients I interviewed had received some form of chemotherapy and/or radiation therapy as part of their treatment protocols. At the time these children were treated, the five-year survival rate for children with cancer was roughly 62 percent (Raymond 1988, Monmaney 1988). The current overall survival rate has increased to approximately 77 percent (National Cancer Institute Cancer Facts 2002). Although these odds are better than the flip of a coin, these families felt lucky that their child survived treatment.

A patient must remain cancer-free for a period of five years after treatment has ended before he/she is labeled cured because of the high risk of recurrence or secondary occurrence during this time period. Even after this period has passed, however, both doctors and patients fear that the treatments the patient received (chemotherapy and radiation therapy) may themselves cause secondary cancers later in the patient's life. These families recognized the cruel irony of their situations. Fearing that a toxic environment had contributed to the development of their child's cancer, the parents had to allow the doctors to inject and/or bombard their child's body with toxic substances in order to save their child's life. They recognized that the price for the child's survival now may be the development of another cancer down the road. The parents viewed chemotherapy and radiation therapy as both heroes and villains, friends and foes, like so many of the technologies that are a regular part of our lives. We create an environment full of poisons, adopt a lifestyle that exposes us to various harmful substances, and then create toxic medical treatments to battle the harmful effects of this environment and lifestyle.

Returning Home to a Toxic Environment

When their child was first released from treatment, the parents worried about three possible events: (1) the child's reexposure to the original carcinogen(s), (2) a recurrence of the same cancer, and (3) the development of a secondary cancer from the treatment regimen. In this section, I will discuss how the parents assessed their child's risk for the first of these events based on their interpretation of the cause of the disease.

Months before and, in some cases, years before the child was released from the hospital and from treatment altogether, the parents had begun to create a home environment characterized, to the degree possible, by a low probability of reexposure to the original culprit carcinogens. When possible, the carcinogen(s) that had been identified as the cause of the disease was removed from the house. The hospital maintenance worker quit her job, another mother changed the smoke detectors in her house, the employee at the wood-treatment plant showered at the plant before going home, and the dairy farmers no longer spray pesticides close to the house. But in some cases, parents identified a carcinogen(s) over which they had no control: for example, "the winds from Harrisburg and Three Mile Island." In fact, six of the families specifically referred to living in a "cancer belt." How did the families balance their desire to return home and to put the illness experience behind them after treatment was completed with their fear of the child's possible reexposure to the culprit carcinogens?

For these families, "home" was a vision of a safe haven, not a dangerous waste dump of toxic chemicals. In fact, the setting of four of the families' homes was almost idyllic—the rolling farmlands of central Pennsylvania— nothing at all what would come to mind when we imagine a harmful, noxious setting. But it was not the beautiful landscape the family desired. At home, the family would be reunited again: fathers and mothers and all the children. Happy memories of the good times the family shared in the home prior to the disease foreshadowed the happy times yet to come.

> I couldn't wait to get home and neither could [child's name]. I couldn't wait to sleep in my bed again, see my friends, have a cup of coffee in the kitchen. And [child's name] wanted to play with his brothers and sisters so badly. He missed them so much, even [sibling's name] who teased him so much.

The routine of their precancer lives would be reestablished. They would once again go to the old schools, parents would shop at the old stores, and they would wave at their old neighbors. After such a long period of illness and uncertainty about the child's prognosis, the family was anxious to get back into a set of familiar and comfortable behaviors. The desire to go home was very great.

The parents also felt that they had to go home for a number of practical (conflicting) reasons even if the environmental dangers might still be present to some degree. For one thing, they had to consider the feasibility of finding employment in other areas of the country that were not also in cancer belts. Like the subjects in Brown and Mikkelsen's study, these parents believed that there was "no safe place" (1990, 3) to run to since the culprit environmental carcinogens were everywhere in our society, the result of our economic development.

> Where was I going to go with the family? Where could I go and take the skills that I have and not work in some place where these same carcinogens were? There was no better place to go to if you asked me.

There was also the challenge of funding a move even if there was a safer place. After years of treatments, most parents were deeply in debt and many of them had had to seek assistance from funding agencies to pay the hospital bills.

There were also other social and personal considerations involved. A great pull to stay existed because of family ties. Five of the families were living in the same area in which the parents had been raised. The surviving child's grandparents, aunts, uncles, and cousins lived nearby and the families did a considerable amount of visiting with them. How could they move away from the people who mean so much to them?

The parents also had to consider the needs of the survivor's siblings who had continued to establish roots in the home community while the former patient was in treatment. The siblings often relied on these roots to anchor them during the unstable time caused by the absence of the parents and sick sibling from the home. How could the parents justify uprooting them? Some of the siblings interviewed said that once the survivor's treatment had ended, they believed that the crisis was over, and that the parents now had to "make up" for their physical and emotional absence. They wanted to be spoiled—they wanted their parents to get involved in their lives again, to catch up on all the news they had missed.

The families' desire and need to return home was undoubtedly great, but the question remains: How could they return home knowing that they could not make the home environment carcinogen-free when they believed that exposure to these carcinogens led to the child's development of cancer? The parents found themselves once again torn between conflicting values. The parents valued the health and safety of the former patient, but not only did they have to fulfill their roles and duties to the child who had been ill, they also had to fulfill their obligations to their employers, their other children, their families, their friends. How did the parents manage this conflict?

Examining certain elements of the parents' theories of etiology helps us understand their resolution. We can recall that five sets of parents cited above believed that their child had been exposed to the carcinogen(s) while in utero. Therefore, the risk of recreating the *exact* conditions that originally caused the child's cancer was nonexistent for these five families. Although the child may be reexposed to the one or all of the culprit carcinogens, he/she would never again be as impressionable or as vulnerable as he/she had been in utero. Therefore, the parents could return home with the survivor, remove all the carcinogens that could be removed, and "try not to worry about" the carcinogens over which they had no control. The parents, therefore, could go home despite the fact that the environment was not carcinogen-free in part because of their particular interpretation of the timing of the child's original exposure that defined him/her as in a vulnerable but nonreplicable physical state.

For the other two families who believed that exposure occurred while the child was an infant and toddler, they also took some comfort in the notion that their children, now much older, were no longer as vulnerable as they had been when they were so young. Like the other five families, these parents took comfort in the belief that they had sufficiently reduced their child's risk of reexposure when they removed all of the removable culprit carcinogens.

Having taken these steps, the parents no longer worried about reexposure but about the risk of recurrence and of a secondary occurrence. Their theories of etiology did not appear to help them deal with these worries. Assessing the child's risk of recurrence involved an ongoing reinterpretation of the treatment process. The parents continually questioned whether or not their child had received enough treatment. Had all the cancer cells been destroyed, or were some still hiding somewhere in the body, ready to grow unbounded in the absence of treatment? These questions plagued the parents' minds especially during the first year posttreatment. After a year the risk of recurrence drops significantly, so the families who were past the first-year mark were much less worried about this risk.

Assessing the risk of a secondary occurrence (the development of a different cancer as a result of the treatment modalities) also involved a reassessment of the treatment process. The parents who saw their child "go through hell and back again" were much more worried about this risk than the parents whose children seemed to tolerate the treatments with few and/or minor side effects. Those whose children seemed to suffer greatly from the treatments feared this was an indication that the treatments had destroyed or harmed the child's healthy cells as well as their cancer cells. As time went on, however, and their child developed no new symptoms, the parents pushed these fears into the recesses of their minds so that they could live their lives without obsessing about an uncertain future.

These families faced many fears when returning home with their child but due to a variety of constraints on their lives, they had to go home. In order to feel some control over their child's destiny, the family took steps to reduce the carcinogenic components of their homes and yards. They changed some of their behaviors in order to avoid ever having to face another diagnosis of pediatric cancer. But these families did not go after big business or government to file a complaint. They did not become political activists, move, or change their jobs. They had long accepted the toxicity of their environment, and even after that environment proved more toxic than expected, they responded by taking additional measures to minimize their own personal exposure. They saw this response as their responsibility, as part of the deal we have all made for a certain way of life. Would their response have been different if a more obvious cluster of pediatric cancer patients had been identified in the neighboring communities? If the offending substance had been chemical runoff in their water supplies rather than the ethereal winds from Harrisburg? Perhaps then we would have seen the kind of political activism that Brown and Mikkelson (1990) witnessed.

Conclusion

How safe should our environments be? Were these parents right when they attributed the cause of their children's cancers to our toxic world? Maybe, maybe not. Although the "true" cause of these pediatric cancers remains uncertain, what is certain is that the long-term risks associated with living in the path of the winds of Harrisburg are unknown, and that the type of research that could possibly provide the answers is complicated, costly, and never adequately done (Nelkin and Brown 1984, 149). Why then do we accept the risks associated with new technologies before we are sure that the benefits are worth the cost? In most cases the benefits are immediately obvious and desirable while the risks may seem vague and invisible.

It is also true that we live in a world in which specialization makes us feel trapped. How can we comment on areas of technology about which we have no understanding? We are limited by our own experience and expertise, bound by our own understandings. We know too little about production processes, the effects of chemicals on the human body, and the cost in terms of health and safety of every little new gadget and item that hits the shelves. But by participating in the culture, by buying into a certain lifestyle, we feel like we are passively accepting the risks that others have generated for us. We do not have enough information to reject certain technological developments in the name of health and safety. And there are many obstacles—limited time, energy, and accessibility—that make gathering this information almost impossible.

People spend more time and energy taking care of today's business than planning for the future. Workers are more concerned about wages and benefits than they are with job safety (Brown 1985). The information about the risks associated with our chemical world that we get from the mass media typically portrays the risks as manageable (Raymond 1985). We face a host of competing demands on our time and energy that force us all to cut corners and make trade-offs. We buy processed foods loaded with additives because we cannot shop for fresh food everyday. We drive because it is not feasible to walk. Technology marches on and we jump on the bandwagon. But few of us would want to return to a time when we had to chop our own wood.

Human beings are also extremely adaptable, perhaps to a fault. We find ways to live and harmonize all the various conflicting forces in our lives. As discussed early in this chapter, we live everyday with the contradiction that we desire both health and risk. Although an observer may see a life as a series of conflicts, pressures, and strains—a balancing act of sorts—people tend to experience their lives as coherent wholes. We can be parents, and children, and employees simultaneously, trading off one obligation to fulfill another and switching back when other forces dominate. We can change our behaviors and even our opinions when we are talking to our children as opposed to talking to our friends. We fulfill many roles and fill the scripts rather adeptly even when the roles demand contradictory views.

People also have an uncanny knack for imposing order where there is chaos, for only with a feeling of control, of some sense of mastery over our world, can we motivate our participation in that world. For example, the families in this study pulled information about cancer from a variety of resources and with a jumble of bits and pieces, composed rational, coherent, and therefore believable causal theories that helped them feel as though they had some control over the risks they faced. The information was both broad enough to appear comprehensive but personal enough to be manageable, not unlike what other researchers have found (cf. Renn 1992, 65–66). Acting on their local environments empowered these actors. Had they not been so successful at establishing a sense of control, they may have had a much harder time going home.

But all this adaptability, and all these trade-offs may result in us tragically realizing one day that the risk was too costly, not just for the randomly scattered sick children in central Pennsylvania, but for all human beings. We may run out of quick fixes for the problems our technology continually creates. And it may be at that point, when we all are suffering in our poisoned bodies, that we decide that the price for all that technology was too high. Hopefully we will not have to wait that long.

PART III

COMMUNITIES

7

Permitting Poison
Public Participation, the Criteria for Action, and Environmental Justice in the Case of Dioxin

KAREN HOFFMAN

All socioeconomic groupings tend to resent the nearby siting of major (incinerator) facilities, but middle and upper socioeconomic strata possess better resources to effectuate their opposition. Middle and higher socioeconomic strata neighborhoods should not fall within the one-mile and five-mile radius of the proposed (incinerator) site.
—Consultants report for the California Waste Management Board, 1984

(Z)oning boards and planning commissions are typically stacked with white developers. Generally, the decisions of these bodies reflect the special interests of the individuals who sit on these boards. People of color have been systematically excluded from these decision-making boards, commissions and governmental agencies . . .
—Robert Bullard, *Confronting Environmental Racism*, 1993

Environmental justice demands the right to participate as equal partners at every level of decision-making including needs assessment, planning, implementation, enforcement and evaluation.
—Principles of Environmental Justice,
First National People of Color Environmental Leadership Summit, 1991

. . . (E)ach federal agency shall conduct its programs, policies, and activities that substantially affect human health or the environment, in a manner that ensures that such programs, policies, and activities do not have the effect of excluding persons (including populations) from participation in, denying persons (including populations) the benefits of, or subjecting persons (including populations) to discrimination under, such programs, policies, and activities, because of their race, color, or national origin.
—Executive Order 12898, Federal Actions to Address Environmental Justice in Minority Populations and Low-income Populations, ex-president Bill Clinton, 1994

A comprehensive approach to identifying and addressing environmental justice concerns requires the early involvement of affected communities. . . . (I)n efforts to pool all available knowledge, EPA will access and incorporate expertise of local, affected community members throughout this process.
—Environmental Protection Agency, *Environmental Justice Strategy*, 1995

Starting in the late 1980s, the environmental justice movement brought to the foreground of public awareness the fact that low-income and minority communities have been less well protected from industrial pollution than middle class white communities. This movement used mass protests and demonstrations to block continued siting of hazardous dumps, incinerators, and industrial facilities in low-income communities of color. Environmental justice advocates charged environmental regulatory agencies with environmental racism in the form of exclusion of low-income people of color and with not considering pollution problems in areas disproportionately burdened by pollution. Movement spokespersons called for agencies to include and receive direction from the previously excluded as the solution to the problem. Within the environmental justice movement, community organizers cultivated leadership in disproportionately impacted low-income communities of color for members to become involved and give direction in environmental politics.[1]

In 1994, then president Bill Clinton issued an executive order (quoted in the epigraph) that required all federal agencies working in the areas of health and the environment to make achieving environmental justice part of their mission. The president directed the many branches, programs, and offices of the Environmental Protection Agency and the National Institute of Environmental Health Sciences to ensure that they were not perpetuating environmental injustice. These developments inspired both hope and skepticism. I am driven in this chapter and the larger project of which it is a part by an awareness of the distance between endorsing the idea of inclusion and actually meaningfully including those who have been excluded.[2] I examine here one case of residents of a disproportionately impacted area involving themselves in public health and regulatory decision-making. I analyze what resources they found in our public agencies and the prospect of preventing toxic pollution in disproportionately impacted areas through participation by residents of them in the decision-making of pubic health and regulatory agencies in their current forms.[3]

In this case, residents of a heavily industrialized, coastal city in the United States, which I call Springfield, got involved in a pollution prevention campaign.[4] Springfield is a multiethnic city with a high poverty rate, located in one of two industrial areas of a large metropolis. Private companies operate over 350 industrial facilities, including a large oil refinery, chemical plants, and metals manufacturers. Springfield residents got involved in the campaign through community organizing efforts made by the Clean Air and Water Network, an environmental group that works on pollution prevention and has been sympathetic to the environmental justice movement and responsive to its call to work together with and in support of disproportionately impacted communities.[5] In the mid 1990s, working in alliance with several other environmental health and antitoxics organizations in the region, the Clean Air and Water Network was initiating a campaign to stop the production of dioxin.[6] This Dioxin Prevention Alliance decided to try to work together with residents of the neighborhoods near the dioxin sources, including those in Springfield. Already involved in pollution politics in Springfield, the Clean Air and Water Network began community organizing around dioxin there.

Dioxin is a group of "persistent organic pollutants" (POPs), toxins that accumulate rather than passing through organisms or breaking down. At miniscule exposures, dioxin can disrupt biological reproduction, development, and immunity. The World Health Organization's International Agency for Research on Cancer and the U.S. Department of Health and Human Services' National Toxicology Program have classified dioxin as a "known human carcinogen" (IARC 1997; NTP 2001). According to a U.S. EPA draft report on dioxin's health effects, the background levels of dioxin-like compounds found in the general population may cause a lifetime cancer risk as high as one in one thousand. This level is one thousand times higher than the risk level that is generally considered "acceptable" by regulatory agencies (one in a million). Dioxin is also associated with endometriosis (Rier et al. 1993; Cummings et al. 1996; Yang and Foster 1998), reduced fertility (Murray et al. 1979), reduced sperm count (Gray et al. 1997a), birth defects (Gray et al. 1997b), learning disabilities (Schantz and Bowman 1989; Seo et al. 1999), diabetes (Pazderova-Vejlupkova et al. 1981; Henriksen et al. 1997), and immune system impairment (Burleson et al. 1996; Gehrs et al. 1997; Gehrs and Smialowicz 1998; Ross et al. 1995; Tonn et al. 1996). According to EPA estimates, the amount of dioxin in tissues in the general human population is near levels that cause adverse effects (http://www.epa.gov/ncea/pdfs/dioxin). This toxin is passed from one generation to the next through the placenta and through breastfeeding. It is produced in specific locales as a preventable, unnecessary, commercially unusable by-product of industries that bring together chlorine and organic matter at high temperatures. Its effects are felt both locally and remotely, as this substance can travel through the air hundreds of miles away from its source. The effort to eliminate dioxin production is nationwide and the effort to ban the larger group of POPs is international.

I present here an abbreviated overview of the development of collaboration between the Springfield residents and the Clean Air and Water Network, and move quickly to a detailed discussion of the interactions of the Springfield contingent of the dioxin prevention campaign with government health and regulatory agencies. Examining the dynamics between the Springfield residents, relative newcomers to environmental advocacy, and the relatively more seasoned activists on the staff of the Clean Air and Water Network, is crucial to thinking through the idea of inclusion of the excluded as a solution to environmental racism and inequality. I give that topic my full attention elsewhere (Hoffman in progress). Here, I focus on interactions with government health and regulatory agencies.

As recounted to me by community organizers in the Clean Air and Water Network, this group connected with Springfield residents by making presentations at neighborhood meetings across the city about dioxin, its health effects, and local sources.[7] In addition to many defenders of the local refinery and other polluters against environmental regulation, the community organizers also found a broad base of awareness of toxic pollution and support for the dioxin prevention campaign. Some of the Springfield residents knew about dioxin through relatives in Lakeview, a small Southern town in a heavily industrialized area with a number of dioxin sources, including a large vinyl production and four hazardous waste incinerators associated with the vinyl industry. The town was founded by Blacks after the Civil War, prior to being overrun by the vinyl industry, and is predominantly populated by low-income African Americans today. Lakeview is also unincorporated and, therefore, without a strong political voice in local politics.

Racism carried out in the name of medical science in recent history in the U.S. has given African Americans good reason to be skeptical of any kind of medical testing.[8] Alongside of any skepticism African Americans overrun by the vinyl industry in Lakeview may have felt, it seems they also felt they had something to gain by finding out the level of dioxin in their blood. Tests yielding high levels might convince regulatory agencies to limit dioxin in industrial sources, and to provide health services and medical monitoring that Lakeview residents were fighting for. Testing also offered the possibility, however remote, of assistance in relocation from Lakeview, as the corporation that owns the large vinyl plant in the town previously bought out the homes of some earlier residents in the settlement of a lawsuit over contamination of well water. Some Lakeview residents and lawyers working with them privately contracted to test their blood for dioxin. Finding some higher than normal levels of dioxin, the concerned group asked the federal Agency for Toxic Substances and Disease Registry (ATSDR) to do further testing.

ATSDR is one of few government health agencies that can test for dioxin. According to its website (http://www.atsdr.cdc.gov), the agency is mandated by Congress "to protect America's health from toxic exposures." ATSDR assesses health effects and risks associated with waste sites, emergency toxic releases by industry, and other sources of hazardous substances. The agency also does health surveillance, applied research in support of health assessments, and education and training concerning hazardous substances. Through its close relationship with the Centers for Disease Control, ATSDR has access to some of the only equipment for analyzing biological samples for dioxin in the United States.[9]

The agency agreed to take a small number of human blood, soil, chicken egg, and human breast milk samples in Lakeview (ATSDR 2000). Residents were waiting for the results of this round of tests when their relatives and others in Springfield were hearing presentations on dioxin at their neighborhood meetings.

A number of the Springfield residents had lived in Lakeview during their childhood. When they learned in the presentations about the persistence and accumulation of dioxin in fatty tissue, they became concerned about their previous exposures in Lakeview as well as their current exposures in Springfield. Through the initial neighborhood presentations, six Springfield residents became active participants in the dioxin prevention campaign.

The more experienced activists in the Clean Air and Water Network were committed to supporting the newcomers from Springfield in making their own analysis and deciding their own goals, in addition to drawing on their own experience in pollution battles.[10] Working together, this Springfield contingent of the dioxin prevention campaign decided on two goals. The first came from the Springfield residents' reaction to learning that they lived near a dioxin source. Like the Lakeview residents, they wanted to know how much they had been exposed to and decided to ask ATSDR to test them. The second goal came from a plan already underway in the Clean Air and Water Network: to ask the Regional Water Quality Bureau to enforce the dioxin limit in the permit of a local dioxin source, an oil refinery in a nearby town, and to take action on a commitment made several years earlier to require that refinery to investigate how to stop producing dioxin in its refining process, with the intention of eventually phasing out of this pollutant.[11]

One of the organizers arranged a meeting with a regional representative of ATSDR. In August 1999 the Springfield residents, as part of the dioxin prevention campaign, met with the ATSDR representative in a community center in a neighborhood just downwind of the refinery, the major local dioxin source.[12] They told him they were concerned about living near a dioxin source. Those who previously lived in Lakeview expressed their worry about that additional source of exposure. The group asked to be tested for dioxin.

The response of the ATSDR representative was that he needed the results of the dioxin exposure investigation being done in Lakeview before the agency would consider testing in Springfield. He and others in the agency wanted to know if the previous investigation yielded useful results before taking on another similar one. He said he could take the initial step of looking up the data available on toxic pollutants released and cancer incidence in Springfield,[13] but could not give the activists an answer to their request for testing.

When the activists suggested scheduling a follow-up meeting, the ATSDR representative was reluctant. He did not know how long it would be before the agency would have any information from the Lakeview investigation. But he agreed to a meeting in December, four months away.

For the Springfield residents, four months was a long time to wait. Their concerns about the pollution that had been around them all their lives had crystallized. They now had a name, dioxin, to put on at least some of that pollution. They believed that they could learn the amount they were carrying in their bodies and, thus, what harm had been done to them all these years. They could then fight for health care services and other compensation for the harm done to them. Excited about their request to ATSDR for testing, the Springfield contingent talked it up to their friends and neighbors while they waited for December to roll around.

In late November, one of the community organizers from the Clean Air and Water Network called the ATSDR representative to confirm the upcoming meeting. The representative said he would not be able to make it. He was still waiting for the report on the Lakeview dioxin exposure assessment and all the federal agency's resources were still tied up there. The Springfield residents were disappointed and angry.

The ATSDR representative had also not sent the pollution and cancer data he had promised. The organizer called him back to ask him to send it and to reschedule the meeting. He again was reluctant and noncommittal. He also mentioned that he had held a meeting on the request for dioxin testing in Springfield with the County Health Department and the local office of the State Health Department, at which it was decided that the role of the concerned Springfield residents would be as an advisory board.

In the eyes of the activists, this representative and ATSDR were blowing it. They had not followed through on promises made. They neglected a meeting they had agreed to with representatives of a low-income, minority community living next to many pollution sources who had made a request for an investigation. And they excluded this group from a meeting at which government agencies decided for them what would be their role. As diplomatically as possible, the organizer told the ATSDR representative that the Springfield residents needed to be included in every meeting, from the start, and that the meeting with him needed to be rescheduled as soon as possible. The ATSDR representative put her off, saying that he couldn't speak for the other agencies regarding inclusion of the Springfield residents and repeating his need to wait for results from the other dioxin exposure assessment.

After the ATSDR representative's reluctance, the Springfield activists were surprised when someone else in the agency called them and proposed a meeting date in mid December 1999. This alternate representative came in the previous one's place with a proposal to set up a meeting with the original representative in February 2000 when, he hoped, a report from Lakeview would be available.

Following this perplexing meeting, the Springfield contingent of the dioxin prevention campaign was abuzz with something the alternative representative had said—that he was sure that residents of Springfield had been exposed to dioxin, living as close as they do to an oil refinery.

In March 2000, the ATSDR representative finally met with the Springfield contingent of the dioxin prevention campaign. Seven months after their original request, he had nothing new to tell them. The results were still not in from the other investigation. There were still no resources available for testing in Springfield.

Although the Springfield activists were determined to be tested for dioxin, they concluded ATSDR had nothing to offer them and abandoned their request to this agency.

What happened when the residents of a city disproportionately impacted by pollution tried to get involved in public health policy regarding toxic substances in this case? They found a health agency that could not answer their request for testing and otherwise had nothing to offer them for addressing their concern about routine dioxin emissions and exposures.

I asked the ATSDR regional representative by e-mail why the agency would not test the Springfield residents and if there was something the agency could do to address their concerns. Regarding testing, he said that ATSDR "does not have good information" about what health problems to expect at particular levels of exposure to dioxin, nor about treatments. Without this information, ATSDR does not get involved. Regarding other ways of addressing concerns of residents of areas in or near industrial zones, the agency representative said nothing.

This agency, which is mandated to collect information about and try to understand toxic substances, disease, and the links between them, does little or no work on and has nothing to say about the chemical mix in the air and the water in industrial zones and exposures and health outcomes of the residents who live near them—not only in Springfield, but also in all heavily industrialized cities. ATSDR's own representative admitted that Springfield residents surely must be exposed to dioxin from nearby industry. Instead of using this information to urge industry and regulators to do all they can to prevent dioxin and the full range of toxic pollution, its policy is to remain silent. ATSDR's silence on this issue tacitly tells industry and regulators to continue polluting, even though they are emitting dioxin, people near and far are being exposed to it, and it is making some of them sick. In ignoring these situations, the agency protects polluters from toxics prevention and precautionary proposals as much or more than it protects public health.

The other way the Springfield residents got involved in the dioxin issue was to join in with activities that the Clean Air and Water Network and others in the Dioxin Prevention Alliance had organized: finding out who was producing dioxin in the area, directly asking them to stop, and asking the regulatory agencies to require them to stop. When community organizing was getting under way in Springfield in the winter of 1998–1999, a decision was coming up at the Regional Water Quality Bureau about the dioxin limit in the pollution permit of Sanmar, one of six oil refineries in the area that line the northeastern shore of San Luis Bay. The Sanmar refinery is about ten miles northeast of Springfield. The activists were concerned about it both because of its dioxin contribution to the area and because the case could set a precedent for how dioxin would or would not be regulated locally, including at the larger refinery in Springfield.

Dioxin had been added to the Sanmar refinery's pollution permit in 1993. In the wake of the dioxin contamination disasters at Love Canal, New York, and Times Beach, Missouri in the late 1970s and early 1980s,[14] the EPA began investigating and inventorying industrial sources of dioxin in an effort to stop further contamination. By 1986, directives to identify and control industries producing dioxin had come down to regional regulatory bodies, including the Water Quality Bureau. Faced with having to set a regulatory standard for dioxin and having no measurements of dioxin levels in wastewater dumped to the Bay, the Water Quality Bureau asked the polluters to test themselves for dioxin. Despite the facts that polluters have a conflict of interest in carrying out this kind of testing, and that dioxin is difficult to detect in the small concentrations that matter, Sanmar detected dioxin. In 1993, the Water Quality Bureau added a 0.14 parts per quadrillion dioxin limit to Sanmar's pollution permit.

The company installed a filtration system, but it did not bring the dioxin level down to the permit limit. In 1995, the Water Quality Bureau cited the company for being out of compliance with its pollution permit. It gave Sanmar four years to comply with the dioxin limit and required the company to investigate how to eliminate dioxin production from their processes.

There were no other technological, end-of-pipe measures the refinery could take. Accustomed to being required to take only this kind of action rather than to do holistic pollution prevention through changing parts of their production process, they made no progress in those four years. Sanmar lawyers and engineers crafted an argument for the Water Quality Bureau to raise the dioxin limit. Although their dioxin level was not down to the permit limit, they claimed, it was lower than what is found in urban surface run-off, water that flows off of streets and other surfaces into the Bay. They pointed out that the refinery is unique in that it mixes surface run-off with wastewater and claimed that run-off is the source of the dioxin in the wastewater. Until there is a plan for controlling dioxin in run-off, Sanmar lawyers argued, the company should not be made to make more drastic and costly process changes. Claiming that the company had acted in good faith by installing the filter and had done all that they could, Sanmar managers asked the Water Quality Bureau to raise the dioxin limit to the level they had achieved.

Although the company's claims about the small and unimportant amount of its dioxin discharge were not substantiated, the Water Quality Bureau was compelled by the company's reasoning. Its staff took some measurements of dioxin in surface run-off. Their interpretation of the results pointed in favor to the Sanmar argument.

No one examined the refinery's role in producing the dioxin in the run-off in Sanmar's wastewater discharge, neither its emissions of dioxin to the air and deposition on ground, nor emissions from automobiles that burn gasoline contaminated with dioxin and dioxin precursors in the refining process.

In the weeks before the public meeting at which the Water Quality Bureau would make a decision, its staff circulated and solicited comments from all interested parties on a written proposal they planned to make to the bureau: to extend Sanmar's deadline for complying with the dioxin limit by one year. The rationale of the proposal was that before the Water Quality Bureau could require the refinery or any other polluter to further lower their dioxin discharge, its engineers needed more information. Engineers at the Water Quality Bureau and other agencies that regulate water quality calculate permit limits by identifying all of the different sources of any given pollutant that end up in the water body, and the amount of the pollutant that the water body can handle and still preserve all of its established uses (for example, drinking water supply, swimming, and fishing). The engineers then divide the latter amount among the polluters (http://www.epa.gov/owow/tmdl/intro.html# definition).

The Regional Water Quality Bureau staff held that the Regional Air Quality Bureau would need to be involved in generating this information much more centrally than the Water Quality Bureau, as the dioxin in urban surface run-off falls out of the air. Additionally, the staff stated that the Environmental Protection Agency would be taking the lead on producing this information and would set dioxin limits within the next twelve years. From my perspective, twelve years is too long to allow more dioxin pollution to accumulate in the bay or anywhere, but the Water Quality Bureau staff argued that it made no sense to force costly changes at Sanmar before then.

The dioxin prevention activists were dismayed to see the Water Quality Bureau change its position so radically since 1995. The activists wanted a stricter limit, or at least enforcement of the current limit. They could see that Sanmar had no other end-of-pipe, technological solutions, but they wanted the limit enforced so that Sanmar would need to holistically examine its dioxin production, including its air emissions and deposition on the ground. According to the Dioxin Prevention Alliance, there was much more that the refinery could do through process changes to lower and even eliminate dioxin in wastewater, in air emissions, and in run-off if they wanted or were required to make the investment. They understood the Water Quality Bureau's proposal as a tactic of dodging responsibility by pointing to other sources, air emissions and run-off. They perceived the Regional Air Quality Bureau and the federal Environmental Protection Agency to be doing the same thing. The activists saw strategic omission of the fact that dioxin in run-off originates in oil refineries, among other industrial sources, and from cars burning gasoline that is contaminated with dioxin and/or its precursors in oil refining. In their written comments on the proposal submitted to the Water Quality Bureau, the activists agreed that there is a larger problem involving air deposition of dioxin and run-off, but drew a different conclusion: now is the time to address this problem; it should be addressed holistically—even if that means air emissions need to be lowered to meet a water pollution limit—and regulators should start with known dioxin sources, such as the Sanmar refinery.

In contrast to the request to ATSDR, not all of the Springfield residents who got involved with the Dioxin Prevention Alliance actively participated in the proposal to the Water Quality Bureau. Everyone agreed that the intervention was a good idea, but others in the Dioxin Prevention Alliance who had been working on it for a long time went first and delivered the most extensive public comments at the meeting at which the bureau would make a decision. Two Springfield residents who already had experience in activism and public speaking gave comments at the meeting. Some of the others from Springfield attended the meeting; some participated only through hearing others report on it.[15]

Here I present an account of the Water Quality Bureau meeting. I include enough detail about the meeting to demonstrate not only the decision made, but also how it was made, as well as what newcomers to regulatory politics, including myself, experienced there.[16]

On the day of the Water Quality Bureau meeting, in June 1999, the hearing room was packed. Whereas with the request for dioxin testing, only the Springfield contingent of the Clean Air and Water Network and ATSDR were involved, many parties on both sides of the issue had an interest and came to weigh in on the refinery permit decision. The Water Quality Bureau long ago had created an orderly structure to handle this kind of situation. Everyone who wants to comment on the issue at hand signs up on their way into the meeting. The staff of the bureau gives its report and/or proposal. Then speakers say their piece, restricted to a certain number of minutes depending on how many speakers sign up.

The chairwoman of the Water Quality Bureau, Amy Screpsi, began the meeting by calling on Helen Choy, a staff engineer, to present the proposal. Helen stated the proposal to put the decision off for one year, as had already been circulated among interested parties before the meeting and described above. Her rationale was that since the dioxin in Sanmar's discharge is not coming from the refinery (a fact that would be disputed by the dioxin prevention activists), it was not the Water Quality Bureau's jurisdiction, nor responsibility. She also mentioned that EPA would be setting a dioxin limit within the next twelve years and that bureau enforcement of Sanmar's permit limit, therefore, might create double work for the refinery. For the bureau staff, then, the main issue in this case was whether or not the refinery was responsible for the dioxin in its discharge, not the fact that the refinery is a source of dioxin that could be prevented.

Next the bureau chair gave the floor to Sanmar general manager, Joe Marella. Joe did not come alone. He brought a team of three experts to the floor with him. After introducing them, he spoke in support of the Water Quality Bureau staff proposal. He presented no evidence, but claimed that refinery operations had nothing to do with the dioxin in its wastewater, and that it was coming from surface run-off, which the refinery mixes with its process water.

Before relinquishing the floor, Joe offered to have any questions from the bureau answered by Dr. Fred Weber, the "board-certified toxicologist" he had brought with him who, he announced, is "internationally known for his expertise in toxicology, risk assessment, and environmental engineering."

Chairwoman Screpsi praised Sanmar's efforts to lower the levels of dioxin in their water pollution and bureau member Leon Hughes agreed to Joe's plan to have experts speak in support of allowing Sanmar to continue polluting at the current levels. He asked Dr. Weber if he concurred with the bureau staff's analysis that the source of dioxin in Sanmar's wastewater is surface runoff.

Weber agreed.

"It's aerial," he elaborated. "We have a lot of dioxins in us because of airborne emissions from miscellaneous sources. Refineries are thought to be a source, but they have been thought to be a diminimous source. It deserves more evaluation, for sure, but . . . I think EPA's concluded it's just not high on the radar screen.

"We see this pretty much all over the country," Weber continued, implying that refinery and other industrial emissions are not a significant source of dioxin, but presenting no evidence.

"(U)rbanized areas have high surface concentrations. . . . Things aren't that much different if there's an industrial emission or not . . ."

"So we ought to get the same reading off a parking lot in a shopping center?" asked Leon.

"Oh, a lot of shopping center parking lots are a lot worse," answered Weber.

"Is it true," Leon lead, "that even the fire that I build in my fireplace for a romantic evening is putting dioxins in the air?"

"Sure," Weber answered. "All combustion, especially of logs, will give you dioxins in the ash. . . . (T)he chlorines are . . . in the wood. . . . (I)t's in the bark. . . . A lot of people believe bark serves as an absorber of at least some portion of the airborne chlorine and chlorinated chemicals. . . . (There are) hundreds, thousands of analyses of fireplaces and ash and the gaseous emissions. If you review the analysis, . . . you will see it was the second biggest producer in (the region) of dioxins and furans. I don't know if it's true, but I did read that."

The main issue the refinery manager and the hired expert highlighted was that Sanmar is not the source of the dioxin in its discharge and that other sources are more relevant. The refinery manager surely brought Dr. Weber along to lend scientific credibility to the Sanmar position. How odd, astonishing, and—one would think—ineffective it was, then, that neither of the men supported these claims with evidence. The Water Quality Bureau members made no comment on the lack of evidence. Nor did they ask Weber any questions about the source of chlorine in tree bark.

Bureau member Sam Ehrlich moved to end the discussion with Sanmar management and experts with praise for the oil refiner, "I compliment you on your moving forward with scrubbers and stacks. . . . (I)n another year, I would like to hear how we're doing there, because that's a great step forward, and a very difficult step. . . ."

Nearly an hour into the proceedings, praise for Sanmar, and all the time the company representatives wished to use, the chair gave the floor to the first of fifty odd speakers who wanted the Water Quality Bureau to use its authority to stop dioxin production and opposed the delay of the compliance deadline.

The main issue for the activists was that dioxin is highly toxic and bioaccumulates, that too much dioxin is getting into San Luis Bay, and that Sanmar is a source of dioxin and could and should prevent this pollution. The activists worked to assert this issue as the main one in the meeting and urged the Water Quality Bureau to make its environmental and public policy decision on this basis and to take action.

Teresa Duncan, a county supervisor, was the first speaker called who opposed the Water Quality Bureau's proposal and articulated the dioxin prevention position.

"(T)here is no question but that dioxin is getting into the bay and is, at least some amount of it, emanating from Sanmar. Action is necessary to remove it from each of these sources, and any dioxin from Sanmar in water or air emissions is too much dioxin.

"Dioxin is deadly. We all know that. We know that refineries produce dioxin and we know that Sanmar produces dioxin and that it has been in violation of the limit. Simply requiring Sanmar to investigate options for eliminating it is a no-brainer. . . .

"We know that the environment is being polluted with harmful, deadly chemicals. The prudent thing to do is to err in favor of the public and on the side of caution to eliminate sources of pollution. This is the perspective that the public relies on from boards like ones you and I serve on. . . . Thank you."

Next, Chairwoman Screpsi called Pete Glasser, the lead researcher and advocate in the Clean Air and Water Network's Dioxin-Free Industries Project.

Pete's approach to persuading the Water Quality Bureau was to use its own data to dispute its claim that the dioxin in the company's wastewater did not come from its own processes. He argued that the evidence does not support Sanmar's conclusion that there is less dioxin in the refinery discharge than in urban run-off. Pete also pointed out that, in addition to dioxin in its discharge water, some amount of the dioxin in Sanmar's wastewater is initially emitted into the air by the refinery, then falls on the land and runs into the refinery's waste stream. In other words, Sanmar contributes to the dioxin in run-off. He urged the bureau to make Sanmar take responsibility for the dioxin in its wastewater.

Pete further pointed out the unsound basis of the company's conclusions by stating that there is no evidence for the claim that refineries create less dioxin than cars and wood stoves. There are no measurements of dioxin coming from cars and wood stoves in the area and no examination by a government agency of the total amount of dioxin emitted from all refinery processes. Regarding cars as a dioxin source, they run on gasoline manufactured by refineries, with dioxin precursors that create dioxin when combusted.

There was another new and extremely relevant piece of support for this position that Pete wanted to introduce, an EPA memo to the Water Quality Bureau and other interested parties, sent by fax only the day before, stating that cars, trucks, and wood burning are much less significant dioxin sources than industrial sources. Because this analysis by EPA scientists was released after the deadline for comments at the Water Bureau, Pete planned to introduce it by cross-examining the recipient the day of the public meeting. Before concluding his comments, he mentioned that he wanted to ask questions of witnesses at the appropriate time.

Pete concluded his presentation by stating that Sanmar is in violation of its water pollution permit. It contributes to a health threat that has been named a high priority by the EPA.[17] The Water Quality Bureau should keep the permit limit, it should not delay the decision, and it should enforce its previous order for Sanmar to search for ways to eliminate dioxin.

The Water Quality Bureau responded defensively to Pete's critical position. Bureau member Stacy Freeman denied that the bureau had ever "ordered zero dioxin."

Prepared for this fight, Pete quoted the 1995 Water Quality Bureau order, "'This alternative should consider the feasibility of eliminating dioxin-generating processes.'"

Tom O'Reilly joined Stacy in the effort to dismiss Pete's criticisms of the bureau staff's proposal, "Mr. Glasser . . . , we've come to believe that this is really largely an air problem."

Pete assured Tom that the Clean Air and Water Network was working on air sources, but that it is also a water problem.

"The food chain exposure is the problem, not inhalation," Pete countered and explained that the dioxin is initially released into the air, but ultimately ends up in the aquatic food chain, via deposition and run-off.

Chairwoman Screpsi entered the fray, rhetorically pushing the responsibility off of the Water Quality Bureau and onto the EPA, "Mr. Glasser, . . . as you know, we are waiting now for orders . . . from the EPA . . . as to what the official limit shall be. It is a complex and broad-based problem. (It's) pandemic throughout the United States, not exclusive to San Luis Bay."

The chairwoman claimed that the Water Quality Bureau could not take action because it needed to wait for the EPA.

Pete argued that the Water Quality Bureau had the authority to act and that the Air Quality Bureau and the EPA were at the same time trying to shake the responsibility. He pressed the Water Quality Bureau on whether it would continue with the existing order for Sanmar to investigate options for eliminating some or all of the dioxin.

"Mr. Glasser, I think our joint goal is toward an elimination of dioxin."

"Then why would you not want to study it when you have an existing requirement to do so?" Pete asked.

"Because the EPA and the State Department of the Environment are studying it in microscopic scientific detail, far beyond our capacity to do that," Amy replied, exasperated.

Chairwoman Screpsi had expressed implicitly, yet clearly, in these comments the Water Quality Bureau's criteria for action. These criteria had not been presented, neither explicitly nor implicitly, in the staff proposal, nor at any other time in the meeting. The chairwoman reasoned that the work of setting dioxin permit limits—calculating how much the bay can assimilate, identifying the contributing polluters, and allocating the allowed amount among them—is beyond the capacity of the Water Quality Bureau. The relevant criterion for action, the one that was not met in this case, was that the agency should already have resources available for the task. The basis of the bureau's decision was not the danger posed to bay ecology and public health by high levels of dioxin in San Luis Bay. Instead of first considering what was the right thing to do, and then finding the resources to do it, the Water Quality Bureau first considered whether or not it had the resources to do the job.

Pete took issue with Amy, "No one is studying how Sanmar can eliminate dioxin. That is your part of the puzzle."

"Thank you for your participation" the chairwoman seethed, dismissing Pete from the floor. "We'll move onto the next speaker."

Pete protested, "I want to ask questions of witnesses, as is my right, at the appropriate time."

The Water Quality Bureau lawyers stated that whether or not Pete could cross-examine was up to the discretion of the bureau. Seeing that he was about to be shut out, Pete tried another avenue of introducing the new material from the EPA.

"In that case, I would like to introduce into evidence a letter that I understand was faxed by EPA to the bureau yesterday. I was told EPA would be here, but apparently they aren't."

"We cut off comments on June third. Because somebody faxed us a letter yesterday does not allow it to be put in the record," replied the executive officer, Sharon Kemp, using her power to prohibit rather than authorize the presentation of obviously relevant, critical information.

In a sea of gasps from the audience, Pete left the floor.

The next speaker was Stephen Girard, lawyer for San Luis Bay Watch, a bay pollution watchdog group, and long-time colleague of Pete and lawyers at the Clean Air and Water Network. Stephen directly raised the issue of political will to deal with dioxin, in contrast to the red herrings the Water Quality Bureau had presented. He began by rephrasing as a question the claim made by bureau member O'Reilly and by Sanmar: Is dioxin in San Luis Bay the responsibility of the air quality regulators, rather than the Water Quality Bureau?

"Madam Chair, members of the bureau, I believe the . . . rationale that the staff has provided for the proposed amendment sidesteps the opportunity that the bureau has to control dioxin releases at Sanmar. Referring to Mr. O'Reilly's comment about this being an air problem, I think we have in the record the fact that the Air Quality Bureau has said it is not an air problem. They've, in fact, passed on it, despite the large amount of dioxin coming out of Sanmar's stacks.

"Whether you are talking about wastewater or you're talking about air releases, Sanmar's processes are a clear source of dioxin to the bay, which is, of course, within your authority and your jurisdiction, and you have ample authority to go after sources coming out of stacks. Your authority extends to the placement of pollution in a manner that's going to get into the water."

This idea startled the bureau.

"Give him extra time," the Chairwoman interrupted. "(It's) a critical issue . . . I would like a statement from the staff, does the Water Quality Bureau have the authority to rule on stack emissions?"

After some discussion, the bureau's legal counsel concluded, "It probably isn't what the legislature had in mind."

Stephen continued, "It's quite clear, despite the lawyers not having written it out, that the statute says 'may.' Anything that *may* be discharged, things that are put in a position that they're going to get into the water, you can cover with state water quality law. So you have the opportunity to take up the reins and use them. . . . We are getting dioxin out of the Sanmar facility, as well as any number of other sources, but this is one clear source, and it is going into the environment, into the bay, into the fish, it's going into the parking lot we heard mention of, and running off into the bay, it's going into, I guess, the bark of trees, it's getting deposited there by these discrete sources, and your authority extends to them. . . . A lot of effluent is in the air before it actually hits the water, so this just perhaps takes a little longer to get there. But there's nothing philosophically different from controlling that pipe, from a pipe that's discharging water into the bay.

"We urge no action at this time on the proposed amendment to the Cease and Desist Order. No one's proposing end-of-pipe treatment from anywhere in the room that I can hear of. Everybody's talking about pollution prevention, trying to get to the sources and eliminating them, which is really, I think, really the only way we're going to get a handle on dioxin. . . . I don't think the fact that we have some potential new standards out there is a relevant fact to this . . . I would ask you, instead of going with the amendment, instruct the staff to either revise the amendment or come up with a proposal where you're asking Sanmar to go to all the sources and do pollution prevention."

"So thanks for your time, and if you have any questions."

Stephen's statement cleared away any question of jurisdiction in the path of the Water Quality Bureau's limiting dioxin.

"Next speaker," called the chair.

Next up were four women who would speak about their experience with cancer and endometriosis, illnesses that are associated with dioxin, and argue that the knowledge that dioxin causes these and other painful, debilitating and, often, terminal, diseases, and that Sanmar is a definite source of dioxin, is a strong basis for taking action. These speakers' comments reiterated points made in earlier comments; I recount them here to show the differentiation and depth of the dioxin prevention constituency.

Diane Lucas, a registered nurse, representative of the State Nurses' Association, and member of the District Board at a local hospital, spoke about her patients on a gynecology oncology floor.

"I take care of women with cancer. Cancer causing chemicals are not an academic discussion for myself, my coworkers, and my patients. . . . (W)e see lots of pain and suffering, and we see plenty of women who die on our floor. For us the equation is simple. Dioxin is an identified carcinogen. Carcinogens cause cancer. Sanmar is a known producer of dioxin. And Sanmar, as a good corporate citizen in the area, should look at ways to eliminate dioxin that they release. Not to do so is inhumane to all of the people who live in the San Luis Bay area. Therefore the State Nurses' Association urges no action on the issue that's before us today."

There were no questions from the bureau.

"Michele Callum," called the Chairwoman.

Michele introduced herself as the public policy advocate for the Women's Cancer Support Center and a woman living with cancer. Her argument was similar to Diane's, continuing the call for action based on already available knowledge.

"These are the facts. One: the EPA has determined that dioxin, which is linked to cancer, has seriously compromised San Luis Bay water quality and that it is a high priority safety item because of its human health risk. Two: Many cities and counties in the bay region have passed resolutions to move the area toward dioxin elimination. Industrial polluters should be compelled to move in the same direction. Three: Sanmar is far exceeding its discharge limit. Four: Sanmar cannot escape responsibility by saying that the dioxin comes from diesel fuel and motor oil since the dioxin in the fuel comes from the refining process . . .

"As a member of the Water Quality Bureau, you are charged with protecting the health of the bay's waters and we who live near its shores. . . . (I)t is your job to eliminate (dioxin). . . . The precautionary principle demands today that . . . you resolve any doubts in favor of public health. That weighs in favor of not changing the permit. The Women's Cancer Support Center and the hundreds of women we serve living with cancer urge you to do the right thing, the lawful thing, by requiring that Sanmar comply with your order, reduce its dioxin discharge, and look for ways to eliminate dioxin from its processes. Thank you."

Next, another breast cancer survivor, Janis Hayes, explained to the Bureau that although it is not known if dioxin was a factor in her cancer, the possibility is much too great to be ignored. She described her horror, not only of losing her breasts, but also learning that while she had them she had nursed her children with them and, in so doing, gave them a lifetime dose of dioxin in that vulnerable and formative developmental stage. Like the others, she urged the Water Quality Bureau to keep the limit and move toward zero dioxin.

Carol Jensen, one of the community organizers working in Springfield, followed. She brought endometriosis—one of a host of diseases often overshadowed by interest in cancer—into the discussion of health effects.

"We talk about a lot of technical, complicated things, but for those of us who have diseases that are linked to dioxin exposure, the problem is simple. . . . (H)uman suffering . . . and dioxin pollution (are) preventable. If there is a way to eliminate it, it needs to be eliminated. . . . You have a known dioxin source that is violating the law. I urge you to uphold the law and get them to work towards elimination."

Last in the line-up of activists came two speakers from Springfield. The first was Gary Combs, the executive director of the Springfield Anti-Toxics Task Force. An African-American, Gary was one of only two people of color participating in the meeting. "Good morning, Madam Chair, members of the Water Quality Bureau. I'm here to encourage you to stick with the original order and require that Sanmar pursue the elimination of dioxins. As you've heard . . . , when we're talking about dioxins, we are talking about a deadly chemical substance on a spectrum where a little bit is too much. So we encourage you to go forward . . . in your wisdom and require that Sanmar comply with the order."

"And I would caution you to be wary . . . of the science . . . when it is coming from one of the parties that are accused of violations. I have learned that lesson . . . from . . . companies in my area telling us that we don't have to worry about emissions from their facility because they stop at the fence line. If that is science, I would seriously question that. . . . (M)y community has come to trust Mr. Pete Glasser and his scientific expertise over the years. We certainly support Mr. Glasser and his work on dioxins and the positions that he took before your bureau. Thank you."

"Thank you, Mr. Combs. Phyllis Thompson, please," called the Chairwoman.

Phyllis Thompson—an African-American woman, and the second of only two people of color participating in the meeting—was born in Lakeview. Her family moved to Springfield during her childhood, first to a housing project adjacent to a chemical company, and then to a subdivision directly downwind of the large refinery in the city. That subdivision was one of many built in the open space around the city and county in the postwar years—the one that was marketed specifically to Blacks. Phyllis had become involved in environmental politics when her sister died of cancer at the early age of forty. She had participated in a campaign for a community inspection and pollution and accident prevention agreement with the local refinery in the late 1980s, but then fell out of activism when her mother was diagnosed with lupus and emphysema a few years later. She only recently had gotten involved in environmental activism again through the Clean Air and Water Network's presentations on dioxin at Springfield neighborhood meetings.

Phyllis stood at the podium, "I'm passing pictures around because I want you all to see my aunt—"

"You're going to have to speak up," interrupted bureau member O'Reilly. "That is my aunt," Phyllis stated more loudly.

"I'm reminded you'll have to introduce yourself, please, for the record," interrupted Chairwoman Screpsi.

"My name is Phyllis Thompson," Phyllis started anew. "I live in Springfield. My mother has emphysema, she's never smoked a day in her life. And she has lupus. My sister died of cancer, and she had lupus also. . . . What I am saying is mostly all those people in those pictures are dead. . . . The point is dioxin kills. It's in the air, it's in the water. . . . We are in a crisis. . . . Sanmar has to eliminate dioxin. . . . The other refineries have to eliminate dioxin. Plain and simple. I would hope . . . you all sitting in a position that you can do something with protecting people's health . . . that you will not amend the permit, but go ahead on and do the investigation of zero dioxin. . . . Thank you."

That afternoon, the Water Quality Bureau voted unanimously to allow Sanmar to exceed its dioxin limit for another year. One year later, neither the Water Quality Bureau, the Air Quality Bureau, nor the EPA, which had named dioxin in San Luis Bay a high priority, had taken charge of addressing the problem. After another public meeting similar to the one I have discussed here, the Water Quality Bureau voted unanimously to raise Sanmar's dioxin limit to the amount the refinery was discharging, as the company had requested, and to do nothing to address the problem of dioxin in San Luis Bay.

What, then, happened when residents of this disproportionately impacted area got involved in the regulatory process? They found a regulatory agency that would not use its authority to stop the production of an extremely toxic substance that bioaccumulates and is already present at background levels that cause health problems. They found a regulatory agency that weakened its own earlier dioxin limit for the refinery.

The Springfield residents and others in the Dioxin Prevention Alliance witnessed the Water Quality Bureau make this important decision that affects the ecology of the bay and the chances for health and sickness, and life and death, of those who eat its fish, based on its current availability of resources. The bureau first considered the costs of taking action, rather than first deciding what is the right thing to do given the scientific information about the extreme toxicity and persistence of dioxin and the high levels of it in San Luis Bay, and then looking for the resources to do what is right. The agency made its determination based on cost rather than threat to bay ecology and public health.

Instead of admitting that dioxin in the bay is a serious problem that needs to be addressed and that the Water Quality Bureau does not have enough resources to determine dioxin permit limits, the agency directed attention to a red herring, the larger puzzle of other sources of dioxin and the idea that the amount Sanmar creates comparatively is small and unimportant. The staff presented this red herring in technical terms so that no one but engineers and others trained in that technical language and way of thinking could intervene. This move claims authority through technical knowledge and language; it says, "trust us, we're experts," "leave it up to us." The Water Quality Bureau then further tried to justify its inaction by claiming that more science is needed (see the chairwoman's statements that the bureau is waiting for orders from the EPA, which is studying the problem in microscopic scientific detail, above), when the relevant science is already done. The tasks involved in putting dioxin limits in pollution permits require empirical observation and best estimates (of dioxin levels in the bay, water discharges, air emissions and deposition, and surface run-off and of the relative contribution of each source) that may be considered scientific or technical. But the scientific crux in making the decision about what to do consists of the knowledge of the toxic and persistent character of dioxin and the excess of it in San Luis Bay.

Whether as direct participants or interested observers, Springfield residents witnessed the Water Quality Bureau use the power embedded in its rules and procedures to silence critics and authorize advocates for criteria for action that harm rather than protect public health and ecology, protecting private profit instead. They watched the bureau ignore any need for accountability to a growing and differentiated constituency concerned about dioxin pollution in the region.

By 1986, directives to identify and control industries producing dioxin had come down to regional regulatory bodies, including the Water Quality Bureau.

The bureau was supposed to have been limiting dioxin since that year. Toxicologists have known of dioxin's health hazards and how to avoid producing them since before the chemical industry boomed in the postwar period, mass-producing and -dispersing this toxin (Baughman 1977). Engineers working in the regulatory system should have been aware of this information throughout the development of the regulatory system. Yet after thirty years of developing that system—which includes more than ten years and millions of dollars spent to study dioxin exposure and health risk at the EPA[18]—what newcomers to regulatory politics from a disproportionately impacted area found was that the Water Quality Bureau and other regulatory agencies are still not limiting dioxin in a way that protects human health and the environment.

What can be learned, from this case, about inclusion of residents of areas that are disproportionately impacted by pollution in public health and regulatory decision-making as strategy for preventing pollution there and as a solution to environmental racism and inequality? Essential as inclusion of residents of disproportionately impacted areas in decision-making processes of health and regulatory agencies is to democracy, inclusion in agencies, in their current forms, does not necessarily lead to change. Inclusion of any critic in health and regulatory agencies, in their current forms, does not necessarily lead to change. Advocating for or agreeing to inclusion of the formerly excluded without critically examining health and regulatory agencies' practices lets those agencies off the hook. Advocates outside and inside public agencies need to specify what will count as meaningful inclusion and, in order to do that, we need to know what happens in those agencies, including and more broadly than when low-income, minority newcomers from disproportionately impacted areas participate. What agency protocols and practices block meaningful inclusion and preventive, precautionary changes? How were those protocols and practices produced? How are they perpetuated, and how might they be transformed?

In the case I have discussed here, criteria for action in both ATSDR and the Water Quality Bureau limit the scope of problems each will address. The criteria for action in each agency undercut the preventive and precautionary proposals made by members of the public—low-income or not, minority or not, and disproportionately impacted or not. In ATSDR, the criteria that block the agency from recommending that dioxin producers stop producing dioxin are that the agency needs to know what health problems to expect at what levels of exposure, and needs to have treatment advice. In the Water Quality Bureau, the criterion that blocks proper regulation of dioxin is the need already to have a budget for it.

Administrators and engineers first produced these limiting criteria for action over twenty years ago in the case of ATSDR, and over thirty years ago in the case of the Water Quality Bureau, when they were beginning to build these agencies. The criteria solidified in their limiting form through the process of implementing pollution control laws and building the agencies—in part because of limited resources allocated for these initiatives. Instead of developing a vision of adequate, socially just protection of public health and the environment from toxics and seeking the resources to bring that vision to life, agencies adapted to their limited allocated resources. In any case, low-income people of color from disproportionately impacted communities were not included in the production of the criteria for action. Nor were other critics interested in environmental justice, precaution, and prevention. Polluters, on the other hand, at least in the case of regulatory agencies, had some degree of input into the criteria for action through their necessary participation in the permitting process. Criteria for action made in the past with little or no public input are actively used today and continue to limit the scope of the work of health and regulatory agencies in the present. In order for there to be meaningful democratic inclusion in agency decision-making in the present, and to change the uneven landscape of environmental and public health protection, these criteria need to be opened up, reexamined, and revised with the input of residents of low-income, minority, disproportionately impacted communities, and other critics interested in environmental justice, precaution, and prevention.

A reexamination and revision of health and regulatory agencies' criteria for action needs to acknowledge their currently very limited capacities of health and regulatory agencies—regarding not only dioxin, but all toxic substances—and then work to expand them. An in-depth look at the solidification and reproduction of the criteria for action in health and regulatory agencies would be a useful starting point for plotting how to transform them.[19]

8

Chemicals, Cancer, and Prevention:
The Synergy of Synthetic Social Movements

MAREN KLAWITER

Death and disease were configured quite differently at the end of the nineteenth century than they were at the end of the twentieth. In the United States of a century ago, contagious diseases such as pneumonia, typhoid, tuberculosis, and diarrhea represented the greatest threat to human health and survival. Cancer, on the other hand, was of only marginal importance, in both absolute and relative terms (Department of the Interior Census Office 1896). By the 1930s, however, cancer and contagious diseases had switched places in the official statistics. Cancer was now the second leading cause of death (behind heart disease) and contagious diseases had moved several rungs down the ladder. This trend continued during the second half of the twentieth century, as age-adjusted cancer incidence and mortality rates continued creeping upwards and the specter of life-threatening contagious diseases continued to recede.[1]

Cancer, of course, is not one disease but many, and while the incidence and mortality rates of several types of cancer (e.g., stomach, uterine, cervical, colon) actually diminished in the United States during the post–World War II era, age-adjusted incidence and mortality rates for most types of cancer (e.g., lung, breast, brain, prostate, colorectal, etc.) grew. Between 1971 and 1993 alone, the overall incidence of cancer increased by 18 percent and the mortality rate grew by 7 percent (National Cancer Advisory Board 1994, 10).[2] In the case of lung cancer, a consensus regarding the reason for the dramatic increases emerged within a broad spectrum of "expert" communities—scientific, medical, public health, public policy—and was shared by the lay public. In most cases, however, no consensus has emerged regarding the cause, nor even the extent, of the slow but steady growth in the rates of occurrence. Breast cancer is one of these cases. Between 1950 and 1990 the age-adjusted incidence of breast cancer increased by 53 percent (National Cancer Advisory Board 1994, Appendix D) and during the last decade they have continued to climb at the rate of about 0.6 percent a year (Clegg et al. 2002).[3] During that same period of time, despite the incorporation of radiation and chemical therapies into the standard treatment regimen, and despite improvements in early detection technologies and the spread of population-based screening, breast cancer mortality rates increased by four percent (Centers for Disease Control and Prevention 1994). During the 1990s, U.S. breast cancer mortality rates finally began to drop. In 1990, the age-adjusted death rate for breast cancer was 18.9 per 100,000. By 1999 the death rate had dropped to 15.3 per 100,000 (National Cancer Institute 2002, Table IV-3).

Increases in the incidence and mortality rates of cancer in general, and breast cancer in particular, however, were not the result of the state's neglect or its lack of interest. The primary way in which the state addressed the "enormous cancer burden" (National Cancer Advisory Board 1994, 9) was through its investment in cancer research. The federal budget for cancer research grew dramatically during the last decade, but even before that, the state was heavily invested in cancer research. President Nixon signed the National Cancer Act of 1971, for example, which declared "War on Cancer" and mandated that the NCI, with the advice of the National Cancer Advisory Board, "plan and develop an expanded, intensified, and coordinated cancer research program encompassing the programs of the National Cancer Institute, related programs of the other research institutes, and other Federal and non-Federal programs" (National Cancer Advisory Board 1994, 9). Between 1970 and 1972, the NCI's budget doubled, from $181,454,000 to $378,794,000, and it grew steadily throughout the decade, topping off at $937,129,000, almost double the size of the budget of its closest competitor in the National Institutes of Health, the National Heart, Lung and Blood Institute.[4] By the end of the 1980s, the NCI budget exceeded $1.5 *billion.*

But even before the passage of the 1971 National Cancer Act and the development of the National Cancer Plan, cancer "control" and cancer research were on the state's agenda. As early as 1922 the U.S. federal government was sponsoring two small cancer research groups—one at the U.S. Hygienic Laboratory in Washington, D.C. and the other in Boston (Baker 1977, 651). The most important step occurred in 1937, however, when the National Cancer Institute was created over the protests of the scientific and medical communities—the first and to this day still the most powerful of the twenty-seven health and disease research fiefdoms that comprise the National Institutes of Health.[5] Although the NCI received modest funding during the first twenty years of its existence, its budget grew by more than *one hundred fold* between 1946 and 1957. Between 1940 and 1946, the NCI's budget hovered between $530,000 and $570,000. But in 1948, riding the rising tide of postwar enthusiasm for scientific research, the NCI's budget soared to $14,500,000 and by 1956 it had grown to $24,978,000. Between 1956 and 1957, the NCI's budget doubled again, from almost $25 million to $48 million. Clearly, the NCI was one the primary recipients of the postwar investment in biomedical research (National Institutes & Health 2001, 256).

Nor, contrary to contemporary popular opinion, was *breast* cancer, in particular, given short shrift in the budgeting priorities and program planning of the NCI. For example, one, if not the, most important research focuses of the NCI during the postwar era was chemical research (Endicott 1957, 275) and by 1957 the NCI's Cancer Chemotherapy Program was receiving 41 percent of the NCI's total research budget (Baker 1977, 653). The Cancer Chemotherapy Program screened thousands of chemicals; usually they were submitted by private industry—chemical companies in particular—for evidence of anticancer activity.[6] Within this program, mammary tumors were one of only a small handful of tumor-types (lung and colon were the others)[6] against which chemicals were tested if results from the early screening tests looked promising (Goodman and Walsh 2001, 95). Breast cancer was not ignored within the NCI's Cancer Chemotherapy Program. Later on, following the passage of the National Cancer Act of 1971, one of the first major NCI initiatives was the Breast Cancer Detection Demonstration Project (BCDDP). The BCDDP, which was a joint venture between the NCI and the American Cancer Society, was a project (not a controlled study) designed to promote mammographic screening to healthy women. Although the design and implementation of the BCDDP generated a great deal of criticism and controversy within both expert and activist communities, the state's investment in the "control" of breast cancer cannot be discounted. This did not change with the infusion of additional resources and attention.

Even *before* President Clinton established the National Action Plan on Breast Cancer in 1994, and *before* the passage of the NIH Revitalization Act of 1993 (which increased breast cancer research funding within the National Cancer Insitute), and *before* passage of the Department of Defense (DOD) Authorization Act (which established a breast cancer research program in the DOD and appropriated $210 million for its first year), and before the Breast and Cervical Cancer Mortality Prevention Act of 1990 (a program administered by the CDC designed to provide poor and uninsured women with access to breast and cervical cancer screening) breast cancer was receiving a *larger* portion of the National Cancer Institute's research budget than, for example, a men's disease like prostate cancer, despite the rough comparability of breast and prostate cancer incidence and mortality. In 1983, breast cancer-specific research received $47.7 million from the NCI whereas prostate cancer-specific research received only $10 million from the NCI. That same year, research on lung cancer—a disease that impacts more men and women and kills more people each year than breast and prostate cancer combined—received only $35 million from the NCI. By 1987 breast cancer research funding had grown to $70 million whereas research for prostate cancer had actually declined slightly to $9.9 million.[7]

More significant than the absolute amount of funding for cancer in general, or the proportion of funding set aside for the production of knowledge about breast cancer in particular, was the way that cancer was constructed by the state as a social problem and institutionalized within the state as an object of scientific inquiry. The state did not, by any means, operate as a monolithic entity, nor did it proceed according to a single logic, nor was it necessarily consistent over time. But it is nonetheless possible and, I think, helpful (at least for the purposes of this analysis) to reduce the complex history of cancer's construction and institutionalization within the state to two principal models: the biomedical and the environmental.[8] In the spirit of further simplification, then, I propose that we conceptualize the principal differences between these two approaches in the following manner. The *biomedical model* begins with the disease, produces knowledge about the biology of cancer, and seeks to develop cancer cures and more effective (often chemically based) treatments. The *environmental model,* on the other hand, begins with the toxic substances and suspected carcinogens, produces knowledge about processes of carcinogenesis, and seeks to regulate, reduce and eliminate our exposure to these (often chemically based) hazards. In the *biomedical model* cancer prevention, increasingly, is being conceptualized as "chemoprevention" whereas in the *environmental model,* cancer prevention is conceptualized as the creation of a safe environment.[9]

The *biomedical model,* as already noted, has primarily focused on understanding cancer as a biochemical process and developing better screening, detection, diagnostic, treatment and, more recently, risk assessment and prevention technologies. At the federal level, the biomedical model has been institutionalized within the National Cancer Institute, the Centers for Disease Control and Prevention, the Food and Drug Administration, and more recently, the National Center for Human Genome Research.

One of the most important developments in biomedical cancer research during the postwar era, which I have already mentioned, was the NCI-sponsored chemotherapy program. The most promising results of these efforts are typically transferred to the pharmaceutical industry, often through cooperative agreements between specific companies and research agencies known as CRADAs (Cooperative Research and Development Agreements). The pharmaceutical companies, usually after some amount of additional research and development, then apply for FDA approval.[10] Many, if not most, of the cancer chemotherapies currently on the market are the product of public-private partnerships.

The *environmental model,* as noted, primarily has focused on the study of chemical carcinogens and on the regulation, reduction, and/or elimination of human exposures to toxic chemicals, industrial processes, and their by-products. Within the state, research in the area of carcinogenesis has been conducted through the National Institutes of Health—first in the Environmental Cancer Section of the National Cancer Institute and later, beginning with its establishment in 1966, in the National Institute for Environmental Health Sciences

(NIEHS). In 1950, 35 percent of the NCI's grants were awarded in the area of carcinogenesis, and cancer therapy received only 18 percent of the grants (Baker 1977, 653). Between 1956 and 1957 the proportion of total NCI grants awarded to carcinogenesis dropped from 29 percent to 16 percent. That same year the proportion of grants awarded to cancer therapy research grew from 33 percent to 41 percent.

Workplace safety has been a major component of the environmental approach to cancer, emphasizing the creation of a safe working environment through the regulation of dangerous substances, industrial processes, and labor practices and the development of safer means for storing, handling, and disposing of toxic substances. Pioneering research in the area of carcinogenesis was conducted by Wilhelm Hueper, a German immigrant, whistle-blower, and maverick who got his start working for the chemical company DuPont before being fired in the 1940s for his whistle-blowing activities concerning worker safety and exposure to toxic chemicals. When the Environmental Cancer Section of the National Cancer Institute was created in 1948 Hueper was hired as its first, and, as it turns out, only director.[11] Hueper gave key testimony in support of the precedent-setting Delaney Clause (section 409 of the Federal Food, Drug, and Cosmetic Act), in 1958, which outlawed the use of carcinogens in processed foods—prohibiting, for example, pesticide residues found to induce cancer in humans or animals. The Environmental Cancer Section was abolished upon Hueper's death in 1964. In 1966, the National Institute of Environmental Health Sciences was created as a separate agency within the NIH. During the 1970s, the environmental model was further institutionalized within the state through the creation of the Environmental Protection Agency (a regulatory agency), the Occupational Safety and Health Agency (a regulatory agency), and the National Institute for Occupational Safety and Health (a research agency).[12] The bulk of the government's investment in cancer control, research, and regulation, however, has been channeled through the NCI and, within the NCI, biomedical approaches have received the lion's share of funding and attention.[13]

During the 1970s, the salience of cancer as a social problem grew in intensity. It was politicized along both its biomedical and environmental dimensions by whistle-blowers within the cancer research establishment and clinical medicine, on the one hand, and by the women's health and environmental movements, on the other. Within the medical and scientific research establishments, the whistle-blowers included George Crile (discussed in Lerner 2001), Samuel Epstein (1979), and Ralph Moss (1980). Outside these rarified spaces, the journalist Rose Kushner (1975) and the feminist poet Audre Lorde (1980) published important works criticizing the medical and scientific research establishments. But the whistle-blowers would have been blowing in the wind were it not for the receptive audiences that had already been primed by women's health and environmental movements. There was no noticeable bridging of frames, however, nor was there significant organizational overlap between the biomedical and environmental fields of activism.

When the breast cancer movement burst onto the national political scene in full stride and in full color in the early 1990s, it was the National Breast Cancer Coalition (NBCC) and its biomedical agenda that captured the media's imagination and the lion's share of attention. Outside the NBCC, however, feminist cancer and breast cancer activists were pursuing the environmental angle from a number of different directions.[14] In Long Island, in Massachusetts, and in the San Francisco Bay Area, potent syntheses of breast cancer and environmental activism gained momentum. This chapter examines that synthesis and the political synergies it produced, paying particular attention to the dilemmas faced by the environmental wing of the breast cancer movement as it sought to challenge the chemical and pharmaceutical industries and their tight interlinkings, without abandoning biomedicine.[15]

Beginning with an historical analysis of how the feminist cancer and environmental justice movements coalesced around the concept of the "cancer industry," organized around the discourse of cancer prevention, and synthesized the strengths of both movements, I briefly take a closer look at three campaigns and organizations (three "cases") situated at the juncture of these two movements. I argue that environmental justice campaigns in the San Francisco Bay Area faced a different set of circumstances than did feminist cancer and breast cancer organizations involved in environmental activism.[16] These differences were the result of the polysemous character of synthetic chemicals and the dual subject position of feminist cancer activists.

Unlike environmental justice activists, who could work solely within the environmental model—starting with the toxic chemicals and industrial processes and seeking their regulation, remediation, and elimination—environmental activists coming from the feminist cancer and breast cancer movements lived in both worlds, and were sometimes caught between them. This led to a set of difficulties and dilemmas, but also, to a series of dynamic political strategies that show promise for successfully bridging and institutionally linking the biomedical and environmental axes.

Synthesizing the Feminist Cancer and Environmental Justice Movements

The feminist cancer movement was born in the San Francisco Bay Area in the late 1980s and early 1990s. Although from the very beginning, feminist cancer organizations in the San Francisco Bay Area framed cancer as an environmental issue, until the middle of the decade, feminist cancer activism concerning the environment took the shape of public education through speeches, organizational newsletters and, at least in the case of the Women's Cancer Resource Center, through the way that they trained and educated new groups of volunteers. Until the mid-1990s, however, feminist cancer and environmental justice organizations moved within separate and largely nonoverlapping political fields.[17] Beginning in the fall of 1994, however, that all began to change. A new group, the Toxic Links Coalition, synthesized feminist cancer and environmental activism. That synthesis created a synergistic reaction that resulted in new campaigns, organizations, and coalitions. It also infused preexisting projects and organizations with new energy and broadened their networks. It was when the feminist cancer movement hooked into the energy, experience, networks, resources, and organizing acumen of the local environmental justice movement, however, that new ideas, campaigns, and coalitions around the issues of cancer and the environment really came to life and began to achieve real political impact.[18]

This transformation was facilitated by the release of a report by the Northern California Cancer Center (NCCC), entitled "Breast Cancer in the Greater Bay Area." The report revealed that the San Francisco Bay Area had the highest incidence rates of breast cancer in the world. The issue of high cancer rates was not a new one, of course, nor was the strategy of dramatizing and publicizing high rates in order to grab people's attention.[19] But when the NCCC released their report in the fall of 1994, it was seized upon, for obvious reasons, by breast cancer and environmental organizations in the Bay Area and used to great political effect. The Breast Cancer Fund, for example, called a press conference to publicize the report and the media began referring to the San Francisco Bay Area as "the breast cancer capital of the world."[20]

The first page of this report contained a chart comparing breast cancer rates among women living in twenty different regions, including Japan, India, Colombia, Israel, France, Spain, Australia, Hawaii, and the San Francisco Bay Area. In visually striking terms the bar chart showed that white women in the Bay Area had the highest recorded rates of breast cancer in the world. Black women in the Bay Area had the fourth highest breast cancer incidence rate of any group of women, anywhere in the world.[21] The interpretation of the table, also situated on the front page, ran under the title heading of "Highest Incidence Rates in the World" and it stated: "Given the available data, white women in the San Francisco/Oakland Area have the highest rate in the world. The rate is about 50% higher than in most European countries and 5 times higher than in Japan."

This article was published in the *Greater Bay Area Cancer Registry Report: A Publication of the Northern California Cancer Center*, a professional publication mailed primarily to cancer researchers, clinicians, and health care professionals. But shortly after this particular issue was published, it made its way into breast cancer and environmental networks and, when the Breast Cancer Fund held a press conference to publicize the NCCC report, it moved into the mainstream media. The public circulation of the "discovery" that breast cancer rates were higher in the Bay Area than anywhere else in the world was used to dramatic effect by the feminist cancer and environmental justice movements.

Higher rates were used as evidence that the environment was to blame. While it might be impossible to trace the chemical exposures and pathways that produced these elevated rates of breast cancer, higher rates alone were evidence of their existence and their significance.

The NCCC was criticized for sitting on data that had been available since 1992 (data covering the period from 1983 to 1987). What was *not* a part of the attack on the NCCC, however, but nonetheless made this sudden "discovery" even more fascinating, was the fact (evident in the report) that *the Bay Area had been the site of the highest documented rates of breast cancer since 1947*. Only when breast cancer became a politically charged issue, however, did these statistics migrate out of professional circles and galvanize action. Their migration and circulation was facilitated, in large part, by the growing level of breast cancer awareness and organizing in the San Francisco Bay Area, along with the growing persuasiveness of the proposal that a plausible relationship existed between the unchecked proliferation of synthetic chemicals and the unchecked proliferation of breast cancer diagnoses.

The Toxic Links Coalition and National Cancer Industry Awareness Month

Late in the summer of 1994 a handful of Bay Area activists convened an informal meeting to network, learn about each other's work, identify areas of overlap, and explore the possibility of working together on issues of mutual interest. These activists came from four organizations: Breast Cancer Action, Greenpeace, West County Toxics Coalition, and the Women's Cancer Resource Center. At their second meeting, they decided to formalize the collaboration and christened themselves the Toxic Links Coalition (TLC).[22] During the next few months, the coalition grew to include a handful of unaffiliated individuals and more than twenty organizations, primarily from the local environmental movement.

At the suggestion of the West County Toxics Coalition, an environmental group organized in opposition to the Chevron refinery located in their neighborhood (in Richmond, just north of Berkeley), the TLC decided to focus its energies on cancer prevention and to do so by challenging the pristine image of narrowly biomedical discourse of National Breast Cancer Awareness Month (NBCAM).

NBCAM was created in 1985 to "promote the importance of the three-step approach to early detection: mammography, clinical breast examination and breast self-examination."[23] By the mid-1990s, NBCAM had been officially endorsed by more than seventeen governmental, professional, and medical organizations, including the American Cancer Society, the National Cancer Institute, the American College of Radiology, and the Susan G. Komen Breast Cancer Research Foundation. Working in concert with these agencies, industries, professional groups, and foundations, NBCAM designed and produced the promotional materials used in breast cancer early detection campaigns and disseminated them via a wide variety of means—public service advertising, speaker's programs, and the placement of brochures, flyers, and posters in churches, beauty parlors, retail stores, physician offices, pharmacies, fitness centers, and so forth.[24]

TLC activists viewed NBCAM's discourse of early detection and its refusal to speak of cancer prevention, the environment, and carcinogens as a campaign of miseducation, obfuscation, and shameless profiteering. In addition to this, however, NBCAM was viewed not only as a symbol of the limitations of the biomedical approach to disease, but as a symbol of the economic interests sustaining the biomedical approach to disease—the pharmaceutical and chemical industries.

NBCAM, it turns out, was not the brainchild of a federal agency, a public health department, a health insurance company, or a private charity but rather, of a chemical company—Imperial Chemicals Industry (ICI), a British manufacturer of plastics, paints, pesticides, and pharmaceutical therapies, among other things. It was ICI that, in 1985, initiated a program designed "to address the lack of public information about breast cancer in the United States." As part of this effort they created a "public service message" featuring Susan Ford Bales and her mother, Betty Ford.[25] The public service message elicited a positive response, and it led to the creation of what is now known as National Breast Cancer Awareness Month, which has taken place with ever-growing fanfare every October since then. ICI's interest in breast cancer, though it might seem puzzling at first, stemmed from their investment in the breast cancer treatment drug tamoxifen, brand name Nolvadex®. ICI held the patent on Nolvadex®, the best-selling breast cancer treatment drug in the world, and the U.S. was their biggest market.

In 1993, Imperial Chemical Industries spun-off, or "demerged," its bioscience business into an independent company, Zeneca PLC, which consisted of Zeneca Pharmaceuticals, Zeneca Agrochemicals, and Zeneca Specialties. NBCAM and tamoxifen went with Zeneca Pharmaceuticals. In 1995, Zeneca Group bought a 50 percent stake in Salick Health Care. At the time of Zeneca's purchase, Salick Health Care consisted of eleven comprehensive outpatient cancer treatment centers, six comprehensive breast centers, and a number of for-profit physician practices specializing in cancer. In 1997 Zeneca Group bought the remaining shares of Salick (including a cancer center just a few blocks down the road from the TLC meeting place), thus adding sole ownership of cancer treatment centers and physician practices to its patent on the most frequently prescribed breast cancer treatment drug in the world. Although pharmaceutical companies had purchased drug-distribution companies and home health care agencies in the past, this was the first time a pharmaceutical company had become, in essence, the employer of physicians in a position to prescribe drugs manufactured by their employer. Zeneca's action prompted the publication of a *New York Times* article that drew attention to this apparent conflict of interest, noting that "Zeneca, the world's second-largest manufacturer of cancer drugs, would now be directly overseeing patients' cancer care" (Rosenthal 1997).[26]

Not all of this had come to pass when the Toxic Links Coalition decided to train their sights on NBCAM and Zeneca Pharmaceuticals, but there was more than enough to work with, and later developments only strengthened and confirmed their analysis of the role of NBCAM within the political economy of cancer and chemicals—the California EPA, for example, had not yet recommended adding tamoxifen to the state's list (under Proposition 65) of cancer-causing chemicals, nor had the World Health Organization classified tamoxifen as a Class I carcinogen.[27] The TLC articulated two main criticisms of NBCAM. First, they argued that NBCAM legitimized early detection programs (mainly mammographic screening) as the only conceivable public health approach to breast cancer. Second, TLC activists argued that NBCAM concealed from the public the fact that multinational corporations, assisted by their allies, were on the one hand, profiting by *causing* cancer—through the pesticides, toxic products, and the "by-products" of industrial processes—and profiting as well from *detecting* and *treating* it. Zeneca Pharmaceuticals thus represented a textbook case of vertical integration, the material embodiment of the cancer industry.

The TLC's first collective action was to set up an informational picket at the 1994 Race for the Cure® in Golden Gate Park. They targeted the Race because its sponsor, the Komen Foundation, was a leading promoter of NBCAM and because the Komen Foundation, like NBCAM, studiously avoided any mention of causes, carcinogens, or the environment in their organizational and event publicity. Shortly thereafter, again, as part of National Cancer Industry Awareness Month, the Toxic Links Coalition staged the first of what became an annual event: the Toxic Tour of the Cancer Industry. This event, which was held in downtown San Francisco, was structured as a one hour tour de force of the local outposts of the global cancer industry. At each stop along the way—including the offices of Chevron, Pacific Gas and Electric, Burson Martseller (a public relations firm), Bechtel (a builder of nuclear power plants), and the American Cancer Society (for its cozy relationship with private industry and its refusal to take a stand against the proliferation of pesticides and other chemical carcinogens), TLC participants engaged in street theater and delivered rousing speeches about the need to shift the focus from early detection to cancer prevention, and from breast cancer awareness to awareness of the cancer industry.[28]

Although the Toxic Tour of the Cancer Industry became the TLC's signature event, probably the single most important event was co-organized by the TLC and the Women's Environment & Development Organization (WEDO), as part of their new "Action for Cancer Prevention Campaign."[29] The event, called the Women, Health and the Environment Community Action Conference, was held August 12–13, 1995 and attended by more than two hundred people from both the environmental justice and women's cancer communities.

The conference was well-timed to take advantage of the public's growing awareness of the high rates of breast cancer in the San Francisco Bay Area. Although the word "cancer" did not appear in the name of the conference, cancer and breast cancer in particular, were the primary focus of the vast majority of the speakers and the dominant lens through which the conference was viewed by the media. The conference program, for example, began with the following question: "Cancer in the Bay Area?" And the press release issued by the conference organizers framed the conference like this:

> Seventeen women's health and environmental justice organizations calling themselves the Toxic Links Coalition (TLC) have formed an unprecedented local campaign to demand answers to the question raised by the NCCC's report on breast cancer in the Bay Area: "Why does the environmentally conscious Bay Area have some of the highest rates of cancer in the nation and perhaps the world?" At the Women, Health and the Environment conference, the front page of the NCCC report was copied onto neon green paper, included in the media packets, and circulated to all the conference participants. The subtitle of the report, "Highest Incidence Rates in the World," was circled in thick black marker with an arrow drawn to the top of the page, pointing to a big fat "Why?"

The first day, which was held in San Francisco's City Hall, was staged as a public hearing on cancer, women's health, and the environment and it was organized around the testimony of a wide array of participants. Nineteen activists representing nineteen organizations provided "expert testimony" to a group of seventeen panelists representing state agencies, public health departments, political offices, and research organizations. The late, great Bella Abzug, Executive Director of WEDO, presided over the public hearing. The next day, the conference moved across the bay to Richmond, a predominantly African-American community just north of Berkeley, located next to a major Chevron refinery. The eight workshops that day once again emphasized the relationship between cancer and chemicals and were organized as follows: (1) Chlorine, Zenoestrogens, and Breast Cancer; (2) Pesticides: The Circle of Poison; (3) Radiation and Cancer; (4) Toxins, Multiple Health Effects, and Toxic-Free Life Style Changes; (5) Cancer in the Workplace–Petrochemicals, Solvents; (6) From Richmond to Bayview Hunters Point: Chevron, Incineration, Toxics, and Power Plants; (7) The Politics of Breast Cancer; and (8) Women's Bodies as a Cancer Battlefield. The community action day concluded with a public demonstration staged at the nearby Chevron Chemical Company plant, where protesters gathered outside the gated facility and demanded that Chevron close an on-site hazardous waste incinerator responsible for releasing dioxin and other hazardous compounds.[30] The two-day conference served as a catalyst for the development of new projects, networks, and organizations, and the strengthening of old ones. Three of these are discussed in the next section.

The Synergy of Cross-Movement Fertilization

The Women, Health and the Environment Conference brought together activists from all over the Bay Area. It strengthened and expanded preexisting networks and relationships and stimulated the creation of new ones. The mixture of environmental justice and breast cancer activism produced a synergistic reaction whose energy was harnessed and channeled in a number of productive directions. In what follows, I highlight three examples of the synergy produced by this synthesis.[31] The first example describes a campaign that was organized in Oakland (across the bay from San Francisco) to prevent the repermitting of a commercial medical waste incinerator whose toxic emissions included deadly dioxins. The second example describes a campaign in Bayview-Hunters Point, a low-income neighborhood in San Francisco, organized to prevent the siting of yet another power plant in their community. The third example, described in greater detail, follows the dynamic growth of Marin Breast Cancer Watch, an environmental breast cancer organization located in Marin County (a region known for its wealthy, white, well-educated, and health-oriented population).

Challenges to Medical Waste Incineration in Oakland

One struggle involved an attempt to prevent a medical waste incinerator located, again, in a predominantly low-income community of color in Oakland, from having their permit renewed by the Bay Area Air Quality Management District. The incinerator was owned and operated by Integrated Environmental Systems (IES) and it had been cited for 164 safety violations since 1990. The IES incinerator was the only commercial medical waste incinerator in the state and it received medical waste shipments from the immediate area and beyond. The main safety issue concerned the production of dioxin from the burning of polyvinyl chloride plastics—the bulk of medical waste.[32] The medical waste incinerator had been operating for fifteen years in Oakland, but there had never been any public input into the permitting process. When the Bay Area Air Quality Management District approved IES's request, the request was appealed by a coalition led by PUEBLO, a grassroots environmental justice organization in a neighborhood heavily impacted by IES's incineration processes. Communities for a Better Environment provided PUEBLO with scientific expertise and organizing assistance. The appeal process became one of the focal points of environmental and feminist cancer activism in the East Bay over the next few years, with protests and pickets and public hearings. On September 2, 1997, the *San Francisco Chronicle* wrote an editorial titled "Dioxin Concerns in the East Bay" that was strongly in support of the local struggle against IES.

Finally, in December of 2001, Integrated Environmental Systems agreed to shut down its medical waste and solid waste incinerators in Oakland.

Challenges to the Siting of a Power Plant in San Francisco

Several months before the Women, Health and the Environment Conference, a small environmental justice organization had formed in Bayview-Hunters Point, called Southeast Alliance for Environmental Justice (SAEJ), and had begun trying to mobilize the community against a new power plant (they already had two in their neighborhood). Because of the momentum that had begun to build against the power plant, the California Energy Commission (CEC) was being pressured to turn down PG&E's application for a new permit. As a result of community concerns about the negative impact of the plant's emissions on their health, the San Francisco Department of Public Health agreed to conduct a community wide environmental and health assessment to determine whether or not residents of BVHP appeared to be unusually unhealthy. Included in their assessment were breast cancer and cervical cancer rates for women living in the impacted zip codes. They discovered that breast cancer rates for African-American women under the age of fifty living in BVHP were 50 percent higher than what would have been expected. Their rates were, in fact, the highest in the city.

Although the San Francisco Department of Public Health did not release their report until after the Women, Health, and the Environment conference (August 1995), word of the report leaked out and the information contained within it was circulated at the conference and announced by a community activist from SAEJ at the end of the first day. A petition to the San Francisco Board of Supervisors requesting a moratorium on polluting facilities in Bayview-Hunters Point was immediately designed, signed, and submitted.

The discourse of disproportionate health risks and higher breast cancer incidence was extremely powerful. Although breast cancer was only one of many health problems in BVHP and certainly one of the rarest, it carried a great deal of political weight. The official release of the DPH health assessment report on BVHP set a number of wheels in motion, one of which resulted in the decision of the Board of Supervisors of San Francisco to overrule the CEC (who issued a permit to PG&E and SF Energy Company) by approving a moratorium on polluting facilities in BVHP.

A second immediate outcome was the establishment of a Health and Environmental Task Force for BVHP, a collaborative project between BVHP residents and the San Francisco Department of Health. The Task Force became a lightning rod for a series of controversies involving community representation, the conflict between "lay" and "expert" knowledges, the politics of epidemiological research and risk-assessment science, and the tension between *studying* the problems of pollution and ill health and *doing* something about them. When, for example, additional studies conducted by the DPH failed to confirm BVHP residents' beliefs that they were being made sick by their toxic environment, they became increasingly angry and distrustful of the DPH's motives and the fairness and goodness of the science behind the studies. Frustrated by the disjuncture between the experientially based knowledge produced by local residents and the epidemiologically based knowledge produced by the San Francisco Department of Public Health, community activists in Bayview-Hunters Point argued for solutions that did not depend upon scientific proof that the toxic environment was causing ill-health. Community activists demanded that toxic sites be cleaned up, that toxic emissions from power plants be better regulated, and that community access to health care be expanded. The battles over environmental health and justice in Bayview-Hunters Point continue to this day.[33]

Environmental Challenges to Breast Cancer in Marin County

The Women, Health and the Environment Conference—and the discourses of risk that circulated in that setting—inspired the formation of an organization in the North Bay called Marin Breast Cancer Watch (MBCW). MBCW was founded in the fall of 1995 by the late Francine Levien and Wendy Tanowitz, two friends who attended the TLC conference and were inspired by it.[34] It was at the conference that Levien and Tanowitz discovered that not only did the Bay Area have the highest breast cancer incidence rates in the world, but Marin County had the highest rates of breast cancer within the Bay Area. Levien had been diagnosed with breast cancer and Tanowitz had not, but both women had histories of involvement with environmental and social justice causes, and both lived in Marin County, a region famous for its natural beauty, its wealth, and its whiteness. The shock and outrage generated by the circulation of this discourse of risk inspired the formation of Marin Breast Cancer Watch.[35] From the outset its purpose was to discover and eliminate the reasons for Marin's high rate of breast cancer.

MBCW started out as a small group of women meeting in Levien's living room, almost like a book group—sharing materials, ideas, and information, and trying to figure out how best to proceed. Of the seven to eight core members during the first couple of years, five had been diagnosed with cancer (breast cancer in four of the five cases) and two were environmental activists with no history of cancer. After meeting for several months in the living rooms of different members, MBCW sought and received permission from Marin Hospital to begin holding public forums at the hospital. In March of 1996, MBCW staged their first public event at Marin Hospital, which they advertised through flyers and announcements placed in local print media. The event was billed as "The Silence is Over!—The Power of Breast Cancer Activism," and the meeting was attended by about seventy-five local residents. Lorraine Pace, a breast cancer survivor and environmental activist from Long Island, New

York, was the featured speaker. Pace, the founder of West Islip Breast Cancer Coalition, pioneered the community mapping projects that resulted in a series of federally funded studies into the relationship between breast cancer and various suspected environmental culprits on Long Island.[36] The meeting was a great success—money was raised, new activists were recruited, new working groups were formed, and a great deal of energy, excitement, and enthusiasm were shared and generated.

From the very beginning MBCW had one purpose: to figure out what was causing the higher rates of breast cancer in Marin County and "end the epidemic." MBCW operated according to the guiding assumption that the answers were to be found in the environment. [37] MBCW pursued three different lines of action with regard to breast cancer and the environment: research, policy, and public education. Regarding research, MBCW started out with the goal of developing a community-mapping project similar to the Long Island project described by Pace—plotting breast cancer cases and environmental threats onto residential maps to see if any patterns could be discerned. This project was eventually abandoned between 1998 and 1999, but quite a number of environmentally oriented community-based research projects were successfully pursued, proposed, and funded. These studies were designed in collaboration with local scientists, universities, and public health departments and are now underway.[38] With regard to direct action and public policy, MBCW involved itself in a number of activities—joining the Toxic Links Coalition, helping form the Marin Beyond Pesticides Coalition, networking with other environmental groups and organizations active in the environmental wing of the breast cancer movement, and testifying at public hearings of various sorts. Marin Beyond Pesticides Coalition, for example, was responsible for a 1999 county ordinance that banned the use of the most toxic pesticides (including those suspected of causing cancer and reproductive harm) on county lands and committed the county to reducing its use of all other pesticides by 75 percent by the year 2004.

Although MBCW was committed to environmental research and activism and had no interest in providing direct services and support to breast cancer survivors and patients, it proved impossible to ignore or exclude the suffering body from the organizing meetings even though it was the political body that they sought to nurture and develop.[39] Each meeting began, for example, with a quick "check-in." Frequently, during the check-in, breast cancer—as a lived and embodied and ongoing experience—seeped in. This might occur in any number of ways—painful and traumatic experiences with reconstructive surgeries, ongoing efforts to seek out nontoxic complementary and alternative treatments, visits to the doctor to make sure there were no new signs of disease, routine mammograms and blood tests, and so on, and almost always some discussion of sadness and anxiety related to worries about the impact of breast cancer on husbands and children.

This bleeding together of the suffering and political bodies carried over into MBCW's forays into public education. Their decision to hold public forums at Marin Hospital, obviously, says a great deal about the conjoining of the biomedical and the environmental. There was no debate, discussion, or hesitation when the idea of holding meetings at Marin Hospital was raised. It seemed like a natural solution with no drawbacks or complications.[40] Consistent with their stated purpose, MBCW organized activities, working groups, and educational forums on environmental issues related to breast cancer. But many of the women who attended MBCW events were former breast cancer patients and many learned of the organization through patient networks and flyers posted at the hospital. For these reasons MBCW quickly developed— and this occurred without any real deliberateness or discussion—into an organization serving two purposes and two, albeit overlapping, populations: environmentalists and breast cancer patients (and ex-patients). Thus, responding to the perceived interests and desires of their constituents, and probably of the core organizers as well, MBCW also organized special lectures and forums on health issues of particular concern to women who were, or had been, cancer patients.

The forum with Lorraine Pace, for example, was followed by a talk by Michael DeGregorio entitled, "Everything you wanted to know about TAMOXIFEN and Breast Cancer but were afraid to ask." This was not a forum on Zeneca Pharmaceuticals and the cancer industry but, rather, a forum structured, in large part, around questions from the audience that were framed as individual treatment issues posed to an expert. The tamoxifen talk was followed by a talk delivered by the associate director from Commonweal, a retreat center for cancer patients, called "Alternative and Complementary Therapies." This talk covered topics such as Chinese medicine, stress reduction, diet, psychological support, and so on. Again, the audience in attendance was seeking answers to their own health and treatment questions. The next few forums featured well-known breast cancer and environmental activists such as Nancy Evans, Sandra Steingraber, and Marion Moses and additional talks that focused on pesticides, electromagnetic fields, the World Conference on Breast Cancer, and the antitoxics campaign, Health Care Without Harm. Interspersed were forums on healthy lifestyles and "strategies for staying alive."

What became increasingly clear, as I followed MBCW's development, was that Marin Breast Cancer Watch approached environmental issues from a very different perspective than organizations solely situated within the environmental justice movement or activists whose only knowledge of chemicals, cancer and prevention came from the environmental model and perspective. Even when MBCW activists tried to bracket the bodily and emotional dimensions of breast cancer in order to focus their energy and attention on the environmental issues at hand, the task proved impossible. Marin Breast Cancer Watch's politics were necessarily derived from its dual subject position and the dual subject positions of its core members and constituents. Their feet were firmly planted in both worlds. On the one hand, they were committed to cancer prevention, environmental research, and environmental activism. At the same time, they could not escape the pull of the disease, their commitment to other women with breast cancer, and the knowledge that they, too, might some day be cancer patients again.

Breast Cancer Activism for the Twenty-First Century: Polysemous Chemicals and Dual Subject Positions

Environmental health campaigns in the San Francisco Bay Area were most successful when they targeted specific chemicals and corporations, organized around clear goals, and advocated for concrete but limited solutions. Such strategies, however, were not viable for feminist cancer and breast cancer organizations. Because these organizations were founded by and for women living with cancer, and women living with the threat of cancer's return, the organizations began from the disease, and from the embodied subject position of cancer patients. A wholesale rejection or refusal to engage with the biomedical approach to cancer was therefore undoable, even if it was, in theory, conceivable. What was required instead was political involvement and engagement in both the environmental and biomedical approaches to cancer. It was this dual subject position, this dual set of commitments and this movement back and forth between the biomedical gaze and the environmental perspective that led the environmental wing of the feminist cancer movement to develop a dual vision of cancer activism.

In this final section, I examine recent developments at the juncture of environmental and biomedical activism by looking at the current agenda and activities of Breast Cancer Action (BCA) in San Francisco. In the last several years BCA, which orginated as a treatment activist organization, has increasingly refocused its commitments and redirected its energies toward bridging between biomedical and environmental research, biomedical and environmental policy, and biomedical and environmental activism. Because of its own history of activism embedded within the biomedical approach to breast cancer, BCA's growing attention to chemicals and the environment, in combination with a similar commitment on the part of other feminist and breast cancer organizations, has the potential to impact a set of social actors heretofore protected and institutionally isolated from challenges from the environmental community. And indeed, BCA is by no means working alone on these issues. Working alongside, as well as in slightly different directions, are a handful of Bay Area feminist cancer and breast cancer organizations such as the Women's Cancer Resource Center, the Breast Cancer Fund, Charlotte Maxwell Complementary Clinic, and Marin Breast Cancer Watch. In the limited space remaining, however, I will focus on three ways that BCA (in collaboration with other organizations) is linking together the two chemical industries (pharmaceutical and industrial) and building bridges between the different histories of institutionalization of the two models of cancer (biomedical and environmental) within the state apparatus.

Continuing in the direction pursued by the Toxic Links Coalition, Breast Cancer Action has continued to promote the concept of the cancer industry by continuing to promote October as National Cancer Industry Month (see Figure 8.1 for their most recent flyer). Extending the campaign still further, BCA developed a "Stop Cancer Where It Starts" campaign—a project designed to encourage and assist local communities in their efforts to petition their politicians to officially declare October "Stop Cancer Where It Starts Month." This campaign followed the successful campaigns initiated by the TLC and its member organizations to convince city and county councils in Berkeley, San Francisco, Oakland, and Marin County to declare October "Stop Cancer Where It Starts Month." BCA drew up a set of steps and guidelines (posted on their website) to help other communities in the efforts to do the same.

Related to the "Stop Cancer Where It Starts" campaign, in February of 2002 Breast Cancer Action and the Breast Cancer Fund copublished a "white paper" (endorsed by a number of local cancer organizations) called "State of the Evidence: What is the Connection Between Chemicals and Breast Cancer?" and they organized an informational hearing on the issue of California state legislators. Policy recommendations put forward in the paper included a "phase out" of toxic chemicals. Due to its success, the California Senate and Assembly Health and Human Services Committees and the Assembly Health Committee scheduled a second hearing on "the environmental causes of rising breast cancer rates." Similar to the first meeting, prominent researchers, academicians, and advocates actively investigating the relationship between environmental toxins and breast cancer will testify at the hearing and submit research and public policy recommendations.

A second arena where BCA sought to shift the relationship between biomedical and environmental approaches to the disease was in the area of research funding and research policy. BCA has advocated that 70 percent of the proceeds from the breast cancer postal stamp be directed to breast cancer research at the National Institute for Environmental Health Sciences (instead of to the biomedically oriented National Cancer Institute). In addition, BCA is calling for the development of a new approach to cancer research, which it proposes calling the Rachel Carson Project, that would be modeled after the Manhattan Project—bringing together the "most innovative thinkers in a wide array of scientific fields" who would be required to sever their ties with for-profit entities, and funding the project at a high level so that scientists would not be required to spend half their time writing grants and receiving piecemeal funding for their research.

Finally, BCA has also been extremely active in the pharmaceutical arena. In this arena, BCA (along with a number of women's health organizations) has

OCTOBER:
National Breast Cancer Awareness Month?

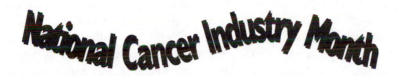

Cancer is big business.
The Cancer Industry consists of the polluting industries, public relations firms, and agencies that fail to protect our health and divert attention away from the need to prevent cancer by finding the causes. Not enough is being done to look into the environmental links to cancer. After all, what profit is there in preventing cancer?

Some who cause cancer also profit from it.
Du Pont produces various pesticides, some of which contain ingredients known to cause cancer. Du Pont also makes drugs to treat cancer. General Electric owns nuclear reactors and sells mammography equipment, both of which create ionizing radiation, a known carcinogen (cause of cancer).

NBCAM: A Public Relations Scam that Reaps Enormous Profits

AstraZeneca is the primary corporate sponsor of National Breast Cancer Awareness Month (NBCAM). They are the American subsidiary of UK-based AstraZeneca PLC, a $15.8 billion international biosciences business including Salick Health Care, Inc., AstraZeneca Pharmaceuticals, and, until fall of 2000, Zeneca Ag Products.

 AstraZeneca dropped its less profitable agricultural arm in 2000, but up until then, they had a complete profit circle:
  • They made agrochemicals, including the carcinogenic herbicide acetochlor.
  • They still own a string of cancer care centers, including doctors, pharmacies, and testing labs.
• They currently make the top selling breast cancer drug, tamoxifen, $573 million/yr. worldwide.

AstraZeneca has final say about the content of official NBCAM materials. It should come as no surprise that there is no mention of carcinogens, or the need to find the causes and a true prevention for breast cancer. Instead, the focus is on "awareness" of breast cancer and the need for women to get their mammograms.

  NBCAM = more awareness = more mammograms = more diagnoses = more tamoxifen sales = more $$$

Figure 8.1

challenged the proliferation of direct-to-consumer (DTC) marketing of prescription drugs, focusing its attention on AstraZeneca's marketing of tamoxifen to healthy, "high risk" women (Klawiter, forthcoming).[41] Tamoxifen (brand name Nolvadex®) was approved by the FDA in October of 1998 for "reducing the risk" of breast cancer among healthy women at "high risk" for breast cancer.[42] The FDA's decision followed on the heels of the early termination of the Breast Cancer Prevention Trial, the clinical trial that, since 1992, had been testing the effects of tamoxifen on healthy women against the effects of placebo. The women's health movement (including feminist cancer organizations) had been critical of the trial since—and even before—its inception and when the trial was terminated early, the drug was fast-tracked for approval, and AstraZeneca launched their advertising campaign, they stepped up their criticism and got organized.

This began to occur in early 2000, when a group of organizations critical of DTC advertising and committed to an environmental approach to cancer prevention began working together on these issues. This collection of organizations became a new coalition called Prevention First.[43] Shortly after its formation, Prevention First produced a flyer (Figure 8.2), which the coalition members circulated via their communication networks (inserting in newsletters, posting on their websites, etc.). The flyer constituted the public launching of their project against the pharmaceutical industry, against DTC advertising of tamoxifen to healthy women, and, more generally, against the notion of prevention in a pill. The flyer begins with a question: "Will Breast Cancer Prevention ever come in a pill?"

The flyer asserts that drug ad campaigns such as those conducted by Eli Lilly and AstraZeneca hurt everyone by generating "misinformation" and driving up the cost of drugs and concludes by identifying the authors of the flyer as health organizations who "maintain their independence from drug companies by refusing to accept funding from them." The column running down the left side of the flyer, labeled "THE FACTS," makes three bulleted claims: drug companies spend twice as much on marketing and administration as they do on research and development, the FDA forced AstraZeneca to withdraw several ads, and "by focusing on pills for breast cancer 'prevention,' the drug ads divert attention from the causes of disease." The Prevention First coalition emphasizes the need to pursue prevention based on the Precautionary Principle instead of prevention organized around the interests of the pharmaceutical industry.

Conclusions

There are a number of conclusions, some more speculative than others, that can be drawn from the synthesis of environmental and breast cancer activism in the San Francisco Bay Area. The first is that the synthesis of the environmental and feminist cancer movements created a synergistic reaction that led to the development of a series of innovative campaigns and coalitions that accomplished more than either of these two movements would have or could have in isolation. The second is the important recognition that at the heart of breast cancer activists' commitments to environmental activism lies an unresolvable but productive tension: synthetic chemicals are both their enemies and their allies. The third and perhaps more speculative conclusion suggested by this analysis is that beginning with cancer and seeking the chemical culprit is a much more daunting task than beginning with an environmental culprit—a toxic chemical, an incinerator, a power plant, an oil refinery—and

Will Breast Cancer Prevention
ever come in a pill?

THE FACTS

- Several reports have shown that major drug makers spend about twice as much on drug marketing and administration as they do on research and development.

- The Food and Drug Administration has forced AstraZeneca, the maker of the breast cancer drug tamoxifen, to withdraw and correct several ads for its drugs.

- By focusing on pills for breast cancer "prevention," drug ads divert attention from the *causes* of the disease.

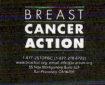

BREAST CANCER ACTION

1-877-2STOPBC (1-877-278-6722)
www.bcaction.org, email: info@bcaction.org
55 New Montgomery, Suite 323
San Francisco, CA 94105

This year more than 192,000 women in America will be told they have breast cancer. The number of new cases increases every year. Billions of dollars are spent annually on cancer research — but the vast majority of that research is on drug development, not on prevention.

Pills touted to "prevent" cancer can at best only lower the risk of developing the disease — and they often increase the risk of other health problems. True cancer prevention requires understanding and eliminating the environmental causes of the disease.

Americans are bombarded with ads for pills to "prevent" diseases like breast cancer. These ads often play down the side effects of the drugs and imply that they will help more people than they actually do. Eli Lilly has promoted Evista® (raloxifene) for breast cancer benefits even though the drug has been approved only for osteoporosis. And AstraZeneca, which manufactures the breast cancer drug Nolvadex® (tamoxifen), has marketed the drug to healthy women, even though it's more likely to hurt than help most of them.

Drug ad campaigns like these hurt us all: they hurt our health by generating misinformation, and they hurt our pocketbooks by driving up the cost of drugs.

A number of health organizations — all of which maintain their independence from drug companies by refusing to accept funding from them — have come together to counter these campaigns. If you're concerned about drug ads you've seen, or if you want to work toward public policy that puts people's health before corporate profit, visit www.bcaction.org.

This ad is sponsored by the Boston Women's Health Book Collective (publishers of *Our Bodies, Ourselves*), Breast Cancer Action Montreal, the Center for Medical Consumers, DES Action, the Massachusetts Breast Cancer Coalition, the National Women's Health Network, the Women's Community Cancer Project, and the Working Group on Women and Health Protection. The coalition's work is made possible through a generous grant from the Richard and Rhoda Goldman Fund.

Figure 8.2

seeking its removal, a finding that points to the political wisdom of the precautionary principle.

Acknowledgments

I thank Monica Casper for her incisive criticisms and thoughtful suggestions on an earlier draft of this chapter.

9
Change of State?
The Greening of Chemistry

E. J. WOODHOUSE

Most contributors to this volume focus on the movement of chemical molecules into communities, into workers' and citizens' bodies, and into political controversies. My method is the opposite: I will be tracing synthetic organic molecules *backwards* to their origins in order to reexamine the social construction of chemistry and the problems associated with it.[1] Some of the origins are literal, historical ones; but I am even more interested in the assumptions designed into twentieth-century chemicals and thereby built into many environmental conflicts. Is it possible, I ask, that what we now think of as chemistry, chemical products, and governmental regulation of chemicals, and even how we envision possible future chemical states, all are products of a governing mentality that deserves searching reexamination?[2]

This work emanates in part from a tradition of political thought associated with Langdon Winner's idea that technology *is* politics (Winner 1977, 1986). How (some) humans design chemicals and other technologies helps establish an enduring framework for social order (Sclove 1995). This sociotechnical "constitution" of everyday life is nowhere written down, of course, and hence is even more difficult deliberately to discuss and renegotiate than is a written governmental constitution. The question arising is this: Might it be technically feasible to draw up, ratify, and implement a very different and better constitution for a reformed chemical state?

This chapter is a preliminary report of a long-term project assessing the implications of a form of chemistry characterized as "green"—meaning "benign by design" (Anastas and Farris 1994). Inasmuch as probably not one nonchemist in a million understands the profound difference between twentieth-century chemistry and the redesigned approach to chemicals that appears to be feasible in the twenty-first century and thereafter, one purpose of this chapter is simply to explain the technical potentials and help liberate our imaginations. A second purpose is to improve our theoretical understanding of the relationship among chemical expertise, the environment, human bodies, and social organizations including nation-states. The lynchpin of this relationship, in my eyes, is to be found in the social structuring of expertise: a revised understanding of chemistry calls into question fundamental features of the social institutions and practices that train chemists and other experts, that deploy and incentivize them, and that mediate between experts and the rest of us. The analysis thus helps illuminate the overall challenges of reconstructing a wiser, fairer technological civilization.[3]

The first sections of the chapter compare twentieth-century "brown" chemistry with the green chemistry that is a potential alternative, providing easy-to-understand examples of the new approach. I then go on to discuss obstacles to chemical greening and strategies for accelerating it. The final sections discuss some of the theoretical implications of the case.

Brown versus Green Chemistry[4]

"Organic chemistry textbooks a generation from now will be unrecognizable compared with today's standard texts," predicts one of the progenitors of what is coming to be called "green chemistry."[5] As the name implies, advocates aim to make humanity's approach to chemicals environmentally benign or "sustainable." With little controversy or publicity, in the past few years a new field has begun to emerge that could turn out to mean a profound transformation in the methods, raw materials, byproducts, and end products of chemical synthesis.

An exaggeration that makes the point is to say that twentieth-century chemistry, chemical engineering, and the chemical industry proceeded according to the following "formula":

- Start with a petroleum-based feedstock;
- Dissolve it, and add a reagent;
- React the compounds to produce intermediate chemicals;
- Put these through a long series of additional reactions,
- Which create millions of tons of hazardous waste by-products,
- While yielding megaton quantities of potentially dangerous final products,
- Released into ecosystems without knowledge of long-term effects,
- Without going through gradual scale-up to learn from experience.

Despite the fact that aspects of the above "formula" appear absurd, especially in light of the public concern over chemicals touched off some forty years ago by Rachel Carson, brown chemistry has remained the basis for textbooks and engineering practice alike throughout the twentieth century.[6] Hardly anyone realized that chemists might adopt a very different approach:

- Design each new molecule so as to accelerate both excretion from living organisms and biodegradation in ecosystems;
- Create the chemical from a carbohydrate (sugar/starch/cellulose) or oleic (oily/fatty) feedstock, instead of using petrochemicals;

- Rely on a catalyst, often biological, in a small-scale process
- That uses no solvents or only benign ones, and requires only a few steps,
- Creating little or no hazardous waste by-products,
- Yielding small quantities of the new chemical for exhaustive toxicology and other testing,
- Followed by very gradual scale-up and learning by doing.

Experimentation with aspects of this second formula has been gradually developing within the chemical research community and even within the chemical industry (Poliakoff et al. 2002). Going under the rubric of green or sustainable chemistry, the organizational heart of the enterprise has been located in a small program in the Pollution Prevention and Toxics branch of the U.S. Environmental Protection Agency. The program there focuses not on Superfund cleanup or other correction of problems already existing, and not on containing future exposures by cleaning up wastewater or scrubbing smoke stacks. Instead, the focus is on prevention of problems before they occur— by redesigning chemical production processes and products at the molecular level to make them radically less dangerous.

Among the progenitors of green chemistry was Stanford chemistry professor Barry Trost, who first proposed the concept of "atom economy" in 1973. Rather than judging a chemical process successful if it produces usable product at a satisfactory cost, Trost argued that those responsible for synthesizing chemicals should aim for elegant efficiency, for using the highest possible percentage of input atoms in the usable output, ideally leaving zero waste (Trost 1991). This seemed a utopian concept when first proposed, but an increasing number of bio-catalytic and other chemical processes now are being proposed that approximate exactly such an outcome.

The brown chemistry formula predominated partly because chemistry did not start out as sophisticated as it gradually has become. Numerous other factors contributed. For example, the chlorinated compounds that have caused so much trouble (e.g., DDT, PCBs) gained impetus from chemical executives' desire to find a use for the excess chlorine created as a by-product of another basic chemical process (Thornton 2000). Then the exigencies of World War I put a premium on finding quick, effective ways to accomplish certain ends, and the resulting means carried over into civilian life via sunk capital, technological momentum, market niches, and habits of professional thought (Travis 1993; Mauskopf 1993; Nye 1993). A not very esoteric example was the cellupaper developed by Kimberly-Clark for bandages (as a substitute for cotton that was scarce during the war), subsequently transmogrified into Kotex sanitary napkins and Kleenex (Vostral 2000).

From World War II came numerous "breakthroughs" including DDT, used by soldiers against body lice and subsequently applied to killing agricultural pests; now banned in most affluent countries, production and use in megaton quantities continues in poorer nations. When petroleum and natural gas feedstocks for chemicals became cheap (and chemically easy), research into lipid- and carbohydrate-based chemistry (from plants) all but disappeared for much of the twentieth century.[7] Additional historical causes for the focus on brown chemistry could be added, but the general point is apparent: Various context-dependent factors led chemists, chemical engineers, and users of chemicals to adopt affordable, doable methods without much inquiry into long-term collective costs. Hence, there never was an across-the-board and deliberate effort to survey chemical knowledge and try to figure out the "best" ways of constructing synthetic molecules. This sort of historically contingent and socially problematic method of choosing among possible technological trajectories is hardly unique to chemicals, of course; for example, there was no significant effort to survey many possible types of nuclear reactors in order to find ones especially suited for civilian use (Morone and Woodhouse 1989).

For the future, however, might chemists and chemical engineers belatedly turn toward more benign approaches to create a greener, if still synthetic, planet? It is not clear exactly how far the idea can be carried into practice, but it appears that the second chemical scenario sketched above may potentially be within the capacities of a revamped chemistry and chemical engineering (Anastas and Warner 1998; Poliakoff et al. 2002).

Examples of Green Chemistry

Examples of recent work qualifying as green chemistry are highlighted by the "Presidential Green Chemistry Challenge Awards" given annually since 1996 by the U.S. Environmental Protection Agency.[8] Included are awards for design of new chemicals that are inherently less dangerous, for creation of safer methods of synthesizing existing chemicals, and for safer solvents. It was the so-called "Reinventing Government" initiative of the Clinton-Gore Administration that created the award competition as part of an effort to reconstruct the state to be less adversarial toward the business sector (Gore 1996; Osborne and Pastrik 1997; U.S. Congress 2001).

The first Alternative Synthetic Pathways Award went to the Monsanto Company for a new technique for manufacturing Roundup™ herbicide in a less dangerous way.[9] Roundup™ is among the less nasty herbicides, and sometimes is described by its advocates as "environmentally friendly." As the award citation put it, in the new process:

> The raw materials have low volatility and are less toxic . . . (and) the dehydrogenation process is endothermic and therefore does not present danger of runaway. Moreover, this "zero-waste" route to DSIDA produces a product stream that, after filtration of catalyst, is of such high quality that no purification or waste cut is necessary. . . . The new tech-

nology represents a major breakthrough . . . because it avoids the use of cyanide and formaldehyde, is safer to operate, produces higher overall yield, and has fewer process steps. (EPA 1996, 2)

The key to the innovation was a new catalysis technology, potentially "applicable to the preparation of many other agricultural, commodity, specialty, and pharmaceutical chemicals" (EPA 1996, 2).

Another award went to the manufacturers of ibuprofen, the well-known painkiller sold as Advil™ and Motrin™. Synthesizing ibuprofen previously required massive quantities of solvents and achieved only 40 percent efficiency (which means 60 percent waste products), whereas the new process achieves nearly 99 percent efficiency. It "revolutionized bulk pharmaceutical manufacturing . . . (by) provid(ing) an elegant solution to a prevalent problem: how to avoid the large quantities of solvents and wastes associated with the traditional stoichiometric use of auxiliary chemicals when effecting chemical conversions" (EPA 1998, 13).

Dow Chemical won an award for using carbon dioxide as the blowing agent for manufacture of polystyrene foam sheet packaging material. The market for such material had grown to 700 million pounds in the U.S. alone by 1995, principally for egg cartons and fast food containers. The Dow technology allowed elimination of 3.5 million pounds of chlorofluorocarbon blowing agents per year, chemicals that contributed to ozone depletion, global warming, and ground-level smog. The CO_2 in the Dow process is derived from existing sources such as ammonia plants and natural gas wells, therefore making no net contribution to climate change.

The Rohm and Haas chemical company developed an improved "antifouling" compound to control unwanted growth of barnacles and other marine organisms on ship hulls. The main compounds used in recent decades to poison would-be fouling organisms have been organotins, which persist in the marine environment and increase shell thickness in shellfish, decrease reproductive viability, and cause other environmental problems. The company's Sea-Nine™ antifoulant biodegrades far more rapidly than previous compounds—with a half-life in sediment measured in hours (compared with six to nine months for the tin compounds). Sea-Nine™ does not bioaccumulate, whereas tin can reach concentrations in marine organisms as high as ten thousand times its original concentration in the paint.

What Chemical State Do Visionaries Anticipate?

What do advocates of green chemistry envision, and what are some examples of research and development forefronts? A "2020 Plan" proposed at a University of Massachusetts Workshop on the Role of Polymer Research in Green Chemistry and Engineering has predicted that within two decades it should be possible to:

- Replace all solvents and acid-based catalysts that have adverse environmental effects with solids, water-based replacements, or other "green alternatives";
- Eliminate nearly 100 percent of emissions in polymer manufacturing and processing, and reduce by more than 50 percent the quantity of plastics placed in landfills;
- Increase energy efficiency by 40 percent or more in the manufacture of polymers;
- Achieve a 30–40 percent reduction in waste (energy emissions, water, and raw materials).

These goals would be approached via "research on alternative manufacturing techniques, solventless processes, new coatings and films, and 'green' separation techniques." Rather than interfering with chemical innovation—not something everyone would fear, but presumably of great concern to industry executives—the workshop participants estimated that the greener processes actually would reduce by 50 percent the development time to produce new polymers, partly by simplifying manufacturing requirements and partly by reducing environmental compliance transactions (2020 Workshop 1998).

One hears pretty much the same sort of expectation from a small but growing number of those at the forefront of chemical research and development. It is reminiscent of what occurred in the field of energy analysis when Amory Lovins' estimates of conservation potentials from what he termed "soft paths" were pooh-poohed by early reviewers but quickly proved sensible (Lovins 1977). Likewise, what would have seemed like chemical never-never land a few years ago now looks increasingly like a safe bet. Emblematic of the shift is the simple fact that whereas chemists once washed their hands in benzene, "Today toxicology is very much a part of the way people do business."

Painter Design and Engineering, Incorporated, advertises that its product is "highly effective, economical and leaves no toxic waste" (Painter Design 2002). Florida Chemical uses terpenes derived from citrus oils to replace petrochemical feedstocks, allowing company executives to claim that E-Z-Mulse™ "is biodegradable and does NOT contain suspect nonyl phenol found in other emulsifiers" (Florida Chemical 2002). Such eco-marketing so far seems to be more common in advertising intended for business purchasers than for ordinary consumers, perhaps because the former, on average, are more informed and more highly motivated. This is true in part because of liability issues including workmen's compensation, unionized grievance procedures, and other workplace health and safety advocacy and negotiation. With the exception of certain firms and with the partial exception of some northern European nations, workers' bodies often are not taken seriously enough by management to make heavy investments or go to unusual lengths in rearranging production; but when a technological breakthrough allows a relatively low-cost change with minimal hassle, managers are reasonably quick to take advantage of it.

This phenomenon has long been at work in more conventional aspects of the chemical industry. In addition to pressure from workers and from government regulators, chemical company executives found that in many instances they could actually save money over the long run by reducing chemical releases because of money saved on raw materials and in disposal of hazardous wastes. Among large Italian chemical firms, for example, between 1989 and 1997 air emissions dropped by 54 percent for sulfur dioxide, 72 percent for particles, 82 percent for volatile organic compounds, and 92 percent for heavy metals. Wastewater effluents likewise declined, but not quite as substantially (Giuiuzza 1998). Smaller firms have not cleaned up their production processes to nearly the same degree, industry spokespersons say, largely because they lack the expertise and financial resources to do so.

What do these and other changes presage for chemicals in coming decades? According to one advocate, Cal Tech professor Francis Arnold, "The future is limited only by our imaginations."

Obstacles to Chemical Greening

How rapidly the change of state can proceed obviously depends in part on whether the optimistic projections prove technically feasible, and, as importantly, on industry executives' perceptions concerning economic feasibility. Movement toward more benign chemicals also will depend on the extent to which government officials put pressure on industry; this will be shaped in part by public interest in the subject, which, in turn, will depend largely on media coverage and on the proselytizing activities of environmental interest groups.

At present, the technical potentials are changing much faster than the social comprehension and response. Even in Europe, most regulatory activity focuses on correction or containment of environmental problems already existing. An exception is the announced plan of the Swedish Chemicals Inspectorate to phase out a dozen especially toxic chemicals, and has some 250 on an "observation" list that pretty clearly are candidates for being banned. Other European nations are moving in that same direction. But even this move is timid compared with the bold possibilities foreseen by a handful of green chemistry visionaries, such as former Greenpeace staff member turned biologist Joe Thornton, who has constructed a detailed argument suggesting that it is technically and economically feasible to phase out virtually all chlorinated chemicals (Thornton 2000).

Systematic inquiry and debate about such a possibility is slowed partly by the way that mass media handle environmental stories. Coverage on television and in newspapers may not be entirely commensurate with the magnitude and scope of the problems, but a greater obstacle is that the focus normally is on symptoms rather than on the underlying problems. Endangered species and habitat loss, spills of hazardous chemicals, toxic torts and their victims, and ordinary air and water pollution capture most of the attention (Allan et al. 2000; Hansen 1993). In the instances where a story deals not with problems but with potentials for solving problems, the emphasis usually is on cleaner emissions, with no consideration of possibilities for more fundamental redesign. In a sense, therefore, media coverage of environmental issues may actually tend to take attention away from possibilities for constructive design of chemicals to make them inherently benign.

Environmental groups likewise generally remain locked into the governing mentality of the 1970s and 1980s: on the one hand, chemicals are inherently villainous; on the other hand, it is politically and economically infeasible to forego the chemicals' benefits. The only viable option, therefore, is treating wastewater, scrubbing smoke stacks, and otherwise trying to keep chemicals away from living organisms. Given the ubiquity of chemicals in contemporary society, the sequestration approach rather quickly runs into difficult obstacles.

Green chemistry advocates accept pollution cleanup and sequestration methods as part of the story, of course, but they entertain a far more radical option: preventing problems before they occur by (re)designing chemicals and chemical production processes so as to come as close as possible to inherently benign. By recognizing that synthetic organic chemistry is highly malleable and that social goals potentially can drive the rearrangement of molecules to serve public purposes, a new governing mentality becomes available that could lead to a reconstructed chemical state.

That there has been some movement toward institutionalizing this social movement within chemistry is indicated by the fact that there now is an annual Gordon Conference on Green Chemistry.[10] The U.S. National Academy of Sciences serves as the venue for a different annual conference covering green chemical engineering as well as green chemistry. The Organization for Economic Cooperation and Development's Chemical Risk Management Program also has begun to tackle the subject. The International Union for Pure and Applied Chemistry focused on green chemistry at its 2001 conference in Brisbane, as did that organization's CHEMRAWN Committee (Chemical Research Applied to World Needs) at an international conference that same year in Boulder. Although scientists and technologists predominate at these conferences, there is some outreach toward interest groups, government officials, journalists, and other nonexperts.

The Green Chemistry Institute cosponsors numerous conferences, and now has more than two dozen affiliate organizations throughout the world (Green Chemistry Institute 2002). The main Chinese technological university, possibly leapfrogging western universities with greater institutional momentum and fixed capital, has recently opened a new building for a green chemistry initiative. A committee of the American Chemical Society is at work attempting to revise chemistry textbooks and curricula. *Chemical and Engineering News* has begun to feature articles on the subject, and the Royal Society of Chemistry has launched the journal *Green Chemistry*.

These many signs of life notwithstanding, as in most social institutions there is in chemistry, chemical engineering, and the chemical industry considerable cognitive, institutional, and other momentum standing in the way of the transformation. This is about as true in universities as it is in industry and government. When a prestigious Australian chemistry chair proposed to his department "a half dozen" good reasons to switch from their outmoded division among physical, organic, and inorganic chemistry to an organizational form more in keeping with contemporary practice, he "provoked outrage" and the best he could obtain was a study committee. Asked to come up with any good reason for maintaining the current substructure of the department, the committee majority responded, "That's the way it's done at Harvard and Chicago." The scientific state of academic chemistry, one might say, is conditioned by the politics of the academic estate, by the status hierarchies, sunk human capital, and even the laboratory equipment designed for earlier trajectories of chemical research and teaching (Bell 1992; Croissant and Restivo 2001; Greenberg 2001).

Additional Examples

One of the hot areas in green chemistry is that of trying to move toward solventless processes, or at least to synthesis pathways and techniques that use solvents less dangerous than benzene and toluene. A promising line of investigation concerns the use of supercritical fluids, particularly carbon dioxide (Kiran et al. 2000). The basics of $scCO_2$ have been understood for about a century, yet until recently there were only a handful of chemical processes utilizing the technique, of which the best known is that of decaffeinating coffee (Williams and Clifford 2000).

Opinions differ on why this has been so. Some point to the capital expense of building equipment to operate at the temperatures and pressures necessary for achieving supercriticality. This seems a bit questionable, in that the pressures involved are only about 4000 pounds per square inch, and the temperatures are within the range often found in industrial practice. Other observers nominate maintenance difficulties and costs as the culprit. Still others argue that safety is harder to assure when dealing with pressurized systems. No doubt there is validity in these claims, but given the life-cycle costs and environmental-social costs of many petroleum-based solvents, it seems pretty clear that a huge number of chemists in and out of industry have for decades not been paying appropriate attention to the potential advantages of $scCO_2$ and other supercritical fluids (SCFs).

A chemistry professor working on SCFs in the UK suggests that the explanation rests partly with the faddish way scientists sometimes approach new techniques. There have been recurrent cycles, he says, in attention to SCF potentials: first the potential is oversold as enthusiasts propose and try out fancy schemes far beyond the existing state of knowledge; then, when these fail, participants and funding agencies make the interpretation that SCF has not worked out, and attention turns to some other hot topic. An obvious alternative would be patient, steady exploration of whatever fundamental questions remain, coupled with modest chemical and other engineering innovations designed to apply relatively simple SCF technology in relatively simple manufacturing and other processes. But such steady attention to a high-priority social task would require agenda-setting processes and linkages between political institutions and research institutions better than those now prevailing (Cozzens and Woodhouse 1995; Woodhouse et al. 2002).

A more modest, successful approach is illustrated by the work of Materials Technology Limited (MTL) of Reno, Nevada, which in partnership with the Navaho Nation operates a facility next to the Four Corners Power Plant in the southwestern United States. As the primary raw materials for manufacturing a line of new products, MTL is using waste fly ash that formerly had to be hauled away, CO_2 from the stacks that formerly was released as a greenhouse gas contribution, and thermal waste heat. Thanks to supercritical technology that turns the CO_2 into a solvent, the company is able to achieve molecular bonding that gives the products improved functionality coupled with lighter weight than competing materials (Jones 1998; Rubin and Tyler 1998).

The firm's founder was unable to get any assistance from the federal government in this start-up venture because "it did not fit into existing environmental programs; and venture capital firms were not interested because the process was deemed too risky." Ironically, the main innovation required in the MTL case was not technoscientific but social: the entrepreneur *set out* to create a new business that would sequester carbon dioxide while utilizing waste products from an existing, but initially unidentified, business. He had no specialized training in SCFs, and merely uncovered their potential while doing research to figure out how to make something out of the materials available. Other green chemistry practitioners report being turned down or downgraded in status because their work seems "too applied" or otherwise not sexy enough.

Staff in Congress and at the Office of Management and Budget in Washington have known too little about the emerging potentials to take the lead in educating their superiors about the ways green chemistry may lead to modifying traditional approaches to environmental regulation. Top administrators at EPA tend not to be very knowledgeable about cutting-edge science, perhaps any science, and the dozen or so EPA staffers most directly working on green chemistry and engineering have been committed to voluntary cooperation with industry, as are most of the chemical researchers I interviewed (and, of course, industry executives).

It is true that harmonious relations have been preserved with industry and that the green chemistry (GC) movement appears to be gaining momentum, if number of conferences and growth in number of interested researchers is an accurate gauge. But with the exception of Rohm and Haas, industry participation at GC conferences has been lackluster, and I have not seen evidence of a massive shift in industry practices. This impression is confirmed at least in part by minimal activity on the subject at the American Chemistry Council (formerly Chemical Manufacturers Association), which has lent its name to several green chemistry conferences, but has not focused real money or attention on the subject as of this writing. In mid 1998, responsibility for one such conference was assigned to a junior staff member in the Regulatory Affairs Division, which apparently was because those with more seniority "did not know how to fit green chemistry into the organizational structure." The organization's members—the largest players in the chemical industry—generally "do not seem very interested in green chemistry."

A number of European government officials have told me they do not find the North Americans' purely voluntary approach persuasive; nevertheless, as of 2002 European environmental agencies had nudged industry only rather gently toward fundamental redesign of chemicals.

A Few of the Implications

Shifting toward a new chemical state almost certainly would require addressing the political obstacles to a shift in governments' regulatory approaches toward the chemical industry. This probably requires creation and diffusion of a new imaginary, a new vision of how to operate a synthetic planet in ways that do not threaten the health or environmental integrity of the natural planet. Yet, it is far from obvious how the old enunciatory community and its governing mentality can be reformed or revolutionized (Anderson 1983).[11]

This is true partly because of the momentum problem introduced above. Chemistry and chemical engineering majors still do not study much about benign design, and chemistry professors left to their own accords have not changed curricula much in this regard in the past decade. In principle, accrediting agencies could force a more rapid pace of curricular adaptation; in practice, however, organizations such as the Accreditation Board for Engineering and Technology (ABET) uphold tradition more than departing from it (Accreditation Board for Engineering and Technology 1991; American Academy of Environmental Engineers 1999). If professional licensing exams for chemical engineers emphasized environmental considerations (which at least in the U.S. they have not), the curriculum might move in that direction. Or if large sums were available for innovations in benign chemical education, recalcitrant faculties might suddenly find room in the curriculum. But brown chemistry's momentum remains strong as I write (Hughes 1969; Staudenmeier 1985; Hughes 1989).

Thus, one Lawrence Laboratory scientist expressed bitterness that the Department of Energy killed his research project after four years despite the fact that it was on schedule to do exactly what he'd promised. He felt "pressured by DOE to obtain industry funding," but found the businesses he thought needed the technology uninterested. And those doing peer review at funding sources such as the National Science Foundation tend to look down on green chemistry proposals as "too applied." "Science politics sometimes are more important than science," a practicing scientist told me during my research, wearing a facial expression suggesting that social scientists would not previously have entertained such a thought. If science inevitably is a human activity that is bound to involve habit, politics, and other controversial judgments, and if the green chemistry case suggests once again that "science is too important to be left to scientists," what would it take to go beyond that clichéd insight?

One direction that seems clear to me is to explore the possibility of bringing to chemical design more of the relatively open, participative, and frank negotiation of democratic politics. Chemical engineering is an inherently political activity, as is all engineering, because it restructures everyday lives of workers, chemical plant neighbors, organisms in the environment impacted by hazardous wastes and plant emissions, and those who come into contact with chemical products (Woodhouse 1998). Arguably, technoscientific research and innovation now exercise greater influence over ordinary people's lives than did government in the centuries when democratic principles first were being applied. If so, is there not ample reason to ask whether and how it would be appropriate to think about democraticizing the technosphere, including that pertaining to toxic-versus-benign chemicals (Mumford 1934; Winner 1977; Sclove 1995).

The case raises interesting and important questions about whether and in what ways more democratic participation in setting scientific agendas arguably could have made positive contributions to shaping chemistry in the late twentieth century. More importantly, it raises questions about where democratic methods might be used in the future to steer science differently and perhaps better (Fuller 2000; Cozzens and Woodhouse 1995). The lessons I tentatively take away from the green chemistry story derive in part from commonplace understandings:

- Very substantial damage to environment, workers, and users of chemicals resulted from the actions of chemists and chemical engineers (in collaboration with others) in the twentieth century;
- Many or most of those technical personnel devoted relatively little attention to investigating, publicizing, or protecting against the risks of the chemical products they helped make available for commerce;
- Nor did most technoscientists seek diligently to find alternative synthesis pathways that would produce fewer waste byproducts of lower hazard;

- Nor did most chemists and chemical engineers seek to develop (or recommend, if already existing) alternative final products that would take the place of chemical products posing risks.

Knowing what we now do about the potential for benign chemicals, one can infer that many environmental and health problems might have been avoided or reduced if scientists and engineers had moved more expeditiously to investigate, develop, and utilize different techniques. What stopped that from happening is partly conjecture at this point, but a few key points are hard to miss, starting with the fact that most chemists and chemical engineers work directly or indirectly for industry, and their careers depend on the continuing goodwill of corporate executives. Both the great successes and the horrible failings of the past century's chemistry can be traced in part to this relationship.

Second, we know that university chemical researchers exercise substantial discretion over their research and teaching, although obviously influenced greatly by other members of their fields. This helps insulate them from undue external influence, except from companies awarding consulting contracts and research grants. The academic freedom also partially insulates them from accountability for those aspects of their work that have impacts outside the university, impacts on the general public and on the biosphere.

Third, we know that the split between scientific and social science/humanities education just about assures that most supposedly educated people will not know much about chemistry (or other sciences). Most of us know next to nothing about reduction, oxidation, methyl groups, ring-opening polymerization, or anything else involved in chemical processes and products. Nor do we know much about biochemistry and the new catalysis-based chemistry coming to the fore. That might be all right, if there were public interest scientists we could count on to represent us competently, with relevant expertise that is relatively independent from established cliques and hierarchies within mainstream chemistry itself. Sierra Club, the Environmental Defense Fund, British Nature, Greenpeace, and other major environmental groups have some scientifically competent staff members, of course, but they are relatively few in number—and disproportionately drawn from biological rather than chemical sciences. The world has nothing approaching the number of public interest scientists that would be needed for competently overseeing the work of experts employed primarily by business (Primack and Von Hippel 1974).

Fourth, partly because of the above, we know that contemporary societies do not have well-designed and fully articulated social institutions for monitoring chemistry and chemical engineering. Nor do most nations have satisfactory institutions for interpreting and deliberating about emerging directions, or for setting priorities in a way that integrates broad public concerns with relevant expertise. In the U.S., for example, the House Science Committee, the appropriations subcommittees, and other relevant committees exercise far more detailed and sophisticated scrutiny than what is available in the British or French parliaments, but Congress nevertheless delegates most decision-making about chemistry and chemical engineering to the National Science Foundation, the National Academy of Sciences, and to the university and industry sectors. That seemed like a fine arrangement to most people for most of the past several generations, but the unwanted legacy from brown chemistry raises serious questions about abuse of the authority traditionally delegated to chemical scientists and engineers and their institutions.

Neither social scientists nor other observers of science have offered penetrating, constructive ideas for how to arrange genuine accountability for scientists and scientific institutions. Science fraud and related issues have drawn a fair amount of attention, leading to tighter auditing, institutional review boards, and other procedural safeguards (Wells et al. 2001). But the reformers have not usually focused on substantive research directions, in part because it is widely assumed that only those within a subfield are in a good position to judge which topics most deserve investigation.

Yet the green chemistry case suggests that in some respects insiders can be exactly the wrong ones to control priorities, because they can be wedded to habitual ways of doing things that suit themselves and their benefactors more than they meet the needs of humanity and the ecosystem. The basic insight of pluralist political thought is that increasing the diversity of participants brings to light important considerations that are accidentally or willfully neglected when decision-making is controlled by those with the greatest stake in the outcome (Lindblom and Woodhouse 1993; Dahl 1998). I see insufficient reason to believe that this principle would not apply to scientific institutions and to the negotiations occurring therein.

Another reason for mounting serious inquiry into the possibilities for broader, more open negotiation concerning the design of chemicals is that the pendulum seems to be swinging too far in the direction of "cooperation" with industry in many nations. "Co-optation" has just about the same spelling, and, I fear, in some cases the same meaning. One ought to worry when public official after public official, and academic scientist after academic scientist, speaks of "forming research agendas based on industry needs," "Industry + university = new science and new process," "environmental improvement and economic growth are not in conflict," and so forth. I am sure that negotiation often makes sense; but blindly relying on business executives and their employees to serve public purposes does not fit with some of our most reliable understandings from economics and political science concerning market shortcomings and the privileged position of business (Lindblom 1977, 2001).

Conclusion

Given the inherent malleability of synthetic chemicals and the myriad, partially conflicting public and private purposes to which they can be put, one might have expected high levels of controversy from the outset of the chemical era. Instead, the modern chemical state has generally been characterized by a strange quiescence, by an eerie acceptance (Edelman 1971). This claim seemingly is belied by the intense controversies over Bhopal, Agent Orange, toxic waste at Woburn and Love Canal, Gulf War Syndrome, and other chemical-political events. In light of what we now know about solvent replacement and other aspects of green chemistry, however, it becomes apparent that neither the famous controversies nor the quieter, business-as-usual regulation of chemicals actually has gotten beneath the surface to problematize matters at a molecular level. The struggles normally have concerned how dangerous dioxin is, or how many people have been harmed—in other words, struggles over medical and scientific knowledge about chemistry-as-usual instead of over the chemistry-that-might-be. The question rarely if ever asked, the demand rarely if ever made: redesign chemical activities from scratch to be inherently benign.

Given that the majority of the chemical industry's activities could have been pursued quite differently, in ways radically less prone to create health and environmental risks, it is clear in retrospect that there has been a dreamy, somnambulistic quality to the ways government officials, consumers, workers, and even environmental interest groups have largely accepted whatever chemical engineers and their employers decided to offer by way of chemical synthesis pathways and products (Winner 1977, 1986). If more people had known of the potentials of green chemistry, they would have been in a position to search for counter narratives to those disseminated by industry and by the mainstream chemistry community (Roe 1994). Having not known to question the mentality governing brown chemistry, however, even environmentalists have been trapped into debating chemical activities within the relatively narrow discourse deployed by the dominant community of chemical practice.

Whereas public policy conventionally is conceived as emanating from government, nongovernmental decisions about technology by technologists and their industrial employers in fact have transformed everyday life in ways more profound than anything governments normally do. Innovations in communication, transportation, manufacturing, household, and leisure technologies lead to fundamental changes in the ways people spend their time, money, and attention. "Innovations are similar to legislative acts or political foundings that establish a framework for public order that will endure over many generations" (Winner 1986, 29). And just about everyone—from the crassest spokespersons for the chemicals industry to the most outspoken environmentalist critics—has bought into the brown-chemistry framework, has looked at the chemical state via the same impoverished governing mentality. If this is to change across the board, ways will have to be found for expert communities not to lock into overly narrow ways of inquiring and thinking.

192 • Synthetic Planet

Governments were involved, certainly, but chemists and chemical engineers arguably were the primary policy makers in establishing the enunciatory community whose discourse and worldview framed how the rest of us approached our roles as toxic victims, environmental activists, consumers, chemistry students, science journalists, government regulators, and industry executives. The result of the narrow thinking within chemistry and chemical engineering was to help form a "nation," an imagined community, whose shared imaginary was oriented around a single, unduly limited version of chemistry and chemical products (Anderson 1983).

If chemists and other experts are to participate more helpfully in the future in nongovernmental (as well as governmental) policy making, nontrivial revisions in the social relations of expertise would be required (Woodhouse and Nieusma 2001). A new sociotechnical constitution for a new chemical state would need to arrange for:

- Many different interests to negotiate via democratic processes;
- Drawing on much more diverse sources of expertise to understand the potentials and problems;
- So as to design nation-state regulatory policies and other social norms and practices that strongly encourage university science and engineering faculty to give very substantial weight in their teaching, research, consulting, and public commentary to chemical ideas and practices highly protective of environment and health;
- And that evoke from industry only those innovations in the design of new molecules that are biologically benign, or close to it, both in terms of manufacturing processes and in terms of final products;
- Thereby protecting the bodies of workers, consumers exposed to chemical products, and living organisms in the environment.

If every step in this process was violated egregiously by the brown chemistry of the twentieth century, some of the violations surely were due to a nearly inevitable naïveté about chemicals that was nobody's fault. However, many of the violations were due to the studied indifference and even willful neglect that is typical of elites making decisions with inadequate accountability—in this case, chemical executives, their technical employees and contractors, their allies in universities, and government officials pursuing wartime successes and peacetime economic competition.

Inasmuch as the chemical state emerged via a complex sociopolitical process, however, it may be more instructive to use our new appreciation of chemistry's potentials to acknowledge how far humanity has yet to go in designing the social relations within which expertise functions. Citizens' ignorance, consumers' nonchalance, educators' myopia, journalists' inadequate training— the list of factors in the overall social construction of contributory negligence is long. It may not be too strong to say that inappropriate chemical expertise and poorly designed intermediary institutions have crippled public under-standing of environmental problems and mistargeted nation-state practices concerning chemical innovation and regulation.

Because equivalent problems apply to some degree to every field of exper-tise, and because experts and their knowledge claims now are implicated in just about every human activity, the overall project of redesigning expertise probably amounts to a partial redesign of human civilization. As important as the design of benign chemicals surely is, therefore, the case of green chemistry could become far more important if it helps put us on the road to the daunting but also inspiring destination of a civilization based more firmly on reasoned inquiry and sensible experimentation, where knowledge is placed in the ser-vice of wisdom more than in the service of the ends favored by twentieth-century brown chemistry.

PART IV

NATIONS

10
Sexual Synthetics
Women, Science, and Microbicides

SUSAN E. BELL

This chapter represents my long-standing interest in and participation in what can very simplistically be called "a women's health movement."[1] A few years ago, when working on the most recent version of the birth control chapter for *Our Bodies, Ourselves for the New Century* (Bell and Wise 1998), I learned about a partnership between women's health advocates and reproductive scientists.[2] In the chapter, I devoted a long footnote to describing the partnership. In subsequent work, I have turned the footnote into a more sustained examination of the partnership because it signals an important transformation in women's health politics, and suggests directions for the twenty-first century. The collaboration was between women health advocates and the Population Council from 1994 to 1997 to produce vaginal microbicides to prevent transmission of HIV and other sexually transmitted diseases. Women's health advocates from around the world, Women's Health Advocates on Microbicides (WHAM), worked in the collaboration to promote their goals in the broadest sense of improving women's health and empowering women politically. Scientists from a nongovernment agency, the Population Council (PC), worked in the collaboration as part of the Council's shift towards combining contraception and disease prevention technologies. The Population Council is well known for its development of Norplant and the Copper-T IUD, technologies criticized by women's health advocates for embodying demographic goals of limiting the size of certain groups (especially poor and minority populations) rather than reproductive rights goals of helping individual women control fertility and improve their lives. I explore the sources of this collaboration and its consequences for scientific practice and women's health activism, and suggest what we might learn from it and use in promoting collaborations like it in the future.

I explore this collaboration in light of transformations in international feminisms that have enabled some feminists to pass from opposition to, to collaboration with, one agency in the population establishment. I link my interpretation to recent work in science studies that considers ways in which users are configured in technologies. I view these developments through a distinctive lens shaped by my experience in the women's health movement over the

197

past twenty-five years. In this work I have had to come to grips with the technoscience of contraception, and with the politics of reproduction and reproductive rights nationally and internationally (Bell 1979, 1994, 1999).

First I place work on microbicides within the context of women's health politics, international feminisms, and science studies. I then consider the social and scientific origins of microbicide research as well as the ways that women centered research is exemplified in and shapes microbicide research. Finally, I describe how the collaboration between WHAM and PC emerged, worked, and dispersed, and consider the implications of this case for the future of collaborations between women's health advocates and scientists.

To some extent I oversimplify my discussion by focusing not on individual scientists and activists but on two groups. The two categories, "women's health advocate" and "scientist," are not mutually exclusive. Were I to focus on individual microbicide researchers and individual women's health advocates, the boundaries between the two groups would blur. For example, some of the microbicide researchers identify themselves as women's health advocates, and might indeed have become scientists as part of a feminist agenda to put disease control and pregnancy prevention in women's hands and to look for methods of disease control that are suitable for multiple forms of sexual interaction (heterosexual, homosexual) that could potentially be used for either contraceptive or noncontraceptive purposes. The groups are neither as distinct from one another as might appear in this chapter nor as oppositional as might be suggested by a simple reading of the text.

International Feminisms

Reproductive health issues have been central to women's health politics for over a century (Clarke 1998). Reproductive rights became a central concern for the second wave of the women's health movement that emerged in the 1960s in North America, Australia, New Zealand, and Western Europe (Norsigian 1996).[3] Over the past decade, the "center of gravity" of women's health politics has shifted to the less industrialized world, and the practice of women's health politics has become increasingly international (Doyal 1996, 47). These transformations have brought together and resulted from women with different material interests, desires, commitments, styles of working, and frameworks of meaning. Under the broad banner of reproductive rights, for example, there are many groups of women following a variety of routes and using different levels and types of resources, to struggle toward a world containing faithful *accounts* of "sex," "gender," and "reproduction," embodied in reproductive technologies, as well as containing the material, cultural, and political *resources* for reproductive freedom (Doyal 1996; see also Haraway 1988).

In 1994, international women's health groups were instrumental in the creation of a new consensus in population policy at the United Nations International Conference on Population and Development (ICPD) held in Cairo, Egypt (McIntosh and Finkle 1995). The new consensus places the rights of women at the center of population policies and decenters demographic concerns from population policies (Girard 1999). The ICPD endorsed microbicide research. Beyond sexuality and health, the new consensus advocates that government population programs "should address issues such as women's rights to property ownership, gender discrimination in employment and pay, and violence against women" (Riley 1997, 40).

The new consensus forged at the ICPD embodies a "women-centered agenda." This agenda "attempts to integrate concerns for contraceptive efficacy into concerns for the overall reproductive health and general well-being of the primary users of contraceptives, that is, women" (Harrison and Rosenfield 1996, 2). Most generally, "the model also takes into account the social, political, and economic context of reproductive health and women's general empowerment and the ways in which each of these complements and enforces the others" (Harrison and Rosenfield 1996, 32). It favors methods "more directly under women's control so as to enhance their autonomy, enable them to shield themselves from sexually transmitted disease, diminish their dependence on the medical system and on the agreement of a partner for use of a contraceptive or anti-infective, and provide them with entirely new access to a range of methods that can be used postcoitally" (Harrison and Rosenfield 1996, 33). What Rosalind Petchesky (1997, 576) calls the "surprisingly feminist content" of this new consensus reflects an alignment between a strong international women's coalition and population and family planning groups as well as a transformation from the language of "health" to "human rights" among women's organizations concerned with reproductive and sexual issues. The Population Council's inauguration of an accelerated program of microbicide research in 1993 represents part of this new consensus (Heise et al. 1998, 2).

An ongoing tension in women's health politics has been between the strategy of working only in opposition to government agencies and international family planning organizations, and the strategy of cautiously working with these agencies (Doyal 1996; Clarke 2000). Women's health advocates have entered these "corridors of power" as workers and campaigners in a variety of settings (Doyal 1996, 49). Those advocating this strategy of engagement argue that it can be—and may indeed be a prerequisite for—achieving reproductive rights. Those critical of this strategy argue that the marginal gains that might result from it will be made at the cost of legitimating historically problematic population policies (Doyal 1996, 48–49). For example, regarding the new consensus developed at the ICPD, alongside of progressive elements are "contradictions that carry negative consequences for women, health, and human rights" (Hartmann 1998, 733). Even though the ICPD endorses the empowerment of women, its proposal for "more efficient government, higher levels of foreign investment, and greater reliance on the private sector and nongovernment organizations, rather than any substantive measures to redistribute wealth in an effort to eradicate poverty" tends to reinforce the economic status quo (Hartmann 1998, 733) and its proposal for empowering women reduces the definition of empowerment to education for girls and reproductive health services for women that are likely "to have the most immediate impact on fertility but the least impact on transforming social and economic relations" (Hartmann 1998, 733). Furthermore, determining whether an apparent "conversion to feminism" among population and family planning groups during and following the ICPD is sincere or merely tactical will take "time and continued vigilance by women's movements" (Petchesky 1997, 576). And, conversely, it remains to be seen whether routine participation in corridors of power such as at the ICPD transforms the goals and tactics as well as the collective identities of women's health advocates in problematic ways (see Epstein 2000).

This chapter traces one effort to enter the corridors of power when women's health advocates on microbicides (WHAM) worked with the Population Council (PC). The goal of their collaboration was to improve women's reproductive health by developing a women-controlled method of protection against sexually transmitted infections. The process for reaching this goal was to bring together those positioned "within" and those positioned "outside" reproductive science to design, carry out, and evaluate research on a new technology.

One of the collaborators was WHAM, founded in 1994 by eleven women's health advocates from Latin America, Africa, Europe, Asia, and the U.S. committed to reproductive rights.[4] Their strategy was to incorporate both the perspectives and concerns of scientists and of women's health advocates in the design and implementation of the research process itself (International Women's Health Coalition).

The other collaborator was the Population Council, a non-government agency founded in 1952 with funds from John D. Rockefeller III (Clarke 1998). Until its entry into the collaboration to produce vaginal microbicides, the Population Council developed only provider-dependent, systemic methods of contraception.[5] It had supported population control research but not research into the prevention of sexually transmitted diseases.

The collaboration was risky for both sides. For women's health advocates, it represented entry into the process of development, diffusion, and continuing evaluation of reproductive technology and into serious dialogue with scientists and philanthropists. For the Population Council, it represented entry into a new area of research in women's reproductive health and into serious dialogue with feminist activists about it. For both, it represented an entirely new form of collaboration.

The collaboration between WHAM and the PC was the first to bring together users and reproductive health scientists in the development of a reproductive technology. It was not the only collaboration, however. Two others that occurred at about the same time, also fraught with complexities and tension, were between AIDS activists and AIDS researchers (Epstein 1996, 2000) and between DES daughters and DES researchers (National Cancer Institute et al. 1999). Neither of these collaborations involved the production of reproductive technologies, although both of them included users and potential users in setting the terms of scientific practice.

Representations of users' bodies have been influencing the development of antifertility vaccines over the past twenty-five years (van Kammen 1999). Until recently, conceptions of users' bodies were produced by reproductive biologists, immunologists, and gynecologists from within their own social worlds.[6] That is, users have provided the material or imagined basis for researchers' conceptions (Akrich 1995; Oudshoorn 1996). Microbicide research, by contrast, reflects the participation of actual and potential users in the conceptualization and practice of reproductive science itself.

Microbicide Research

Microbicides are substances that can substantially reduce transmission of sexually transmitted infections, including HIV, when applied in a vagina or rectum before sexual intercourse (Zaneveld et al. 1996). Some microbicides target specific pathogens, whereas other microbicides have nonspecific action (Stephenson 2000). Microbicides currently being developed could work in a variety of different ways. Some microbides are being developed to kill or otherwise immobilize sexually transmitted pathogens. For example, surfactants—such as nonoxynol-9—are detergent-like chemicals that disrupt the outer membranes of cells and the outer shell of viruses (HIV and herpes simplex viruses). Nonoxynol-9 is a spermicide that has been used for decades in contraceptive creams and jellies. In the laboratory, it is lethal to some sexually transmitted pathogens, including HIV (Bell and Wise 1998). However, it has shown mixed results in clinical trials as a microbicide (Stephenson 2000). A second type of microbicide being developed blocks infection by creating a chemical or immunological barrier between pathogens and a vagina or rectum. Examples include acid-buffering agents that inhibit many pathogens by preventing an alkaline environment or by recreating an acidic environment in a vagina or rectum. Attachment inhibitors, such as dextran sulfate, block the attachment of pathogens to the mucus surface with charged polymers or human monoclonal antibodies. Passive immunization uses monoclonal antibodies (MAbs) to create a barrier to infection, and such antibodies, as well as methods to deliver them directly to the vagina or rectum, are being developed to protect against STD pathogens as well as sperm (Zeitlin et al. 1999). A third type of microbicide prevents infection from taking hold after a pathogen has entered a person's body, such as with antiretroviral agents already approved for systemic treatment of HIV infection (Bell and Wise 1998; Heise et al. 1998; Stephenson 2000).

Microbicides can potentially be produced in many different forms for use in a vagina or rectum (gels, creams, suppositories, film, or sponge/vaginal rings). Vaginal microbicides could potentially be designed as barrier methods having microbicidal and spermicidal effects to prevent both pregnancy and sexually transmitted infections. They could also be designed to allow conception and still prevent sexually transmitted infections; that is they could be microbicidal but not spermicidal.

What we now call microbicides are the kinds of birth control/disease prevention technologies that Margaret Sanger and the early feminist birth control movement initially sought, starting in 1915 (Clarke 1998; McCann 1994). Until recently, microbicide research was marginalized in reproductive biology research, birth control development, and HIV/AIDS prevention (Population Council 1994, 6). Over the past decade it has moved further into the center of research. A combination of maverick advocates among reproductive scientists, acknowledgment of epidemic proportions of HIV/AIDS and sexually transmitted infections, and years of thought and advocacy on the part of internationally oriented feminists, have brought microbicide research closer to the center of reproductive biology, birth control development, and AIDS prevention (see Clarke 2000; and Harrison and Rosenfield 1996, 31). This centering has had impressive results: in 1994, there were twenty candidate microbicides under development, twelve in preclinical studies, and eight in clinical trials. By 2000 there were at least sixty compounds under development, thirty-six "in preclinical development, twenty in or ready for safety studies in humans, and four in or moving into large-scale efficacy trials" (Peter Piot, in Stephenson 2000, 1811). These results reflect "persistence on the part of those already engaged [in 1994], appearance of new entrants into the earliest development phases, and a certain amount of momentum" (Harrison 1999, S52).

According to Adele Clarke (2000) "in the 1990s, some combination of individual women's resistance and the activism of feminist and other women's health organizations [became] consequential" for scientists and policy makers. Centering microbicide research is both signaled and accomplished in actions such as those taken by the World Health Organization, the Rockefeller Foundation, the Institute of Medicine, and the Boston Women's Health Book Collective. At a 1993 meeting of the World Health Organization, an international working group was formed to develop a consensus statement of recommendations for facilitating "the development, production and distribution of safe, acceptable, effective, and affordable vaginal microbicides to prevent HIV infection and other STDs" (International Working Group on Vaginal Microbicides 1996, 2). That same year the Rockefeller Foundation adopted a "Contraception-21" strategy. A central theme of this strategy was to "mobilize and lift up the whole field" of contraceptive research (Fathalla 1999, S7) and to tailor it to the unmet needs of women as they had been identified by women's groups in the developed and developing worlds: first, women-controlled methods of contraception providing additional protection against sexually transmitted infections, such as vaginal microbicides; second, methods of contraception women can use as a back-up when exposed to unprotected sexual intercourse; and third, expanded male contraceptive choices, participation, and responsibility (Fathalla 1999, S7). Beginning in 1993, Rockefeller provided financial support to advance the science, particularly in cell and molecular biology, in these three areas (Fathalla 1999, S9).

A year later, in 1994, the Institute of Medicine in the United States gave prominence to the benefits of microbicides in two workshops reported in *Contraceptive Research and Development* (Harrison and Rosenfield 1996). The workshops reviewed the prospects of the science underlying the development of new contraceptives and the opportunities for private-sector participation in this development. Their attention to microbicides was heavily influenced by the endorsement of microbicide research at the International Conference on Population and Development (see below). In 1998, when I wrote the birth control chapter for *Our Bodies, Ourselves for the New Century*, I listed microbicides as one of the "promising new developments" in contraceptive research (Bell and Wise 1998, 288). This endorsement of microbicides helped to give feminist legitimacy to microbicide research, and simultaneously reflected communications between women's health advocates and reproductive scientists.[7]

Work on microbicides represents a change in policy at the Population Council. Traditionally, the Population Council had supported birth control research and development, but had not supported research in the prevention and treatment of sexually transmitted infections. Recently, in the face of growing need, it has expanded into developing new ways for women to protect themselves against sexually transmitted diseases, especially HIV/AIDS (Population Council 1994, 10). To some extent the source of change in policy was "local." It was initiated by Christopher Elias, at the time a Senior Associate at the Population Council. Elias was a newly hired young biomedical scientist who took on the issue after meeting with and hearing from women's health advocate Lori Heise. Elias was soon joined by David Phillips, another scientist at the Population Council, who was a Senior Scientist at the Council's Center for Biomedical Research. Elias and Phillips were invited by George Zeidenstein, then president of the Population Council, to present a plan to the Board of Trustees. The Board subsequently agreed to support pursuit of "both contraceptive and noncontraceptive microbicidal preparations" (Population Council 1994, 9).

To some extent the source was "global." The larger social and political context encouraged and made the negotiations by Elias and Phillips possible. The Population Council had had problems with earlier methods—Norplant and the Copper-T IUD—which many women had refused to use and against which feminists had organized. In addition, hormonal methods of contraceptives and

IUDs appear to make women more susceptible to HIV and some other sexually transmitted infections (Bell 1984, 1992; Bell and Wise 1998). That is, the systemic hormonal contraceptives promoted by population control advocates since the 1950s may have heightened women's vulnerability to many sexually transmitted diseases, including HIV/AIDS (Alexander 1996; International Working Group on Vaginal Microbicides 1996). Acknowledgment of the growing risk of HIV infection faced by women throughout the world and of serious limitations of contemporary AIDS prevention strategy in meeting women's needs created a scientific context for birth control and disease prevention groups of scientists to try to work together to produce methods combining these two actions/streams of research (Elias and Heise 1994; Heise and Elias 1995).

Elias and Phillips were also informed by worldwide meetings and consultations held in preparation for the International Conference on Population and Development (Population Council 1994, 29). In fact, in its Program of Action, the ICPD endorsed efforts to "to develop women-controlled methods, such as vaginal microbicides, to prevent infection" with HIV (United Nations 1994, ch. 8.33); to develop microbicides "which may or may not prevent pregnancy" (United Nations 1994, ch. 12.12); and to incorporate "users' in particular women's perspectives and women's organizations . . . in all stages of the research and development process" (United Nations 1994, ch. 12.16). In their collaboration together, WHAM and the Population Council put into practice the research strategies recommended by the ICPD Program of Action concerning the development of vaginal microbicides. The same combination of forces that led the Population Council to change its policy has made activists and other scientists more willing to work together on reproductive technology development (Heise et al. 1998, v).

Connecting Women and Science

Women's Health Advocates on Microbicides (WHAM) was a group of eleven women from eight countries in different regions of the world that worked collaboratively with the Population Council on all phases of microbicide development and testing (Population Council 1994; Heise, McGrory, and Wood 1998). WHAM was created by the eleven women in May, 1994, when all of the initial founders attended "Partnership for Prevention," a meeting sponsored by two women's health organizations—the International Women's Health Coalition and the Pacific Institute for Women's Health[8]—and the Population Council to initiate an ongoing consultative process between women's health advocates and scientists about the technology of vaginal microbicides (Population Council 1994, 1). The "Partnership for Prevention" was the first of two international meetings that brought together women's health advocates, social and biomedical scientists, and policy makers from around the world.

The Partnership for Prevention meeting was the first example of a strategy encouraged by the World Health Organization and the International Women's

Health Coalition. Three years earlier the two groups had jointly recommended bringing together reproductive scientists, program planners, and women's health advocates for an intensive exchange at an early phase in the development of reproductive technology (Population Council 1994, 5). Planning for it by the International Women's Health Coalition and the Population Council was informed by meetings and various consultations around the world in preparation for the International Conference on Population and Development, which brought tensions about reproductive technology development into sharp focus (Population Council 1994, 29). Planning for the Partnership was also shaped by meetings initiated in 1991 by the Population Council to build momentum around the idea that microbicides could and should be produced as part of a global strategy against HIV/AIDS (Population Council 1994, 6). Lori Heise, who at the time was Director of the Pacific Institute for Women's Health, turned her attention to microbicides as part of her work on violence against women. Heise helped provide an explicitly feminist analysis in a Population Council working paper that simultaneously catalyzed action within the Council and the broader scientific community, and amongst women's health advocates (Population Council 1994, 7). While Heise's work helped to set the conceptual and strategic boundaries for the Partnership, Adrienne Germain, who was at the time vice-president of the International Women's Health Coalition, identified women's health advocates to include in the Partnership meeting (Heise, personal communication, October 4, 1999).[9]

At the eight day long meeting of the Partnership for Prevention, conference participants met with a wide range of scientists involved in microbicide research and development, with senior staff from USAID, the Food and Drug Administration, and the National Institutes of Health, as well as with women's congressional and lobbying groups. This partnership "was the first step in building greater understanding and mutual respect among women's health advocates and Population Council staff and scientists in regard to the technology of microbicides" (Population Council 1994, n.p.). For example, scientists were surprised when they learned that women's health advocates were often suspicious of scientific research (Population Council 1994, 16). The meeting gave the two groups an opportunity to address this concern collaboratively. In his contribution to the report of the 1994 meeting, David M. Phillips, Senior Scientist at the Center for Biomedical Research at the Population Council, wrote that "the role of [women's health advocates] is especially critical in light of the great gulf that separates biomedical scientists of the western world from women of the developing world" (Population Council 1994, 11).

WHAM members brought a women-centered perspective to the collaboration. Amparo Claro, coordinator of the Latin American and Caribbean Women's Health Network proposed two strategies to create a participatory, democratic, and respectful approach to microbicide research. One strategy would be for scientists to begin a dialogue with local networks and members of a community early in the research process by identifying women's health advocates in health centers where trials might be conducted and sending project lists to these health advocates and local organizations requesting input and collaboration. Another strategy would be to write a job position for a women's health advocate into study proposals. Both of these strategies would "establish open and meaningful communication with the study participants which would provide, for the scientists, more accurate and complete reactions to the product" (Population Council 1994, 14).

Establishing open and meaningful dialogue with potential study participants would also strengthen the ethical dimensions of research. Drawing from her experience with Empower in Chiang Mai, Thailand, WHAM member Liz Cameron proposed ways to develop clinical trials that are both scientifically rigorous and ethically defensible. Scientists seeking to conduct research on "vulnerable" populations such as sex workers should begin the study design process by learning about the details of everyday life for women in these populations. Women sex workers are often the targets of HIV prevention research because they are at greatest risk of HIV. Finding ways to join with the sex-worker community instead of merely doing research on them would be mutually beneficial. The working conditions of women who work in brothels, for example, leave them unprotected from exploitation and abuse by brothel owners and researchers. Thus, "regardless of informed consent, use of women who work in brothels in clinical trials is unethical because the women themselves don't grant consent" (Population Council 1994, 20).

According to Muriel Harris (Population Council 1994, 24), director of the Society for Women and AIDS in Africa, in some communities women's status depends on childbearing, and so a non-contraceptive vaginal microbicide is urgently needed. The simultaneous development of vaginal microbicides with and without spermicidal effects is a way for science to acknowledge and respond to the multiple positions of women worldwide. Beyond building flexibility into microbicides along these lines, Harris illuminates the need to address "*both* longterm or *strategic* gender needs of women . . . as well as meet the immediate *practical* need for women-controlled technologies" in developing protection against HIV and other sexually transmitted diseases (Population Council 1994, 25).

The partnership between WHAM and the Population Council broke new ground and proceeded slowly and cautiously.[10] Throughout this intensive eight-day consultation "the women met frequently as a small group and discussed their emerging concerns and impressions" (Population Council 1994, n.p.). Tensions in women's health politics concerning the strategy of engagement were mirrored and played out within WHAM. Some of the women in WHAM belonged to reproductive rights groups that were sharply critical of the population establishment, and were in an oppositional relationship with agencies included in it, such as the Population Council. To address this tension, WHAM wrote a "Statement of Group Principles," warning that its work with the Population Council on microbicides did not constitute an unconditional endorsement of the Population Council. WHAM reserved the right "to independently evaluate and interpret the implications of research findings for women's lives."

In their joint reflections on the meeting, Population Council bioscientist Christopher Elias and International Women's Health Coalition activist Adrienne Germain wrote that three short term goals had been met. Participants had "fostered considerable sensitivity and insight among participant scientists regarding the realities of women's lives ... increased the abilities of the women's health advocates who participated by increasing their access to accurate scientific information ... and furthered the dialogue between women's health advocates, scientists, and program planners on issues that affect women's sexual and reproductive health" (Population Council 1994, 31). The collaborators tried to incorporate both these social-political and technical concerns into the design of studies. For example, they committed themselves to pursuing two longer term aspirations. First, they wanted "to ensure that the Population Council's current commitment to microbicide development [resulted] in the availability of vaginal products that are safe, effective, and meet women's needs." Second, they hoped "to develop an effective example for future reproductive health technology development that engages women as active partners in all aspects of the product development process" (Population Council 1994, 31).

In a second set of meetings, in April 1997, a larger group of "fifty-five advocates, scientists, policy makers, and industry representatives from fifteen countries across Africa, Asia, Latin America, Europe, and the United States" explored key practical and ethical dilemmas raised by clinical testing of new microbicides (International Women's Health Coalition 1998). They planned research projects for sites in the South (less industrialized world) as well as the North (industrialized world). Research protocols for the proposed studies would mix scientific, logistical, and ethical matters in evaluating potential sites and populations for clinical trials of efficacy (Phase III). For example, to help protect against potential exploitation of vulnerable women, these trials would proceed only after consulting with members of the local communities and potential trial participants in each site. Study participants would include diverse populations, not primarily sex workers as had been the emphasis in previous microbicide trials (Heise et al. 1998, viii). This would increase the generalizability of results and share the burdens and benefits of microbicide research (Heise et al. 1998, 52). Recommendations also included giving periodic updates on the progress of microbicide science to women's health advocates and consulting with them on selection of research sites and design of clinical trials.

The day after the second set of meetings ended, in April 1997, members of WHAM met to reflect on the meeting and to look ahead to opportunities and needs for future engagement in microbicide research.[11] In their view, the landscape had changed over the past three years: many more actors had entered the arena, a number of efforts were moving from the laboratory to the field, and HIV- and contraceptive-related funds were being directed to microbicide research. The need and opportunity for advocates to work on microbicides was expanding and changing. WHAM decided to dissolve as a formal entity focused exclusively on the Population Council but to continue to work as part of a wider, more flexible network. Decentralization would encourage each individual and group to pursue "that aspect of the microbicide agenda closest to its strategic interest and ability" (Heise et al. 1998, 52). Members of WHAM agreed that the larger cause of microbicide development would be better served by taking advantage of local opportunities, regional connections, and the needs of the field.

These local opportunities, regional connections, and needs of the field have been expressed in several ways. In 1998, supported by a start up grant from the Rockefeller Foundation and contributions from some participating companies, a few former members of WHAM joined with reproductive scientists and biopharmaceutical company representatives to form the Alliance for Microbicide Development, a consortium established to catalyze the development of microbicides (Harrison 1999, S39–S40). The Alliance seeks federal (U.S.) funding for microbicide research through federal legislation. It is also working to facilitate the exchange of scientific information and collaboration and to streamline the research and development process. The first organizational act of the Alliance was to form an advocacy committee. According to the Director of the Alliance, Polly F. Harrison (1999, S47), "there was broad consensus across the Alliance that its first order of business was to formulate a policy agenda, a knowledge base, and a network of health and research advocacy groups to serve as the foundation to evoke meaningful change in the U.S. public sector," such as securing significant increases in budgetary allocations. Women's health advocates chair the Advocacy Committee of the Alliance, which focuses on public education, advocacy, and constituency building amongst national and local U.S. women's health groups, international grassroots organizations, high level public-sector research entities, and industry (Harrison 1999, S47). In this way, women's health advocates retain a central voice in the Alliance.

As part of its commitment to advocacy, the Alliance launched a Global Campaign for STI/HIV Prevention Alternatives for Women at the Twelfth World AIDS Conference in 1998. The Global Campaign is led by some former WHAM members. Its goal is to increase access to prevention technologies other than the male condom by directing public and private investment in women-controlled methods of STI/HIV prevention, including microbicides (Harrison 1999, S47). The Global Campaign is circulating a "Petition for Greater Investment into STI/HIV Options for Women," calling on the U.S. government, the European Union, and other governments to accelerate research into topical microbicides and female condoms (Heise n.d.). In 1999, the campaign received funding from UNAIDS; within two years it grew "into a major global organizing effort, with more than seventy partner groups worldwide" to educate the public, build constituencies, advocate for legislation, and to ensure scientific accountability (Global Campaign for Prevention Options for Women). To date, the campaign has among other things, successfully secured or "rescued" $26 million for research; organized a Microbicides Advocacy Day in March 30, during which researchers and activists visited members of U.S. Congress to promote investment in microbicide research; achieved unprecedented visibility in scientific and community programs at the Thirteenth International AIDS Conference in Durban, South Africa; and placed articles in popular press and scientific journals about microbicides (Gottemoeller 2000; Global Campaign for Microbicides, "Looking for Mrs. McCormick"). In 2001, the Microbicide Development Act was introduced in the U.S. House of Representatives and Senate to create a "Microbicide Program" at the National Institutes of Health, to require the expansion and coordination of federal research activities, to authorize necessary funds for research, and to require regular reports to Congress on progress of the coordinated initiative (Global Campaign for Microbicides, "Legislative Message").

In 1999, several members of the Global Campaign launched a fund raising initiative, titled "Looking for Mrs. McCormick," to support microbicide advocacy and to advance the mission of the campaign. The title evokes the story of Katherine McCormick, a wealthy philanthropist who worked in 1951 with feminist Margaret Sanger to provide funding for early research on what subsequently became the birth control Pill. On its web page, the Global Campaign states "We are looking for Mrs. McCormicks of the new millennium—visionary women and men who will take matters into their own hands and provide the critical funding that will advance science and make microbicides a reality" (Global Campaign for Microbicides, "Looking for Mrs. McCormick" http://www.global-campaign.org/dom/lookingdom.html).

Other former members of WHAM have been participating in consultative meetings in Thailand and South Africa to exchange views and build consensus about future microbicide trials being planned in those countries (Heise et al. 1998, 52). The meetings in Thailand and South Africa exemplify a gradual move (beginning in the early 1990s) away from confrontation and distrust of each other towards attempts at communication and collaboration between women's health advocates and contraceptive scientists—research institutions (and individuals) heeded advocates' call for greater input into the technology development process by consulting with women's health advocates and hosting forums for exchange (Heise et al. 1998, v). Both of these meetings made special efforts to include women's health advocates, from Thailand and South Africa respectively, working in collaboration with scientists, private industry representatives, and policy makers.

Reflections

The WHAM/PC effort was an extremely important step in the history of dialogue among women's health advocates, social scientists, and biomedical researchers. It was the first time that staff of an organization like the Population Council asked women's health advocates to offer their views on the research and development process of a biomedical innovation from the outset, and that women's health advocates turned to this strategy for reproductive rights. Whether the consequences of collaborations such as this can lead to reproductive science that is more democratic and results in microbicides that are more flexible and user-friendly remains to be seen. As Clarke (2000) observes, "the 'cultures of science' which have been reproduced by five generations of scientists is cumulative—previous discourses remain lively as resources into the future—hegemonic and difficult to displace" even by those who are self-consciously attempting to replace them.

Microbicide research is beginning to secure more attention and more funding. In 2000, the Bill and Melinda Gates Foundation awarded $25 million for microbicide development. With these funds, CONRAD (a program founded in 1986 as a cooperating agency of the U.S. Agency for International Development) established the Global Microbicide Project "to help develop new microbicidal agents that specifically address the needs and perspectives of women" (Global Microbicide Project 2001). Microbicide research is only beginning to move from the laboratory to the field and women's health advocates have been working inside the world of contraceptive research for only a few years. The democratizing practices initiated by WHAM/PC are continuing and being transformed into a wider, more flexible network of actors, in a transforming and transformed global environment.

Microbicide research collaborations have the potential to produce high-quality, flexible medical technology and thereby to improve women's health through clinical interventions. Effective clinical interventions such as microbicides "can often hope to efface the embodied manifestations of social inequalities" (Farmer 1999, 15). Women in different social locations, with different needs and desires, can potentially prevent sexually transmitted diseases with microbicides. However, effacing the inequality of outcomes with clinical interventions "is not the same as eliminating the underlying forces of inequality itself" (Farmer 1999, 15). In other words, "for women most at risk of HIV infection, life choices are limited by racism, sexism, political violence, and grinding poverty" (Farmer 1999, 88).

Efforts to produce microbicides, as important as they are, must be linked to efforts to empower women—especially poor women. This includes efforts to gain control over "land, systems of production, and the formal political and legal structures in which lives are enmeshed" (Farmer 1999, 91). Making microbicides, making science more democratic, and making societies more equitable should be interconnected practices.

11

Chemicals and Casualties
The Search for Causes of Gulf War Illnesses

PHIL BROWN, STEPHEN ZAVESTOSKI, MEADOW LINDER,
SABRINA MCCORMICK, AND BRIAN MAYER

We begin by asking the question: Why can't the health effects of chemicals in our environment be understood by simply "following the molecule?"[1] This question implies that we can trace the path and effects of disease-causing molecules, much as we would follow scientists in a laboratory or other scientific enterprise. "Following the molecule" stems from the notion of "following the scientist," as in Latour's (1979, 1987) "actor-network" approach. Latourian studies of science-work require paying attention to the combined, interactive technical and social aspects. By seeing how scientists work with their materials in the laboratory, we should be able to achieve an ethnographic account of their work that cuts through the surface layer of what they simply *say* they are doing. Further, this should cut through what *others* are saying. Some have criticized the Latourian model for its "executive approach," whereby only top-level leadership is observed (Clarke 1987). Latour (1999) responds to such criticism by suggesting that objects share the same characteristics that science studies examine in scientists; the normative values held by an object express a "social history of things and a 'thingy' history of humans." In Latour's (1999) recent formulation, the values held by objects tell a narrative with equal vigor as do the scientists themselves. From our point of view, to "follow the molecule" is to follow the nonhuman actor—the molecule—wherever it goes, and then study where it lands.

Following the molecule can also mean the kind of story that Sandra Steingraber (1997, 176–79) and others tell of persistent organic pollutants (POPs) traced to the ends of the earth, where they could not exist as a result of local use. Through what Steingraber terms *chemical nomadism,* "poisons dumped and plowed into the earth are fed, molecule by molecule, into the air, where they redistribute themselves back to the earth and into our food supply." Even that kind of following the molecule does not provide scientists with enough evidence of health effects, however. The CDC body burden study (CDC 2001), the first of its type, may offer such a potential for following the molecules into our bodies.

Following the molecule is an analytic injunction for the social scientist: follow the molecule and you will find where it goes—into bodies, government agencies, medical records, chemical sensors, and commissions to study the molecule. This approach leads us to sites that may or may not have been explored. Most interestingly, it leads us to sites of contestations about molecules, which we can study (Clarke, personal communication). In this sense, the injunction is a methodological tool for the sociologist. But we add to this a more realist "truth-seeking" tool: if medical scientists and epidemiologists could indeed follow the molecule, they would have a better chance of finding out the causes of Gulf War–related illnesses. As we show in this chapter, there are major obstacles that prevent the routine practices of normal science that would allow for such a search.

In the Gulf War, molecules were widely prevalent (through chemical weapons, radioactive ordnance, and preventive medical procedures), and theoretically we should be able to trace their action. But the problem of these molecules, and their potential implication in various Gulf War–related illnesses (GWRIs), is a case of a contested environmental illness. This contestation stems from the initial conflicts over the government's denial that such illnesses existed, its more recent imposition of a stress-related explanation, and the disputes over exposure and symptom measurement. After providing some historical background, we introduce a theoretical framework that we believe helps explain why environmental illnesses are almost always contested. In fact, across the broad range of occupational and environmental diseases we see disputes about what molecules are responsible. When multiple chemicals are implicated, as they are in GWRIs, chemicals interact, chemical structures change, and molecules migrate, further complicating efforts to "follow the molecule" from exposure to illness.

Since such ambiguous situations foster conflict, it becomes easy for interested parties to disagree on which molecules should be followed, and how they should be followed. We observed these disagreements in our examination of the contestations over GWRIs. As we demonstrate, the Pentagon's and Veteran Administration's (VA) initial reaction was to deny that there were any molecules to be followed, instead pointing to stress as the cause of GWRIs. Once sufficient evidence surfaced that chemical exposures took place, veterans, scientists, and involved government agencies began disputing which molecules should be followed, and how. We also demonstrate how these disputes led the media to focus on GWRIs more as a political issue than as a medical/scientific one.

We define "contested environmental illnesses" as diseases and conditions that engender major scientific disputes and extensive public debates over environmental causes. By environmental, we mean toxic substances in people's immediate or proximate surroundings, which have health impacts. However, in the case of GWRIs, the grouping of "environmental" factors often includes inoculations and other medical treatments.[2] It is hard to disentangle the iatrogenic effects from other environmental effects, and indeed, some research focuses on the combinations of these and more traditional, toxic exposures.

Nor do we include local infectious disease potential, such as leishmaniasis from sand flea bites, though a number of veterans have been interested in this possibility. Throughout, we emphasize the importance of lay disease discovery and knowledge production, how diverse interests shape medical knowledge and social policy, and how as a result of these conflicts, science and government often fail to provide adequately for the public health.

Methods and Data

Methods include content analysis of government documents (Congressional hearings, Institute & Medicine (IOM) reports, reports from the Department of Defense (DOD), VA, and other federal agencies) and the scientific literature in medical and epidemiological journals; print media analysis; ethnographic observations of the 1999 and 2001 Federally-Funded Gulf Research Conferences, and (on thirteen occasions) of the Boston Environmental Hazard Center (BEHC, a VA-based center for GWRI research, operated collaboratively by the VA Medical Center and the Boston University School of Public Health); and twenty-one interviews with researchers, officials, and veteran activists. Researchers were selected on the basis of their involvement in the BEHC and related VA programs. Veterans were selected on the basis of participation in the BEHC's Community Advisory Board, referrals from those members to others, as well as some activists participating in the 1999 Gulf War Research Conference. Unreferenced quotes come from our own interviews and observations. Media analysis consisted of searching for articles (1991–1999) dealing with environmental causation of Gulf War-related illnesses in the *New York Times, Washington Post,* the three major newsweeklies, and general circulation science magazines (*Science, Science Digest, Scientific American, Discover,* and *Popular Science*). These articles were examined for how they dealt with environmental causation, as well as enumerated to gauge the extent of public interest.

Historical Background

Following service in the Gulf War of 1991, many U.S. military personnel began experiencing symptoms such as nausea, loss of concentration, blurred vision, fatigue, lack of muscle control and coordination, irritable bowels, headaches, rashes, and other ailments that they had not experienced prior to service in the Gulf. Slowly, veterans experiencing these and other symptoms began connecting their service in the Gulf to their failing health. The VA frequently denied care, claiming either that the symptoms were undiagnosable and therefore did not qualify for compensation, or that they were diagnosable but not logically related to Gulf service. Angered by the VA denials, many veterans began to speak out about their conditions and the perceived origins of their illnesses. As media coverage increased, veterans around the country began to realize fellow servicemen and women were likewise afflicted. Since the Gulf War, approximately 70,000 have sought treatment for service-related illnesses, and an estimated 2.7 million people (veterans, family members, and civilians) are eligible for some form of Gulf War era VA benefits. The VA finally began providing care in 1994 as a result of legislation requiring the VA to award compensation benefits to chronically disabled Gulf War veterans with undiagnosed illnesses. Yet veterans continue to report that the VA is not taking care of them for Gulf-related problems.

In addition to providing medical benefits and compensation for sick veterans, the government[3] began to fund research investigating the possible causes of veterans' illnesses. Possible chemical exposures include sarin gas, mustard gas, smoke from oil well fires, pyridostigmine bromide, depleted uranium, pesticides, DEET (N,N-diethyl-m-toluamide) in flea collars worn by soldiers to protect against insects, anthrax vaccines, and other antidote tablets. Plagued by poor data, disputes over how to study Gulf War health effects, and a long list of possible chemical exposures that could be to blame, research has resulted in no effective treatments of GWRI symptoms, and no clear understanding of their causes. Nevertheless, annual federally funded research on GWRIs has, per year, continued at the cost of $7.1 million in 1994, $17.3 million in 1995, $18.8 million in 1996, $34.2 million in 1997, and $37.9 million in 1998.

Theoretical Background

Our answer to the question "How can the health effects of chemicals in our environment be understood by simply 'following the molecule?'" in short, is that chemicals, and especially the molecules that comprise them, move within and across bodies, and they interact with other chemicals and manifest themselves in ways that confound traditional science. More specifically, our answer focuses on the operation of the scientific process within the social institutions engaging in the social construction of diagnosis and illness (Brown 1995). This social constructionist perspective argues that sufficient medical and scientific research will not always unequivocally establish the presence and etiology of disease. In fact, in cases where the disease and/or its putative cause are politically controversial, often no amount of scientific and medical research is sufficient to unequivocally define the disease or identify its cause. Following the molecule leads you to the sites of contestation, but does not guarantee scientific consensus.

For virtually all environmental and occupational diseases, a broadly acceptable social definition, a new consensus on the part of experts, and often a social movement, are each and all often necessary to achieve a general belief in the existence of the disease and its environmental cause. Michael Reich (1991) conceptualizes the process where toxic victims turn personal troubles into social problems through three stages: (1) making their issue into a public problem by identifying the disease and its social origin; (2) organizing collective action to seek redress; and (3) mobilizing political allies since a victims' group alone cannot do all that is necessary.

As people and groups move through these stages, they engage in "popular epidemiology" (Brown and Mikkelsen 1990), the process in which sufferers and their allies identify environmental health effects and help frame and conduct research. People engage in cognitive and ideological shifts called "frame transformations," especially in the development of an "injustice frame," where people stop thinking in terms of "accidents" or personal responsibility, and shift responsibility onto corporations and governments (Gamson et al. 1982; Snow et al. 1986).

When people and groups mobilize in this fashion, they often find themselves in opposition to a generally accepted belief system concerning the existence and causes of disease. We term this general belief system a "dominant epidemiological paradigm" (DEP). The DEP emerges from a diverse set of social actors who draw on existing stocks of institutionalized knowledge to identify and define disease, as well as determine its etiology, proper treatment, and acceptable health outcomes (see Figure 11.1). While there are often competing belief systems for any scientific issue, there is usually a dominant one at a given point, even if that changes over time.

The discovery of a potential environmental health risk may arise from government, research, or other actors (e.g., journalists), but it is typically laypeople who push it further. For example, most states collect cancer data but do not take action when abnormal cancer rates and/or clusters are discovered (Greenberg and Wartenberg 1991). In that case, it takes activists or others to discover the data and push the issue. In other instances, scientists happen upon a disease first, only to have a disease group and/or the government latch onto the findings in order to support their causes. In yet other cases, investigative journalism might turn up patterns of illness previously undetected.

In all cases, however, the process leads to a dominant explanation for the disease. This need not be a regressive explanation: the dominant explanation of the appearance of West Nile Virus in various East Coast areas in summer 2000 is not likely to engender dispute, even if the insecticide application is contentious. In many cases, the explanation put forth by the DEP fails to make links between a contaminant, an iatrogenic treatment, or another problem of human/social action. That failure results in inadequate recognition, treatment, and prevention. For example, when we look at all forms of cancer, we find that the DEP explanation for local excesses of cancer is an argument that utilizes probability theory to dispute the existence of clusters, claiming that these are random occurrences in the normal distribution. This explanation in itself precludes searching for a source of environmental causation.

While laypeople are generally the most important human actors, in some circumstances, forward-looking physicians, public health scientists, and their

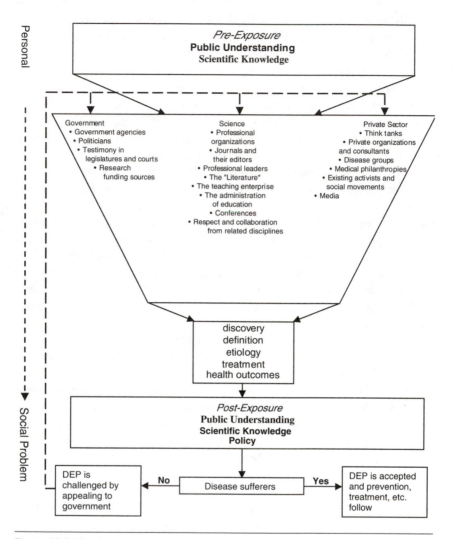

Figure 11.1 The dominant epidemiological paradigm's process of disease discovery, definition, etiology, treatment, and outcomes

organizations may themselves be significant champions of a challenge to the DEP. For example, the early efforts to link tobacco and lung cancer were spearheaded by medical and public health experts, even though later efforts at strict regulation were headed by lay activists.

When disease victims' needs are not met by the DEP's conceptualization of their illness, opposition to the DEP grows. Often, victims' needs are not met because of the preexposure state of policies, public understanding, and scientific knowledge. Following the struggles with various government, science, and private sector organizations, an altered version of the disease may emerge. Ideally, this version's conceptualization of the discovery, definition, etiology, treatment, and outcomes of the disease leads to greater scientific knowledge, new policies, and greater public understanding. However, because of the DEP's nature as a paradigm, even the most passionate efforts of challengers are often insufficient to alter the DEP. The combination of embedded institutional tendencies and practices, cultural belief systems, routinely accepted ways of knowing, and vested interests serve to perpetuate the existing understanding of the disease. The DEP persists through the privileged position of those who define it and subscribe to it, and by subsuming under itself any counter-explanation offered by those who oppose it. Figure 11.1 shows that there are an enormous number of locations of generally accepted knowledge, locations that are unlikely to change due to citizen queries, normal science, or self-realization on the part of actors.

We trace the formation of the DEP for Gulf War-related illnesses by examining the roles of the government, science, media, and activists in creating, perpetuating, and in some cases challenging, the DEP. With GWRIs, the DEP emerged during the period when many in power argued that these diseases and conditions did not exist or, at best, were the outcomes of war-related stress. The construction of a stress-based DEP, in turn, discourages attempts to follow the molecules that may actually have been at the root of GWRIs. Veterans and some of their scientific allies have strongly opposed this version of the DEP for what they see as its tendency to "blame the victim." While we cannot firmly conclude that such pressure has had a dramatic effect, we can see how the DEP has begun to shift: the possibility of environmental exposures, in conjunction with stress, is now being considered as a possible cause of GWRIs. A 2000 Institute of Medicine report (IOM 2000), for example, recommends new research on stress-environment interactions. Though many veterans would prefer no federally funded research on stress at all (National Gulf War Resource Center 2001), official acknowledgment of the need for a better understanding of stress and exposure represents a minor victory. Some researchers are even beginning to suggest that veterans' symptoms, which are now widely recognized as real, should be viewed as similar to other multisymptom diseases and conditions (e.g., Engel et al. 2000).

In its process of change, the DEP can be understood from the social constructionist explanation of social problems (Best 1989; Spector and Kitsuse 1977). Our approach to social constructionism also borrows from Latour's (1987) notion of "science-in-action," which views the production of scientific facts as the result of mutually conceived actions by scientists in the workaday life in the laboratory, combined with both scientists' efforts to promote their work and the impacts of nonhuman actors such as molecules, apparati, and technologies. We also draw on the stages involved in the social construction of diagnosis and illness—identification and diagnosis (the social discovery of disease), the experience of illness, treatment, and outcomes (Brown 1995). Finally, our approach to constructionism borrows from the framing perspective of social movement theorists (Gamson et al. 1982; Snow et al. 1986). For example, we focus on veterans' attempts to frame their illnesses as both a result of service in the war and as sufficiently serious to warrant treatment. We also use the framing perspective to examine the media's interaction with the DEP.

Though the media are categorized under the "private sector" heading in Figure 11.1, they play a unique role as a battleground on which the DEP is contested. As a result, we examine the media's framing of GWRIs in order to determine its role in the construction of the DEP. We also emphasize the media's proclivity for monocausal explanations to social problems (Spencer and Triche 1994; Stallings 1990), the simplification and noncritical acceptance of science (Nelkin 1995), and the framing of issues in a manner that maximizes personal relevance to the media sources' consumers (Seydlitz, Spencer, and Lundskow 1994; Spencer and Triche 1994). Finally, we also draw on Downs' (1972) classic discussion of the issue attention cycle in which media coverage of a topic passes through five stages: the pre-problem stage, alarmed discovery and euphoric enthusiasm, realization of the cost of significant progress, gradual decline of intense public interest, and the post-problem stage. Building upon Downs' notion of an attention cycle and Stallings' critique of the media's coverage of risk, we argue that the media's coverage of GWRIs reflects a cycle which eventually moves away from a focus on disease etiology to a focus on the presence and extent of chemical exposures in the Gulf.

The Government's Role in Following the Molecule

The "government" component of the DEP includes the activities of government agencies and politicians, testimonies in legislatures and courts, research conducted by government agencies, and the government's funding of extramural research. The role played by government agencies in hindering attempts to follow the molecules at the source of GWRIs is best illustrated by the Department of Defense (DOD). Although Pentagon personnel were aware of the possibility of chemical exposures in the Gulf, as demonstrated by predeployment vaccinations and instructions given to soldiers in the event of chemical or biological weapon presence, the DOD was not adequately prepared to handle exposure information or exposure outcomes. The government's lack of preparedness has inhibited a timely and orderly response and, as we will discuss later, left scientists with insufficient and inadequate data. In terms of Figure 11.1, preexposure DOD policies specifically resulted in inadequate data on types of exposures, place and time of exposures, and predeployment health.

Missing Information

A significant barrier to following the chemical molecules coursing through the bodies of veterans is the paucity of data tracking who was where at what time, and what exposures may have occurred. Whether or not this information exists and/or is being concealed remains to be determined. Veteran activists and researchers we spoke with all identified the denials and disputes over exposures as one of the major barriers. One veteran remarked that, "From a political standpoint the biggest job for us is getting the government to recognize the findings that they don't want to hear about." For example, concerning the very tardy public disclosure about the demolition of a nerve gas depot at Khamisiyah, the Pentagon said that no exposures occurred, thereby denying veterans and researchers information vital to the investigation of Gulf War illnesses—and, in fact, denying that there were molecules to be followed.

When the President's Advisory Committee (PAC) asked the Pentagon to turn over the extensive logs of exposure data from the Gulf, the Defense Department was only able to locate thirty-six of an estimated two hundred pages (Shenon 1997). Whether or not the missing logs are part of a larger Pentagon cover-up, the lost information spells serious problems both for researchers and veterans. Without exposure data, researchers are left to hypothesize blindly about what combinations of chemicals veterans might have been exposed to. This is a significant limitation, both slowing the research process and casting doubt on the validity of any findings. Furthermore, as we will discuss later, the rumors of a government cover-up spread rapidly, drawing the media coverage away from the issues of the veterans' illnesses.

Insufficient pre- and postdeployment health data on exposed individuals have posed an additional obstruction. In the absence of this information, claims by the DOD that sick personnel must have been sick before they left, and counterclaims by veterans that they were not, simply cannot be investigated. Researchers are left with the arduous task of retrospectively determining predeployment health status. In lieu of medical records, scientists must rely on self-reported predeployment health, an approach typically criticized for its lack of reliability and validity. Finally, inadequate scientific understanding has limited the discovery of GWRIs. Emerging research suggests that pyridostigmine bromide, a nerve gas antidote which most soldiers received, may have penetrated the blood brain barrier under common conditions of heat stress. These and other findings concerning interaction effects illustrate how a lack of preexposure scientific understanding has made postdiscovery understanding of GWRIs more difficult.

Military Hierarchy and Miscommunication

The hierarchical military structure has appreciably affected the communication of information between parties. Tracing the path of molecules as they were released into the environment and absorbed by the bodies of soldiers in the Gulf requires disclosure of each marker on that path. However, the military hierarchy has impeded those communications, both during and after the military engagement. While in the Gulf, chemical weapons alarms sounded daily.

According to one interviewee who served as a ranking officer during the conflict, soldiers were trained to don gas masks upon hearing these alarms. Military commanders later told Congress that many were false alarms, as communicated by Defense Intelligence Agency and CIA officials. However, because that information was not sufficiently communicated down the chain of command, soldiers believed they were being exposed to lethal chemicals on multiple occasions. Though the stress resulting from the perception of multiple exposures lends support to the stress explanation, it does not rule out the possible interaction of stress and chemical exposures

Disputes among government agencies also revealed communication failures. Information dissemination about the destruction of the Khamisiyah munitions depot in Iraq is a case and point. After admission by the Pentagon that sarin gas shells may have been present in some bunkers, it was revealed that the military knew of their presence prior to the destruction. While the CIA claims they informed top DOD officials, the DOD denies any prior knowledge. That dispute aside, it is clear that soldiers who carried out the bombing were not aware of the potential hazard, even if they had a general awareness that the Iraqis had chemical weapons.

The bureaucratic and hierarchical nature of the military also discourages members from acknowledging the serious risks of military duty, openly discussing their illness, or blaming the military for its cause. Military culture is internalized in veterans, usually diminishing their willingness to become activists. Socialized to accept risks associated with war, and even receiving hazardous duty pay when chemical or biological weapons exposure is a possibility, many veterans are not concerned with the exposures. What upsets them is the military's refusal to recognize their illnesses and to provide adequate care. As one activist commented, "Health-wise you can't do anything about what the soldier was exposed to. I mean, that's what we got the hazardous duty pay for! But, you can do something about how we respond to it and the medical care programming steps that should be in place and have access to do something about."

Like the veterans of the Gulf War, Vietnam veterans, bound by honor and perhaps patriotism, defended the government on the grounds that risks had to be taken in war and that they accepted those risks when they enlisted.

Government Framing of Chronic Effects of Chemical Exposures

In addition to obfuscating the process of following the molecule, the government has continually acted to redefine the effects we should expect to see from the molecule. The government insists that chronic effects occur only if severe acute effects to exposures were documented in the Gulf. The government has maintained, despite some veteran protests to the contrary, that there were few, if any, acute health effects. By insisting that acute symptoms are a prerequisite to any long-term health effects, the government effectively establishes that veteran illnesses cannot be the result of chemical exposure in the Gulf, thereby discrediting their complaints. This also opens the door for explanations consistent with the stress-based DEP, while countering veterans' attempts to characterize their illnesses as environmentally induced.

The belief that acute illness must first be present to define chronic illness stems from both political resistance and from the lack of preexposure scientific understanding of the effects of the multiple chemicals and other substances to which veterans were exposed. In the case of Vietnam veterans, there was a narrow set of herbicides and their chemical components (with special emphasis on dioxin), and health effects of exposure were already known. Consequently, there was no question about which molecule to follow. Nevertheless it took twenty years for the government to recognize eight defined illnesses related to dioxin exposure, due to the political nature of the problem rather than the scientific aspects. This is additional evidence of the difficulties facing researchers investigating GWRIs. If government resistance prevented recognition of illnesses connected to Agent Orange, which were both horrific and highly publicized, it is conceivable that veterans afflicted with GWRIs face an even longer delay in compensation.

Conflicts between DOD and VA

Although the VA often failed to care adequately for Gulf War veterans, sympathetic clinicians faced obstacles due to DOD's denials of exposure. Health officials confronted with veterans' claims that their ill health was due to chemical exposures during their service in the Gulf sought confirmation from DOD officials. Since DOD's stance, until 1996, was that no chemical exposure had occurred, these health officials returned to the vets to tell them they were mistaken:

> There are a lot of smart people in the government with lots of abbreviations after their names from very prestigious schools, and they're very bright. And so when Gulf war veterans would say, "You know, I was exposed to sarin in the Gulf," the people at VA would very diligently follow up with the appropriate people in the Defense Department, and the Defense Department's line at that time was "there was no sarin in the Gulf." So VA would come back to the veterans and say "Sorry, Joe, you weren't exposed to sarin." And the veteran is looking at this person like they're crazy, and saying "wait a minute, I was in the Gulf, and you were never even a vet, no less in the Gulf. How could you possibly tell me what I was or wasn't exposed to?"

Research scientists we interviewed also pointed to examples of government hindrance in pursuit of the substances causing GWRIs. One researcher we interviewed illustrates the framing activities of government agencies in the following comment:

I actually think that DOD does a phenomenal public relations job . . . of shifting the blame from actions that they're probably involved with to being the VA's fault. I mean, if you look at the history of Agent Orange, you'd think that the VA caused rather than help[ed] to treat it in veterans. And if you look at Gulf War illnesses the whole first five years of this era were characterized by challenges to the VA's [not] doing enough to treat these veterans. Well, it would help if we could figure out what they are exposed to in order to prescribe the treatments. That was never said. So I think the VA actually had taken a leadership role and has produced great science, or as good as it can be.

As this interviewee points out, the various involved government agencies maneuver to present themselves as either less culpable for the causes of GWRIs, or less responsible for their treatment. In either case, their actions further hinder scientists', activists', and social analysts' attempts at following the molecules that might be at the root of GWRIs.

Science's Role in Following the Molecule

As actors involved in the construction of the DEP, scientists have various ways of influencing disease identification, definition, treatment and outcomes. Ideally, scientists aim to uncover the empirical reality that helps us understand the cause of an illness and thereby enables us to prevent and treat it. To do this, we would expect them to follow the molecule in order to see the location and action of potential disease-causing substances. But as the previous interviewee's comment demonstrates, scientists' work in uncovering empirical reality is always influenced by the biases of the scientific discipline and by the other human and nonhuman actors who transform the empirical reality into a complex social and political problem.

Scientific Specialization and Insularity

The missing information and miscommunication caused by the government is compounded by a lack of communication stemming from the structure of the scientific and medical communities. According to all the researchers we interviewed, there is no dialogue between the researchers performing studies on Gulf War illnesses and the physicians who are treating the veterans. When asked about the interaction between epidemiologists studying Gulf War illnesses and physicians treating them, one epidemiologist replied:

I know in the veterans' eyes it's a real issue. They have a lot of complaints about their medical treatment and their clinical care that they come and voice to us. But as a resource center we're not directly responsible for taking care of them clinically and so we, I tried to help and direct them into proper channels within the clinical care side of it, people that I know here. But there is a division or separation and so we could spend our whole life trying to clinically get them treated.

Consequently, when speaking with their patients, clinicians do not know what questions might provide clues to potential etiology or even those questions that might illuminate better modes of treatment. As a result, patients do not receive the best possible care, and information valuable to research efforts is not gathered.

Some insularity is partially caused by government procedures. For example, the VA funded several research centers to do dedicated work on GWRIs, yet did not provide ongoing channels of collaboration and discussion. Insularity is also caused by the privatized nature of much scientific research— researchers work in an environment of competition for funding and for findings. Consequently, efforts may overlap and funds are not allocated efficiently. The lack of coordination between parties (researchers, veterans, clinicians) further retards research results. Further, if research continues without many definitive findings, there will likely be a decline in funding and a decrease in research interest. Without that support, researchers might begin to focus on other interests. The fear that funding for GWRIs would dry up likely prevented many scientists from even getting involved with GWRI research, in addition to an original lack of interest on the part of many people. Others who did get involved, as was the case with one researcher we interviewed, had established research careers in other areas and could afford to gamble on GWRIs even if answers might never be found.[4]

A reluctance to cross disciplinary boundaries and to incorporate innovative methodologies into research designs also curtails findings. Scientists who attempt to work outside the accepted parameters of their discipline fear being discredited and risk the loss of funding. Researchers we interviewed often spoke of research group meetings in which epidemiologists debated with toxicologists or neurologists over which items should be included on questionnaires. Because there are so many exposures, there are many potential approaches, methods, and hypotheses, and no consensus on which should be pursued.

This issue of instrument design and question choice clearly indicates that there is no singularly "objective" science happening. In short, the 145 studies receiving federal funding at a total cost of $133.5 million between 1994 and 1999 have been conducted by scientists from such a broad array of disciplinary backgrounds and assumptions, that it is no surprise we still do not have a concise definition of GWRIs, much less an understanding of their etiology or how to treat them.

Single Syndrome or Multiple Diseases

Early in the social discovery of Gulf War–related illnesses, the notion of a single *Gulf War Syndrome* was a touchstone for gauging who was sympathetic to veterans' complaints. Veterans and a significant number of sympathetic scientists and physicians believed there was a single syndrome, while much government attention focused on disproving its existence. This single syndrome perspective stemmed from early impressions by veterans that their diverse complaints might be a single disease, as well as from the continuing belief among a small number of researchers that there is a single Gulf War Syndrome. When a set of odd symptoms occurs among a specific population, there is a tendency to believe that a new syndrome has been found. The identification of a syndrome helps the afflicted parties and the physicians who treat them by demarcating a mysterious occurrence of symptoms, and hopefully aiding in the pursuit of etiologic explanations. Although some researchers, sympathetic to the veterans claims, gave early support to the notion of a single syndrome, most no longer support the idea. Most now believe that there are diverse health effects stemming from assorted exposures. Yet with the small, lingering belief in one or several disease complexes, we even see disputes over both cause and illness definition among those researchers who are seen as advocates for veterans.

For example, in our interviews with researchers, many mentioned the research of epidemiologist Robert Haley at the University of Texas Southwestern Medical Center. Haley claims to have established an association between various chemical exposures and three symptom clusters. Haley and colleagues' (1997) three distinct syndromes include one characterized by thought, memory, and sleep difficulties; a second that includes confusion and imbalance as well as more severe thought problems; and a third comprised of sore joints and muscles and tingling or numbness in the hands and feet. Haley traces the syndromes, which are variants of organophosphate-induced delayed polyneuropathy (caused by cholinesterase-inhibiting chemicals), to the use of flea collars, insect repellant, and antinerve gas pills.

Though none of our interviewees spoke negatively of Haley, all who mentioned his work spoke skeptically of it. As one researcher explained to us, "I personally don't find Haley's work key. I think that [there are] so many doubts about his work that I don't think it's personally convincing, although it's certainly interesting [and] provocative on multiple exposures and a combination of exposures."

Researchers we interviewed also expressed skepticism of Haley's work because it is funded by a foundation run by Ross Perot, rather than mainstream scientific foundations employing peer review of grant proposals:

> The dilemma with foundations is you get into things . . . like Haley or
> Perot wanting to give money to a certain group because it's his pet

group. And that appears to give scientific credibility, and then there's a question of do they peer review it? . . . I guess that's the question, what's the level of review that would go on and isn't that important in a new area? In other words the rigor under which it's scrutinized.

It is important to note that while Haley's proposals may escape such official peer review, his articles are indeed published in major peer-reviewed journals. From Haley's point it may be quite reasonable to secure such funding, given the government's tendency to fund research that is not looking for environmental health effects. As one veteran activist explained to us:

Ross Perot got involved for the right reasons. He was contacted by sick Gulf War veterans and . . . he's always had a soft spot in his heart for people who serve in the military. . . . So he got involved for the right reasons. But where it sort of got off track was, these veterans had already made up their mind as to what made them sick, the ones that he met with. So he funded research to essentially validate their claims. . . . And you know other researchers collectively and in the aggregate just aren't really impressed with Bob Haley's work, his methods and his findings.

Debates surrounding Haley's work illustrate the process by which challenges to the DEP are countered. Haley, who challenges the DEP by denying that stress is the cause of GWRIs, is attacked by colleagues who see his methodology as flawed (Landrigan 1997; Gray et al. 1998). In an interesting exchange of letters to the editor of the *Journal of the American Medical Association*, (*JAMA*) Haley praised a study by Fukuda et al. (1998) for finding two of the three syndromes Haley and colleagues (1997) had identified, but criticized Fukuda's methodology as the reason for not confirming the third syndrome identified by Haley. Fukuda and his colleagues (Reeves et al. 1999, 329) replied by noting that "our study was never intended to replicate or confirm the findings of Haley et al. We are skeptical of his study findings and conclusions because of substantial study design flaws already described by others."

The exchange in this issue of *JAMA* also illustrates the ongoing debate over the role of stress. While Fukuda and his colleagues remain open to the possibility that stress is involved, they depict Haley as having a vested interest in denying any role for stress:

[W]e agree with Haley that our findings do not necessarily implicate a psychological basis for symptoms reported by Gulf War veterans. However, unlike Haley, we do not have a particular etiology to champion. Given the nature of war, it remains probable that psychological factors have an important contributing role in the development of unexplained symptoms in some personnel after all wars. (Reeves et al. 1999, 329)

The exchange of letters also depicts how researchers operate with disciplinary blinders by seeing other's work only as it relates to their own. For example, Hunt and Richardson (1999) responded to Fukuda et al.'s (1998) findings by noting the higher incidence of diarrhea found in veterans who exhibit signs of "multi-symptom illness" compared to those with no signs. They see this as evidence of post-traumatic stress disorder (PTSD) among veterans and cite studies finding that individuals with PTSD have increased rates of irritable bowel syndrome, and that individuals with irritable bowel syndrome have relatively high rates of trauma history and PTSD. These debates among scientists show how hard it is to follow molecules, given the debates on what molecules are present and what health effects they might have.

Obstacles to "Good" Science

As discussed in the previous section, one of the causes of disputes among researchers has to do with methods chosen by particular researchers. These debates have less to do with a given scientist's worth as a scientist, than with the obstacles all scientists investigating GWRIs face. Due to a lack of information from the government regarding predeployment health and exposures during deployment, many researchers have relied on self-reported exposures. The following exchange between Haley and an interviewer for the PBS program *Frontline,* which took place after the interviewer asked Haley about the problem of using subjects' reports of exposure (i.e., perceived exposure) as an actual measure of exposure, epitomizes this problem:

> Haley: Our evidence pretty strongly suggests that chemical weapon, the perception of chemical weapon exposure and interaction, synergistic interaction with pyridogstigmine bromide is a serious risk factor that needs to be explored. Whether there were actual exposures on the battlefield, the evaluation of all the evidence, the political evidence and the intelligence evidence is just so far beyond my expertise I really just couldn't comment on it.
>
> Interviewer: But isn't that the point. There's a difference between perception of a toxic exposure and the toxic exposure?
>
> Haley: We have a very high relative risk, which is a number indicating how strong the association is, with the perception of chemical exposure, synergistic effect with pyridogstigmine bromide which is a very dramatic finding epidemiologically. How that squares with intelligence information is somebody else's call.
>
> Interviewer: But perception of a toxic exposure is not the same as actual toxic exposure. Correct?

Haley: That's correct. Yes. But what you do have to worry is the plausibility of an eyewitness testimony versus the plausibility of intelligence information, and again, that's just out of my area of expertise.

In addition, scientists must choose whether to involve veterans solely as subjects in their research, or as consultants in the development and implementation of research methods. Though "community advisory boards" are now required in all VA-funded studies, some scientists and officials believe that too much veteran involvement in the research process results in a loss of "objectivity." From that perspective, the work of scientists who take on a very pro-veteran point of view and who engage with lay people as coparticipants in the research process may be discredited. Much of the scientific community assumes that involving laypeople in the research process means lowering one's standards of proof or somehow compromising the practice of good science. Researchers who choose to embrace community action models and popular epidemiological methods are therefore subjected to greater scrutiny. A lay advocate we interviewed even suggested that research funding might have been cut to some studies due to lay involvement.

In the quest for legitimacy, scientists are expected to produce results that can be confirmed by their peers and recognized publicly. Yet, many sympathetic scientists doubt whether they will ever uncover environmental causes of GWRIs. This is a barrier to legitimacy and to attracting new researchers to this research area. Researchers' institutional requirements, such as tenure and the need to provide part of their salary through grants, may influence their willingness to study a controversial topic with little promise of great breakthroughs such as GWRIs. This is consistent with the comments of one researcher who surmised that GWRIs do not draw a lot of interest among scientists because they lack the glamour of AIDS or cancer research, for which one would be immortalized for finding a cure.

The institutional and other barriers described previously only add to the difficulty of following the molecules in an already highly complex situation of multiple exposures and multiple symptoms. Trained to specialize in highly unique areas of research, many scientists see Gulf War illnesses from within a very limited framework of understanding. Yet the complexity of GWRIs calls for interdisciplinary collaboration and perhaps even new paradigms. One interviewee stated plainly that she felt there would never be a comprehensive understanding of the causes of GWRIs. As her statement indicates, this is due, in part, to the complexity of the exposures that took place:

> I think there are commonalties, but we are never going to get the exposure models down because I think the exposures are too diverse. I mean, I've just never seen a public health study where you could have possibly multiple exposures. Are there? I don't know. I don't know that there were in the Gulf either but I don't know how you'd prove that there weren't.

Another researcher we interviewed also spoke of the complexity as an obstacle:

> What happens to people who engage in a military conflict when they're removed from their homes, when they witness great horrors, and when you throw into it, from our perspective, some environmental factors? And that's sort of what's interesting. . . . We study things in the way that we know them and the way we're most comfortable. So we're forced to in a way [to] reduce these things to ways we understand and know and know how to deal with. You know, war, like any other social experience, is very complex and it's hard to deal with complexity in a fashion that we're familiar with.

The Media's Role in Following the Molecule

Mainstream media tend to follow a clear set of criteria in determining what is newsworthy. According to Ryan (1991, 95), the story must include "emphasis on events/action, conflict with a possible resolution, strong emotions, identifiable characters, famous faces or powerful institutions, [and] clear impact." We examine how the media frame the story of GWRIs in order to meet these criteria by examining three types of print media: newspapers (*New York Times* and the *Washington Post*), newsweeklies (*Newsweek*, *Time*, and *U.S. News and World Report*) and science magazines (*Science*, *Science News*, *Popular Science* and *Discover*). We collected a total of 180 articles published between 1992 and 1998. Our coding categories were constructed through reading a subset of the total number of articles and identifying recurring themes. We analyzed the data both quantitatively (to determine the frequency and percentage of stories on the Gulf War that discussed environmental causation) and qualitatively (to examine the specific themes).

Our analysis finds that media coverage of Gulf War–related illnesses initially centered on human interest stories. The strong emotions and heartbreaking stories of once healthy soldiers returning from the war feeble and debilitated provided compelling news stories, but ultimately the story could not survive based on these images alone. According to Ryan's (1991) criteria for news stories, an enemy was needed—especially a powerful institution with identifiable characters or famous faces. The government served this function well. Revelations about DOD's withholding of chemical exposure information from the troops enabled the media's transition to a conspiracy frame. This frame, although captivating public interest, resulted in less attention to the sick veterans and to the ongoing scientific research aimed at understanding the veterans' illnesses. In addition, disputes within the scientific community created the atmosphere of unresolved conflict, a media formula for the death of an issue. Our coding of the foci of media stories reveals this shift in coverage (see Figure 11.2).

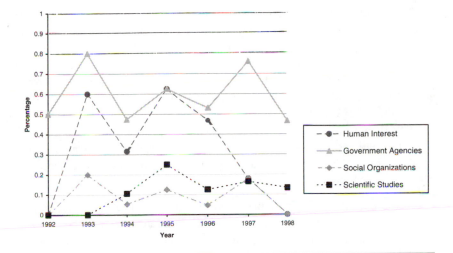

Figure 11.2 Percentages of Gulf War articles dealing with four major categories of concern, 1992–1998

Headlines from the first two years of the GWRI controversy demonstrate the media's attention to the plight of sick veterans and the mystery behind their illnesses: "Gulf Troops Ills Bewilder Doctors" (*NYT*, November 11, 1993); "Triumphant in the Desert, Stricken at Home" (*WP*, July 24, 1994). At the same time, however, *Post* and *Times* headlines reveal the media's skepticism towards GWRIs and evenhanded coverage of early reports failing to find links between GWRIs and chemical exposures: "Scientists Say Evidence Lacking to Tie 'Syndrome' to 1991 Gulf War" (WP, October 10, 1996); "NIH Panel Unable to Pinpoint Cause of Gulf War Syndrome" (*WP*, April 30, 1994); "No Evidence of Gulf Disease, Study Says" (*NYT*, August 1995).

By 1996, however, when the Pentagon admitted some troops were, in fact, exposed to chemical weapons at Khamisiyah, and the science angle on the story had failed to produce a resolution, political coverage mounted. In the *Times*, especially, but also in the *Post*, this led to a shift in story focus. Fall and Winter headlines in 1996 reflect this shift: "Pentagon Health Chief Fights Claims of A Gulf War Cover-Up" (*NYT*, November 3, 1996); "Knowledge of Poison Gas in Gulf War Unlikely to Have Altered Treatment" (*WP*, December 12, 1996); "Data Lacking on Nerve Gas Evidence" (*WP*, December 21, 1996); "Powell Says He Had No Evidence of Toxic Chemicals in Gulf War" (*NYT*, December 3, 1996); "Schwarzkopf Says He Doubts That Chemicals Caused Illnesses" (*NYT*, December 6, 1996). These last two articles also demonstrate how by shifting to the political controversy over whether exposures occurred or not, the media was able to introduce the famous names—an essential criterion of mainstream media stories—of high-ranking military and government officials.

Our findings suggest that media focus on the political elements more than the medical-scientific issues. The distinction between medical and political coverage is most salient in the *Post* and *Times*. David Brown, a physician and reporter for the *Post*, wrote twenty-three of the *Post*'s fifty-nine articles on GWRIs. In the *Times*, on the other hand, Philip Shenon, a Washington correspondent who did not even begin covering GWRIs until 1996, wrote thirty-five of the eighty articles on GWRIs.

This dichotomy in type of coverage is captured in the comments made by David Brown and a *Times* reporter, Andrew Rosenthal, who appeared on the PBS program "Media Matters" (June 13, 1997). Brown, for example, criticized the use of the human interest angle:

Anecdotal reporting is extremely useful in all reporting, because it lends a vividness, a sort of humanness to otherwise abstract subjects. And that's particularly true in medicine. In some of the Gulf War reporting, there was an over-reliance on the validity of the stories of some of the veterans who were reporting illness.

Rosenthal's perspective, on the other hand, seems aimed at justifying the *Times*' emphasis on the political side of the story:

We discovered that there were so many things that we weren't being told; that we had stumbled onto a classic story in which a government agency had made a policy decision that something had or had not happened, without ever even looking at this. And it was just sort of the textbook case of what a newspaper is supposed to do in covering the government. . . . The people who claimed that they had a syndrome resulting from this exposure had no way to have their claim heard, because the government had decided that they were wrong, that they hadn't been exposed, and that the exposure was not relevant to their health problems. So our mission was to focus on the questions of what the government had known, rather than on the end result.

Brown countered Rosenthal's rationalization by adding that "the question about how truthful and how forthcoming the Department of Defense was over the years is a perfectly valid story, and it's an interesting story, and it's an important story. But it just has very little to say about the biological plausibility of various causes of Gulf War Syndrome."

We found media to be an important battlefield on which veterans, the government, and scientists fought over the definition of the DEP. At first the media showed little concern for scientists' attempts to follow the molecules at the root of GWRIs. Later, the inability of scientists to follow the molecule to a definitive explanation made its way into the news before giving way to the conspiracy frame focusing on a government cover-up. Once the political conspiracy frame ran its course, reporters had no interest in covering the inconclusive findings of scientists. After all, the medical science frame for GWRIs failed to offer readers a conflict that had the promise of a resolution, a feature that is one of the mainstream media's fundamental criteria for a good story (Ryan 1991). As a result, according to our interviews, scientists felt their work was never covered adequately by the media, and veterans who felt at first allied with the media later felt abandoned. As well, the government, though its stress-based DEP was never heavily covered by the media, was largely un-scathed from media conspiracy frames when general interest in the story waned.

Activist's Role in Following the Molecule

Veteran activists played important roles, both positively and negatively, in bringing to the government and the public's attention the plight of sick veter-ans who had served in the Gulf. Our interviews suggest that both veterans and researchers felt veteran activism was instrumental in getting the government to acknowledge that veterans were sick and that investigations into the causes needed to take place. One researcher reported:

> That's really what got this thing up and running in the first place was the veterans groups and individual veterans with incredible stories to tell that became public news stories. I would say that without that you wouldn't be getting any of this, you know, the Gulf War related illness work. Wouldn't have done any of this and wouldn't still be doing it.

Another researcher shared similar sentiments:

> I think they've [veterans] had the critical role, I mean the key role. I still think back to when I went to this meeting . . . and there was a panel of GW veterans, some of them with unusual illnesses, who provided very emotional, compelling, and scientific testimony about what happened to them. And I think that that type of involvement and intervention really helped push the agenda . . . I think they were very successful and had it not been for them who knows what would have happened.

Veteran activists worked to frame GWRIs in a way that would be beneficial to sick veterans. One veteran activist, after emphasizing the importance of con-ducting good science, admitted:

> I'd go up to Capitol Hill and say, "yeah we don't know but we're going to have to make a number of assumptions. We're going to have to assume they were in perfect health before they went to the Gulf and that if the population itself is reporting poor health at a greater rate than matched controls, then it was the Gulf." And there's a method to the madness. If there's no nexus between Gulf War service and veterans current health status, the government's not obligated to pay any compensation. The

government's not obligated to treat them for their illnesses. And so our critical role was to try to establish a nexus. So we'd take sometimes shreds of evidence, the little drips and drops of evidence from the science, we'd make more of it than there was there. A lot like lawyers do in court cases. You make the most of what you've got with the evidence.

On the other hand, veteran activists may have also hindered their cause, as explained to us by the same veteran quoted above, who worked for a mainstream veteran service organization:

Where we haven't done a good job I think is when we try to be scientists, or we try to overanalyze the science. The smaller groups, the individuals or the dozens of people in groups have played a very detrimental role because they were so flamboyant and extreme they typically got the sound bites on television and radio and newspapers. Reporters were attracted to them because they had a more compelling story to tell than I did. . . . I was always trying to weigh the science versus what we wanted. I always found that made me more legitimate on Capitol Hill. Our agenda, what we wanted done on Capitol Hill, typically got done. But the media was reporting what these extremists were saying. And some of them were saying that Gulf War syndrome was an infectious disease and that there was an epidemic of birth defects. They frightened the Gulf War veterans population and they told an inaccurate story.

To the extent that some veterans and their activist organizations exaggerated or manipulated scientific findings, they damaged their own reputations. On the other hand, it is the very power of the DEP that leads activists to see science as an authoritative voice that can be used to their advantage. They may have felt that there was no other path than to use arguments based on their understanding of science. But the inconclusive nature of most Gulf War research has hampered their efforts.

Many of the researchers we interviewed provided examples of the ways in which veterans have privileged information about their own exposures and illnesses that can be used in health research. Veterans firmly believe that their knowledge is crucial to understanding the cause of GWRIs, and that they therefore should be brought into the research, treatment, and policy processes. They are aware that their continued action has indeed prompted scientists to look into self-reports of symptoms and exposures. Veterans have also pushed federal and nonfederal researchers to conduct studies on issues they believe are important but which are downplayed, such as the oil well fires and depleted uranium. In addition, veterans' criticism of the dominant stress approach plays an important role in ongoing discussions with the research community. Many initiatives have been made to avoid exposures in future conflicts and provide services more effectively to those exposed in future conflicts. As in other forms of popular epidemiology, affected people have clear ideas of problems and the potential causes, and they press their agenda. Involving lay people can sometimes be a liability in the quest for legitimacy. Nevertheless, in the long run such lay input is crucial to pushing government and science to expand their approaches.

Conclusion

In the process of transforming the problems of Gulf War veterans from a personal trouble into a social problem, much is at stake. This process involves opposition to the dominant epidemiological paradigm, a generally accepted belief system about the existence and causes of disease. The DEP is both a fact and a process, and is subject to ongoing change. But the prevailing systems of scientific, governmental, and military power make it difficult to successfully challenge this DEP. In the case of Gulf War–related illnesses, veterans have been only partially successful at such a challenge. Their efforts at creating a citizen-science alliance have been less well developed in GWRIs than in other contested environmental illnesses, such as breast cancer. While veterans have achieved success in expanding treatment eligibility, they have not fared well in guiding research towards environmental causation. It is possible, though, that veterans' opposition to the stress paradigm has helped spark greater research attention to interactions of stress and toxins, and has legitimated their complaints of physical symptoms. Nor have researchers been that successful in transforming personal troubles into a social problem. Most research has failed to turn up evidence of environmental causation, most notably seen in the recent Institute of Medicine (2000) report. As well, researchers sympathetic to veterans have been unable to generate significant support for veterans as a legitimate group of sufferers. There has, however, been a positive development in the various initiatives to avoid exposures in future conflicts and provide services more effectively to those exposed in future wars. In the last several years, GIs have resisted anthrax vaccinations, and the military has adopted a more cautious and restricted program as a result.

The federal government and the dominant scientific and health establishments have succeeded in withholding information, in preventing the acceptance of environmental causation, and in strengthening their stress paradigm. Perhaps their only concessions have been the pursuit of some research on stress/environmental interactions, and the recognition of the need for predeployment health status reports in future military operations.

A stronger citizen-science alliance would likely lead to a change in the dominant epidemiological paradigm that would be more beneficial to veterans. But such an alliance is not supported by the state, since the state itself is the subject of the controversy. Other federal agencies are presently supporting projects that have some form of a citizen-science alliance. The DOD's breast cancer research program is one example. DOD's involvement stemmed from concern that the Republican capture of Congress in 1994 would result in massive cutbacks in NCI funding. Senator Tom Harkin (D-Iowa) led a successful effort to place considerable funding in the DOD, where cuts seemed less likely. This is primarily nonmilitary research, and it is understandable that the DOD would hesitate to fund research that implicated military chemical usage and breast cancer, especially if GIs exhibited higher cancer rates. CDC, NIEHS, and EPA support university-community partnerships to study and treat asthma, in which lay involvement is very substantial. Since asthma is such a major public health concern, and since the scientific data on air pollution as an asthma trigger is so strong, such public involvement is easier to develop. And unlike GWRIs, there is no threat to military security. Scientists also need to favor a citizen-science alliance, and many scientists studying GWRIs were in the military or the VA, making it hard for them to support an alliance with people who were challenging them. Contrast this with citizen-science alliances on asthma, where laypeople do not find themselves challenging scientists for the most part. The involved laypeople also have to be prepared to fight for a citizen-science alliance. This was less possible with the fragmented veterans movement than with the very powerful environmental justice movement that has made asthma a key issue for organizing.

It is also interesting to ponder how the stigmatizing effect of Gulf War illnesses gets in the way of appropriate research. The Gulf War was a glorious technological feat, a war conducted at a distance with hardly any casualties among U.S. forces, and the presence of many sick veterans would tarnish that vision. The GI's body is simultaneously also the "body politic" in that the soldiers' bodies represent the body of the nation. If the soldiers are sick, then the whole national effort appears less healthy. Other toxic waste contamination episodes may challenge corporations and governmental units, leading to frequent official resistance to searching for environmental causation. But there are few other situations where the whole nation is implicated. This was true with the "atomic veterans" deliberately and accidentally exposed to radiation, and with the Vietnam veterans suffering from Agent Orange exposure. There, too, we saw similar official opposition to dealing with both treatment and research on environmental causation, despite even clearer evidence and a stronger research base.

We are left with a mystery of why so many men and women who served in the Gulf War had so much illness. As with many other environmentally induced diseases, the answers have been thwarted by multiple exposures, incomplete and withheld data, political opposition, and scientific caution. While further scientific advances may help pursue environmental causation in the future, we remain convinced that the political issues of military hierarchy, secrecy, and unwillingness to admit mistakes are central to the outcome. It has not been easy for scientists, epidemiologists, and others to follow the molecule. This would be hard enough anyway, but when people face political and bureaucratic barriers, they never get sufficiently to the biological basis of the molecule itself.

12

The Chemistry of Sovietization
Industrial Solvents and Nationalist Reactions in 1960s Lithuania

DIANA MINCYTE

On a sunny morning of March 21, 1959, a row of fifty heavily loaded trucks slowly started down a steaming fresh asphalt road. Carrying tons of white bricks, wooden beams and metal frames, bags of concrete, and ready-made blocks, the trucks spilled into the remote outskirts of Kedainiai where four ancient Lithuanian villages had just been leveled. The radio incessantly transmitted enthusiastic speeches and marching tunes to entertain helmeted workers moving to their new site, the Kedainiai Chemical plant. For those who were born here, the sound emanating from the distant compound was an ominous sign of the new Soviet regime.

The Kedainiai chemical plant, now "Lifosa," was conceived by a common effort of the USSR Academy of Science, the GIPROKHIM (the Planning Institute for the Chemical Industry), the Lithuanian Board of the Chemical Industry, the Communist Party of the Soviet Republic of Lithuania, and a number of local and Moscow bureaucrats and functionaries. The construction started in 1959 and was finished in 1962.[1] The first ton of sulfuric acid was produced on a memorably freezing cold morning, January 17, 1963, which became known as the official birthday of the Lithuanian chemical industry (Kitriene and Spudulis 1996, 15).

As the Soviet leaders proclaimed, the Kedainiai plant was the first and most substantial step in the industrialization of the primarily agricultural Lithuania, and thus, the country's conversion into socialism (Skupeika 1971, 97). The foundation and the development of this chemical plant was perceived as a strategic move towards freeing the local population from the "shackles" of private property, radical nationalism, and the backward petite bourgeoisie lifestyles of the capitalist system. The Kedainiai chemical plant was to become an agent of the Sovietization of the Lithuanian population.

The idea that science, technology, and industry can be the tools of domination and imperialism is neither surprising nor new.[2] Gyan Prakash, for example, demonstrates that science and local industries served the interests of the

British imperial state by "forging India into a productive, interlocking network of irrigation works, railways, telegraphs, mines, [and] manufacturing" (Prakash 1999, 160). Specific industrial enterprises, communication technologies, and new infrastructures were deeply enmeshed in the re-manufacturing of India. As a result, India was reorganized into a productive colony, or a Heideggerian "standing reserve,"[3] and was rendered as always available and completely manipulable by British imperialists.

In a way similar to the English colonists, Soviet leaders recognized and employed the hegemonizing powers of industrialization. After the death of Joseph Stalin, the Khrushchevian Politburo "softened" its internal policies by moving from active genocide and military suppression of resistance to more elegant and convincing ways to achieve stability and hegemony within the Soviet state (Hill 1987). In the mid-1950s the Soviet leaders launched a new ideological project called the scientific-technological revolution.[4] This revolution rested on the proposition that scientific-technological progress would generate "a major set of advances in 'technique' . . . that transform production forces" (Hoffman and Laird 1985, 11).[5] Such a revolution, the Soviet leaders predicted, would be followed by a transformation in the larger social systems, that would lead toward the desired elimination of the souvenirs of the capitalist mode of production (Fortescue 1986, 20; Savinskij 1972, 12). Even though the scientific-technological revolution was conceived by the cyberneticians and engineers at Moscow's Institute of the History of the Natural Sciences and Technique, who were careful about not making a direct causal correlation between the social order and industrialization, the Soviet government disregarded their further suggestions and consolidated investments in the industrialization of its new "Republics" in the hope of transforming those nationalistic populations into docile citizens.[6]

In Lithuania, the project of chemicalization launched by the Communist Party plenum in May 1958 constituted the essence of industrialization and seemed ideal for the purpose of manufacturing popular consent among the local population (Sumauskas 1963). There are two reasons why chemicalization was expected to be so effective in taming the new Soviet Republic. First, chemicalization was nested within the framework of the scientific-technological revolution that required the elimination of manual labor and replaced "man's direct participation in the production processes by the functioning of his materialized knowledge" (Hoffman and Laird 1985, 8). Chemistry, as one of the most advanced "materialized sciences" at the time, was indeed a sharp turn from backbreaking physical and manual labor to the supervision and control of the chemical processes. Unlike other traditional manufactures such as textile, food processing, construction, or even metallurgy, the chemical industry rested on conceptually different epistemological and ontological grounds. To produce chemicals no longer required man's physical labor, but scientific knowledge and practice (Skupeika 1971, 93). In other words, the chemical industry, as a driving force of the scientific-technological revolution, could take a leap into a qualitatively new mode of production and, by doing so, to fabricate the new social order, of Communism, in Lithuania.

Second, the chemical plant and its products were expected to play a crucial role in the structural-demographic reorganization of the Lithuanian economy. With the application of fertilizers and their concentrates in the local farms, the efficiency of the land was planned to quadruple within five years following the building of the plant (Skupeika 1971). This immediate augmentation of the land's efficiency had to resolve not only the shortage of food in the Soviet Union, but more importantly, was designed to foster a surplus labor force in the rural areas that could then be employed in the growing industrial cities. Since the working class was the heart of the Socialist system, the augmentation of the Lithuanian working class meant the fortification of the Soviet system in the region (Januskevicius 1971). In other words, the chemicals produced at the Kedainiai chemical plant were planned to fertilize the growth of the grain crops as well as *Homo Soveticus*.

Located at the center of the country, approximately 80 miles northwest of Vilnius, Kedainiai was the site of two major rebellions against the Russian Imperial occupation of the Baltics, in 1831 and 1863. According to the archival data, Kedainiai was first mentioned in the correspondence in 1372. Built on the strategically convenient banks of the river Nevezis, Kedainiai was one of the major economic and cultural centers of the Lithuanian Duchess throughout the Middle-ages. In the seventeenth and eighteenth centuries, Kedainiai flourished as an administrative center of the Duke Radvila, which left its mark on the local identity. Its decline started with the war with Sweden when the city suffered immensely in the battles of 1655. The old wooden city was lost in a series of fires from 1774–1781. Prior to falling under Soviet control in August of 1944, Kedainiai was dependent upon the agricultural economy generated by the surrounding farms and villages. By 1974, its population had reached 24,500 (*Lietuviskoji Tarybine Enciklopedija* 1985, 420) and it is still renowned for its cucumbers.

In order to investigate how the Kedainiai chemicals carried out the Soviet plans in Kedainiai and Lithuania in general, it is necessary to take a nontraditional sociological approach that allows us to follow the chain reactions in the real world. This study is, therefore, based on a posthumanist approach that is specifically concerned with tracing the actions of nonhuman agents and their participation in large-scale political projects (Latour 1999; Haraway 1985; Stengers 1997). This posthumanist perspective will engage multiple, self-organizing, and oftentimes confusing developments in the geographic, technological, economic, and political spheres of life that are borne in interactions among chemicals, grains, tractors, cities, humans, and social institutions. Told from this perspective, the history of the Kedainiai chemical plant becomes a product of anthropo-material autocatalysis, what Latour calls a "sociotechnical imbroglio," and a story of connections (Latour 1999). By following the chemical traces, we begin to see the outline of complex socio-industrial systems that constituted the lifeworld of the 1960s in Lithuania.

This chapter explores three specific aspects of Soviet chemicalization in Lithuania. First, I highlight changes in the local landscape and trace the actual physical transformations brought about by the chemical plant, seen as a "success" story. Next, I examine how the chemicals affected the economy—contaminating the integrity of Soviet ideology with capitalist ideologies. Third, I contrast the disembodied and alien Soviet chemistry with embodied nationalist ideologies. In concluding, I show that the chemicalization of Lithuania did indeed bring about some of the intended changes in the socio-geographic structures of the region, but at the same time, the chemicals ran amok and turned against the Soviet regime by contributing to the growing nationalist resistance movements and by spreading consumerist mentalities. This essay thus pushes for an innovative posthumanist ontology that perceives human bodies, machines, imaginations, nature, and economy as an unstable assemblage interacting among themselves and producing fascinating new systems and structures.[7]

The Socio-Geographical Dislocation and Reconstitution of the Kedainiai Area

By 1970, the Kedainiai chemical plant had become one of the largest and most successful enterprises in Soviet Lithuania. In the 1960s, the Kedainiai Chemical plant alone contributed an average of 19 percent of the gross gain of the Lithuanian GNP. By 1965, after the installation of the third set of sulfuric oxidation furnaces, the Kedainiai chemical plant became the main producer of sulfuric acid in the Northwestern region of the Soviet Union. Locally, sulfuric acid was needed for the production of fertilizers, especially for processing phosphate into superphosphate. Within the first two years of operation, the production of granulated superphosphate (18.5 percent P_2O_5) at the Kedainiai plant reached 575,000 tons/year. In addition, the plant manufactured powdered superphosphate (19.5 percent P_2O_5) with a capacity of 200,000 tons/year. Both forms of superphosphate were used as a concentrate for the production of phosphor fertilizer, one of the most effective fertilizers for crops and vegetables. In 1969, the plant started the production of 100 percent amophosphate, another crucial chemical used as a mineral fertilizer, and a mix of mineral fertilizers P:K (14 percent P_2O_5: 14 percent K_2O) (Kitriene and Spudulis 1996). These new mineral fertilizers proved to effectively alleviate natural deficiencies of the soil and to supply the necessary primary nutrients for cultivation.

To sustain a successful operation of this large-scale chemical production, it was necessary to reorganize local infrastructures according to the plant's needs. Even prior to the construction of the plant in 1959, the state funded the improvement of local roads, freeways, and the construction of a transportation artery connecting the plant to downtown Kedainiai with a bridge over the river Obele. In addition, the plant requested the building of a canal between the Nevezis and the Sventoji rivers to ensure an abundant water supply. Finally, to transport raw materials and fertilizers to and from the farthest reaches of the Soviet Union it was necessary to ensure the growth and maintenance of national railroads, and to connect the plants to this network.

In contrast to other roads that were historically embedded in the local landscape, the new roads in the Kedainiai area were designed to serve the objectives posed by the fertilizers' market rather than to guarantee the functioning of traditional social and economic relations. In 1967, the roads connecting the chemical plant to the rest of Lithuania had to carry over 500,000 tons of powdered and granulated superphosphate and sulfuric acid. The distribution of these chemicals became a crucial agent in reorganizing the existing system of local transportation by rerouting the flows of traffic from small towns and villages to the industrial centers (Januskevicius and Miliuniene 1971, 88). As a result of this process of rerouting, the total milage of the roads in Lithuania was actually reduced from 40,200 km in 1950 to 33,200 km in 1965 (*Mazoji Lietuviskoji Tarybine Enciklopedija* 1971, 118). This was due to the fact that the Soviet state chose not to develop many of the local roads. Only those roads that were most efficient and connected to major industrial developments remained on the map. In such a manner, small towns that still maintained their cultural and social vitality among the local population, such as Vosyliskis and Silai, lost their connectivity to the outside world during the Soviet era and, thus, any aspirations for their future (Januskevicius and Miliuniene 1971). In addition, these new roads cut through previously impermeable parcels of private land. The new road from downtown Kedainiai to the chemical plant further disrespected historical landmarks and acclaimed the victory of rationalized and scientific thought over local history. This project of reorganizing the transportation infrastructure, thus, reestablished the presence of a new spatial regime in the region.

The water supply was crucial for the production of superphosphate and phosphoric acid and especially for sulfuric acid. Even though the Kedainiai chemical plant had installed modern contact sulfur oxidation furnaces, it still required large amounts of water to cool down the hot sulfur trioxide gas pipes leaving the three contact furnaces. The contact process yielded high-percent oleum, which also required an additional source of water to bring it to the desired concentration. The closest source of water for Kedainiai was the Nevezis, but this river tended to run almost dry during droughts and late summer. Therefore, to guarantee a consistent water supply to the Nevezis, a dam and a canal were undertaken even before the plant was finished. The new canal was 12 km long and became the most publicized and celebrated project of local water basin reconstruction during the 1960s. The draining of one of the largest rivers in the country directly affected the inhabitants of the Lithuanian towns and cities that were located on the banks of the Sventoji. Once used for transportation and local entertainment industries, the Sventoji now sank almost 3 feet and could no longer be used by larger boats. This change in the water level of the Sventoji also disrupted the ecological system of the Sventoji by slowing down water flow, which resulted in overgrowth of underwater plants.

The expanding networks of railroads were the material arteries that incorporated Lithuania as a territorial unit into the web of economic, social, and political relations of the Soviet Union. For example, for the production of superphosphate, the high-quality radiation-free phosphate rock was extracted in the "Apatite" mines in Kirovsk located in the Kola peninsula (Sagers and Shabad 1990). The railroads connecting Kedainiai with the northern parts of the Russian Federation were vital for this raw material to arrive at its destination in Kedainiai. To neutralize the leftover phosphoric acid from the production of the powdered superphosphate, the plant imported phosphorites from Estonia. The sulfur, as a raw material for the sulfuric acid, traveled all the way from the Razdol Combine, in the Ukraine (Skupeika 1971, 100).

Like the raw materials consumed at the plant, the fertilizers produced there were exported to Belorussia, Latvia, Estonia, and, in later years, to the Ukraine, the Russian Federation, and even Poland (Sagers and Shabad 1990). In 1970, only slightly more than half of the fertilizer products were used by local agriculture, the remaining half was transported to the Soviet breadbasket, the southwestern regions of the Soviet Union, to cultivate crops there. The production of these mineral fertilizers at the Kedainiai chemical plant shaped not only the local socio-geographical landscape by eliminating local roads and building new freeways, but also enhanced communication between Lithuania and the rest of the Soviet Union and boosted partnerships between their industries. The massive trucks and railroad cars carrying fertilizer granules from Kedainiai and mineral rock from the north transgressed all of the former borders between nations.

The most profound and irreversible transformation of the Lithuanian socio-geographic landscape, however, was achieved through the application of fertilizers in local agriculture. The use of superphosphate, and later amophosphate, on the fields considerably increased the productivity of the grain crops grown in Lithuania. For example, after the application of mineral fertilizers beginning in 1965, the annual gross grain yield for the period from 1966 through 1970 grew by over 70 percent when compared to the years 1961 through 1965. Forty percent of this increase was a result of the use of mineral fertilizers while the rest was attributed to the selection of seeds and soil, planting and watering technologies, and the efficiency of mechanized harvesting equipment. In other words, a ton of fertilizer "translated" into an extra 2.7 tons of grain (Lietuvos CSV 1966). This enormous growth in the agricultural production rates of Lithuania "freed" farmers from their jobs and inevitably forced them to move to the city in search of new work (Lietuvos TSR CSV 1965). For example, the application of the superphosphate in the Kedainiai collective farm in 1965 tripled their grain harvest. The next year four farmers out of a few dozen had left the village of Slitkiai for Kedainiai and were employed by the local food processing plant. As this scenario repeated itself throughout the region, the application of superphosphate and amophosphate contributed to the restructuring of the demographics of the Kedainiai area and eventually all of Lithuania.

Moreover, in order to apply these chemicals onto the fields, the new collective farms were forced to obtain heavy-duty fertilizer applicators that required new trucks, tractors, and modern watering systems. In just a decade, from 1960 to 1970, the Soviet Lithuanian collective farms obtained over 73,000 tractors, 9,000 combine harvesters, and over 22,000 lorries. In his report on Soviet Lithuania's achievements, Antanas Snieckus, the head of the Lithuanian Communist Party, stated that this process of mechanization signified the establishment of "a qualitatively new material and technological base" for building Soviet society (Snieckus 1970, 83). Thus, the fertilizers "nourished" the mechanization and cultivation of modern farming technologies that, in their turn, facilitated the growth of large-scale farms. These technologically advanced farms inevitably replaced inefficient small farms and drove their farmers outside of agricultural production. Importantly, the new "fertile" collective farms were now able to fulfill the demands of growing industrial cities and, in doing so, became a solid platform for the development of the Soviet planned economy.

The foundation of the chemical industry and the reorganization of the local infrastructures around Kedainiai had an enormous effect on the every day practices and experiences of local inhabitants. Before the construction workers and trucks filled with concrete and metal frames had showed up, bulldozers had leveled four old Lithuanian villages: Eiguliai, Zabieliskis, Silaineliai, and Zutkiai. The inhabitants of these villages were moved to the city of Kedainiai. On a micro-level, moving to the city meant a break with the country lifestyle and with it the habitual practices determined by close proximity to nature and manual labor. Undoubtedly, urbanization unraveled the fabric of local social networks, but even more so, the new urbanites were forced out of their everyday interactions with the land. A natural connection between a farmer and the land was replaced by an instrumental approach to natural resources. No longer did they directly interact with their gardens, fields, and animals when preparing the food resources for the upcoming year. The labor intensive, but "creative" connection with the land was replaced by eight-hour days of monotonous unskilled work at the chemical plant and endless hours standing in lines to buy food. A symbiotic cohabitation with nature was replaced by a "civilized" life.

On the macro-level, those who were deprived of their isolated private houses and relocated to the monolithic communal apartment buildings constituted a new type of "faceless" Soviet population. Thanks to the Kedainiai chemical plant, the only major industrial development in the area, in just eleven years the population of Kedainiai almost doubled from 10,580 in 1959 to 19,700 in 1970 (*Lietuviskoji Tarybine Enciklopedija* 1985, 421). In 1966,

5,947 inhabitants of Kedainiai were employed by local industry. This constituted 82.1 percent of all labor force in the city.[8] To accommodate this growing
number of new urbanites, the Soviet government funded the construction of
349 apartment buildings, a bus station, a hospital, and a supermarket. Six
routes of public transportation ensured that the workers from different dis-
tricts were able to commute to work. In official accounts of the growth of Soviet Kedainiai, Soviet officials spoke of the "incessant growth of the labor
force" (Sumauskas 1961, 1).

Much like the urban working class, the farmers became yet another category of "laborers." Antanas Snieckus offered reassurance that the new socio-
technological conditions "[have] greatly lightened the farm labourer's work
and changed its character, so that it now more closely resembles industrial
labour" (Snieckus 1970, 83). The farmers were divested of their individualistic
lifestyles and forced to sign contracts with the state in just the same way as industrial workers. In such a manner, both farm and industrial laborers were
now defined in terms of production and reduced to the generic category of
"labor force." Through the workers' employment at the plant, the chemical
industry shaped their living space and location, their food, their health, and
the ways they moved around. The building of the chemical plant on the local
landscape grew into a "compelling disciplinary technique" (Foucault 1975) for
managing the local population.

The purpose of this section is to locate the chemical plant in relation to
geographic, demographic, political, historical, and technological developments in Kedainiai, and Lithuania. In this story, the chemicals and the chemical plant itself have emerged as material agents that imposed an organizational
logic of space upon the local inhabitants, ostensibly in the service of the plans
and objectives of Sovietization. The chemical plant in Kedainiai subsumed the
local resources and rendered them as a reserve for chemical production: the
roads were centered around the plant, the rivers changed their course to supply water for the contact furnaces, and the humans were moved en masse to
Kedainiai to meet labor demand at the plant's refinement department. Moreover, the chemicals inserted themselves into the digestive processes of the population moving from organic farming to fertilized and processed foods, and
simultaneously displacing workers from farms to chemical plants and food
processing enterprises. The Soviet state seems to have achieved its goals of
chemicalization of the region and, most important, structural-demographic
reorganization of Lithuania. This reorganization now allowed the Soviet state
to better survey and manage the local population. The new road and railroad
systems, large-scale collective farms, and state owned urban apartment buildings made the local population more susceptible than ever to the will of the
Soviet regime. The former farmers were no longer seen as autonomous agents,
but became subjects for management and calculation by the Department of
Statistics of the USSR.

This is not, however, the whole story. The insertion of the chemical plant into the local socio-geographical landscape not only materialized the Soviet plans of urbanization and industrialization, but also generated alternative interpretations and bred practices outside of those intended and regimented by the state. As with any other technology, an interaction between industry and humans resulted in vibrantly new and unpredicted chain reactions. For example, the agricultural products that were produced using fertilizers, and filled the shelves of the Lithuanian grocery stores, were perceived by the locals as somewhat "artificial," and even dangerous or dirty. Many people were reluctant to use these fertilizers in their small gardens, preferring to keep their beds "old-fashioned" and "clean." Unfortunately, due to poor soil and few mechanized farming implements, their gardens were inefficient and did not provide sufficient harvests to become a substantial economic alternative to the large-scale collective farms (Januskevicius 1971, 17). Nevertheless, these low efficiency organic gardens have persisted in the region up to this day and should be considered a reminder of other realities and a reaction against the large-scale Soviet collective farms.

Uncontrolled Reactions of Chemicalization: Economic Contradictions

While it seemed to serve many of the Soviet Union's purposes, chemicalization set off a series of chain reactions that the Soviets were unable to neutralize. The emergence of capitalist elements in the Soviet economy was one of the most profound outcomes of chemicalization. Indeed, Soviet ideologists rigorously and incessantly criticized capitalist profit-centered economies and sought to eliminate all forms of private property among the local population. The foundation of the Kedainiai chemical plant, in its essence, however, functioned within the framework of capitalist production relations and was designed according to a market economy. For example, in his work on Soviet Lithuania's achievements and prospects, Juozas Maniusis (1977) suggests that the planned Soviet economy was aimed at unsustainable growth and modernization:

> The main task set to industry in the new five-year period is to meet more fully the needs of the economy. Priority will be given to the development of those branches which stimulate the technological progress of the national economy as well as of those that process mineral and agricultural raw materials. . . . Lithuania's industrial development is being carried on taking into consideration both the Republic's natural and economic conditions and the economic interests of the Soviet Union. (p. 22)

Just like the leaders of capitalist economies, the Soviet planners followed the criteria of increasing the profit margin and "serving the economic interests of the Soviet Union. "As predicted by its designers, the Kedainiai chemical plant brought a profit of almost a million rubles to the budget of the Soviet

Union each year throughout the 1960s and 1970s. In 1967 production at the chemical plant skyrocketed to 67.3 kopecks per ruble of capital investment, making it one of the most profitable industrial enterprises in the Baltic region (Sagers and Shabad 1990). In other words, the plant revealed the running inconsistency of the Soviet system between strictly socialist ideology and capitalist economic practice.

The chemical industry was also an agent of spreading capitalist mentalities in Lithuania. The Kedainiai chemical plant, in fact, played a significant role in the establishment of monetary exchange by enforcing all economic exchange transactions to be performed in rubles and eliminating other traditional forms of exchange. With the coercion of the wage system, the new Kedainees became engulfed by the market economy.[9] They lost their autonomy in defining their own terms of economic exchange and, in so doing, were forced into a new money-value relation to clothes, as well as to food and household goods. The new urbanites now earned money to buy clothes that they used to sew for themselves, and to buy the food that they used to grow for themselves or barter for. In just a decade, the Soviet regime turned the semi-naturalistic exchange system into a uniform monetary market. As Maniusis recognizes, monetary income in the Soviet system became "the basic indicator showing the living standards of the population" (Maniusis 1977, 83). The average income of the worker at the plant amounted to 85 rubles per month in 1968. Even though this was considerably higher than the minimum wage of about 45 rubles per month, a worker could barely afford to buy one pair of shoes and the generic food items for one person for 85 rubles.

Paradoxically, the Soviet project of industrialization produced the opposite of the desired effect of deprivatization and egalitarianism than had been anticipated. High aspirations for communal lifestyles, cosmopolitan values, and an egalitarian society failed to be realized at the local level when the workers were deprived of their connection to the villages. Instead of creating tightly knit local communes, the chemical plant paid the wages that further alienated the worker from their means of production. In his early essay "Estranged Labor" Karl Marx (1964a) contends that

> [W]ages and *private* property are identical: since the product, as the object of labor pays for labor itself, therefore the wage is but a necessary consequence of labor's estrangement. After all, in wage labor, labor does not appear as an end in itself but as the servant of the wage. (Marx 1964a, 117—original emphasis)

In another essay, "The Power of Money in Bourgeois Society" Marx reasserts that "[b]y the *property* of buying everything, by possessing the property of appropriating all the objects, *money* is thus the *object* of eminent possession" (1964b, 165—original emphasis). Monetary exchange, in his reading, is the essence of the capitalist system that alienates the human from his/her labor. It is, indeed, "the agent of separation" (Marx 1964b, 167) of an individual from oneself, from nature, from his/her labor and its product, and even from humanity. An inevitable outcome of this commodification is a prevailing alienation of the worker, "the devaluation of the world of men" (Marx 1964b, 107). Thus, the wage laborers in the Soviet system were not insiders, but outsiders to society, not beneficiaries, but commodities—the faceless labor force. True, it was not the bourgeoisie who exploited and devalued their lives. Nevertheless, the introduction of the unitary wage system had exactly the same devastating effects on the lower classes in the Soviet state as it had in the capitalist system.

From an economic perspective, the fertilizers were also commodities that participated in the local and national markets, as well as agents that significantly transformed the flows of agricultural products and money in the northwestern Soviet Union. The increasing usage of mineral fertilizers directly affected the quality and quantity of the foods, textiles, and medicines that were sold in the local stores. In the Lithuanian food industry alone, the average annual volume of state purchases for the years 1966 through 1970, as compared with the years 1961 to 1965, showed the following increases: grain–nearly 100 percent; potatoes–60 percent; vegetables–80 percent; meat–70 percent; milk–50 percent, and eggs–110 percent (Snieckus 1970). Obviously, through the consumption of these products, the fertilizers were being injected into the bodies and the environments of the citizens.[10] Even though former farmers were reluctant to use fertilizers in their private gardens, the chemicals entered private lives and bodies through the "backdoor" of consumption.

Despite the fact that the production of household chemicals in the Soviet Union remained underdeveloped until the 1970s, it is during the early 1960s when consumers acquired a taste and demand for these products. Because of the disruption in their self-sustaining naturalistic lifestyles during the early years of industrialization in Lithuania, particularly their dislocation into gray apartment buildings, the urbanites started using more consumer goods such as cleaning detergents, disinfectants, plastic articles, synthetic fibers, paints and lacquers. Plastic toys and household appliances, colorful synthetic fabrics, and powerful cleaners became necessary accessories to their modern lifestyles and provided cures for the symptoms and side effects of industrialization (Lantsev 1976). New urbanites were now fully submerged in the chemicalized world; they were eagerly eating, wearing, healing, playing, and washing with the help of the chemicals. The chemicals inserted themselves into the most private zones of the Soviet citizens: their homes, their food, their clothes, and their bodies. This marked the emergence of the second-order chemicalization and the augmentation of a new consumption regime.

Despite the fact that consumerism was incompatible with Soviet ideology, the post-Stalinist officials recognized the importance of a growing consumer market. In his address to the Communist Party plenum in May 1958, Nikita

Khrushchev drew specific attention to consumer satisfaction. His speech was entitled "On the Acceleration of the Development of the Chemical Industry, and Particularly, the Production of Synthetics for the Satisfaction of Consumer Demand and to Meet the Needs of the National Economy" and was the first document that acknowledged consumerism in the Soviet Union and recognized the central role of the chemical industry in it. For the first time in the history of the Soviet Union, a Communist Party leader spoke about the "necessity" of satisfying the consumer market, a concept unheard of among Soviet officials and perhaps central among capitalist concepts. Moreover, the connection between consumerism and chemicalization was not coincidental. The chemicals that were designed as a remedy to the gruesome situation in the Soviet food industry were to be extended to the whole Soviet economy (Savinskij 1972). Khrushchev's decision to address consumer demands was necessitated by a recognition of the failure of Stalin's "iron-hand" policies. This "thaw" of Soviet policies, however, initiated the melting of the ideological integrity of the Soviet system (Gill 1987, 35). The Soviet system continued to proclaim socialism, but fostered an increasing capitalist style. Even as Soviet planners sought to neutralize consumerism through the production of synthetics, the chemical catalysts of consumerism were permeating every aspect of daily life and further circulating consumerist mentalities.

To take a detour into the issue of ideology and chemicals, the fertilizers produced at the Kedainiai chemical plant generated powerful chain reactions in the Soviet economy that eventually eroded the system. The fertilizers used in the Lithuanian fields were, indeed, autonomous and free of Soviet ideology. In their action upon grain harvests, the chemicals went far beyond the treatment of the Soviet economic problems to the contamination of the socialist ideology with capitalist mentalities. Moreover, they forced the Lithuanian farmers out of their self-sustaining lifestyles to brutal urban realities. Instead of the expected growth in support of the Soviet socialist system on the part of the new working class, the new generation of Kedainees adopted capitalist mentalities, consumerist lifestyles, and anti-Soviet positions. The fruit of the fertilized fields did not nourish the contentment of workers in the Soviet socialist economy as much as it infected them with the germ of consumerist desires, thereby destroying the ideological immunity of the Soviet system.

Science and Nationalist Reactions

Gyan Prakash argues that "science . . . authorizes an enormous leap into modernity, and anchors the entire edifice of modern culture, identity, politics, and economy" (Prakash 1999, 12). It is not, however, the emergence of science per se that generated the structural "leap" into modern society, but rather it was a concomitant repudiation of other forms of knowledge that disarmed traditional rejections and alternative forms of social organization than the modern. The chemical industry in Lithuania, as a product of cutting edge chemical science, contributed to establishing the authority of scientific knowledge by devaluing local knowledge.

One of the first steps in the Sovietization of Lithuania in the mid-1950s was the partitioning of the largest university, Vytautas Magnus, in Kaunas, and creating new institutes and divisions of higher education. Even well-established programs in the natural sciences at Vilnius University, and chemistry programs in particular, did not withstand the censure of the Soviet reforms and were closed down. Instead, to train the qualified cadres for the new chemical industry in the area, the Soviet planning institutions initiated the foundation of new chemistry departments.[11] By 1964, six hundred undergraduates and graduates specializing in different fields of chemistry were studying at the newly established Kaunas Institute of Politechnics. The same year, Vilnius University accommodated a department of chemistry with a total of four hundred students. In addition, six other colleges had autonomous programs in both theoretical and applied chemistry (Kitriene and Spudulis 1996). Keeping in mind that the total population of Lithuania was 3 million at the time and that the majority of high school graduates were forced to join the labor force immediately after graduation, this growing army of new specialists in Soviet chemistry embodied the Soviet state's effort to chemicalize Lithuania as well as its attempt to fortify the new hierarchy of knowledge, with Soviet science at the top.[12]

Traditional practical knowledge was fully discredited in this new system. Only the chemical transformations taking place in the highly insulated glass and metal vessels and veiled from the eye of an observer behind the encoded equations and schemes were considered to be genuine knowledge. In the same way, those in white uniforms who knew how to transform the phosphate rock into magic fertilizing crystals deserved higher-ranking jobs in the plant. In other words, the legitimate and respected knowledge resided in the plant's laboratories.

From the perspective of the former villagers, this new and almost mysterious science was alien. It was taught in a foreign language and by outlandish "specialists." In just four years of operation, for example, the staff at the Kedainiai chemical plant were trained by some four hundred consultants from the Ukraine, Belorussia, and the Russian Federation. During the construction of the plant, engineers from the Urals machinery factory, Taganorg Boiler plant, and the coal chemical equipment factory at Slavinsk instructed the local specialists. Consultants from Sumy and Vinnittsa superphosphate plants, from Volkhov aluminium works, from Konstantinovka chemical factory, from Voskresensk chemical combine, as well as from Moscow and Kharkhov visited the plant's compound and instructed the local chemists (Sumauskas 1961; Kitriene and Spudulis 1996).

Workers, on the other hand, were kept outside of these training programs and laboratories. Dressed in gray cloaks, loading and unloading the cars with their shovels, the lowest tier of workers played a minor role in the "progress of

Soviet industry and science." They were deprived of this "powerful" chemical knowledge, and became further deskilled and devalued in the plant. Paradoxically, instead of incorporating the workers into the system and familiarizing them with the science, the system organized itself around the deepening schisms between traditional and expert knowledges. This qualitative shift towards the authority of applied science meant a new "injury" in the worldview of the former farmers. Those who successfully conducted such natural chemical reactions as raising bread with yeast, dying homemade textiles with natural dies, or fertilizing their fields with manure were left outside of Soviet science. The true knowledge was to be brought from the outside, it superceded their everyday knowledge and rendered their ways of living inefficient. On a more abstract level, this meant the loss of the workers' self-esteem and abilities, of their belief in their knowledge, and the stability of their worldviews.

Indeed, the growing estrangement of the former farmer and the urbanite from such public spheres as science, economy, and their own labor were incentives for active resistance. The Soviet discourse of pure cosmopolitanism could not compensate for the profound injuries to the body of the nation. The increasing sense of alienation boosted the search for alternative forms of identity construction and, since nationalism was one of the most consistent ideologies at the time, nationalist movements were able to mobilize the local population. The nationalistic worldview provided a secure shelter for those whose knowledge was discredited and who faced the repressions of the Soviet regime. As Benedict Anderson (1983) has pointed out, shared geographical space, blood, and a common historical imagination constitute the essence of nationalist ideology. In other words, it is the physical connectedness and the imagination of the historical past that makes nationalism such a strong component in modern European identities.

With the fundamental transformation of the local landscape, economic and social relations, and everyday practices and experiences, the newly born citizens of the Soviet Union, even those who had never lived on farms, grew nostalgic about the self-sustaining and "uncivilized" lifestyles of the village. Their recollections and imagination of the pastoral past were inevitably tied to the idea of an autonomous nation state of Lithuania. Since the nationalist agenda was based on the idea of an integrated and customary society that was apparently absent from the Soviet ways of living, it provided a solid platform for strengthening alternative ways of thinking about their history, their relationship to the land, their everyday routines, their tools, their food, their own bodies, and the future of their children.

Nationalism, therefore, recruited its advocates among the local population by offering the most coherent and satisfactory system of values, and by rationalizing acts of resistance. Until 1957, the Lithuanian forests concealed almost 90,000 members of the LLA (Lithuanian Freedom Army) and their associates. Romuald Misiunas and Rein Taagepera (1983) compare this active resistance with "the peak Viet Cong strength in South Vietnam (discounting the North Vietnamese supplements) of approximately 170,000 fighters and supply runners out of a population of 20 million (Misiunas and Taagepera 1983, 81). The Prisikelimo (Revival) that was active in the Kedainiai area consisted of up to twelve active resistance groups of approximately ten men in each.[13] Their guerilla strategies were aimed at "paralyzing the Soviet communication infrastructures, destroying the Soviet secret police, and maintaining order in the area" (Kuodyte and Kaseta 1996, 122). Scattered and doomed, sleeping in the damp bunkers and never leaving the forest, these groups of armed men stood for an alternative reality. The last partisan leader, Arvydas Ramanauskas, was "eliminated" by the Soviet secret police in 1956, making it "safe" for the chemicalization of the country to proceed.

In addition to these military guerilla activities, the forest brotherhoods were able to publish their journals, proclamations, and leaflets at the "forest publishing houses" in the early years of resistance movement, 1944 through 1949. After 1952, however, with the final collectivization of Lithuanian farms having considerably undermined their food, clothing, and medicine supplies, and with the consolidation of the Soviet army in the area, the publishing ceased (Kuodyte and Kaseta 1996). Despite arrests and public executions performed by the Soviet "militia," individual acts of diversion persisted late into the 1960s. In 1958 in Kedainiai, groups of former farmers, students, and school teachers consistently tore down Soviet posters and red flags, distributed anti-Soviet proclamations and flew tri-colored nationalist flags (Kuodyte et al. 1996). The culmination of this resistance was the self-immolation of Arturas Kalanta in Kaunas, just 50 miles away from the Kedainiai plant in 1972. This act resulted in public demonstrations against the Soviet regime and massive unrest in the cities of central Lithuania. These acts of diversion, culminating in a national revival in the 1990s fueled by the urban working class, were a clear indication of the growth of nationalism among the local population. The nationalist revival of the 1990s ultimately led Lithuania to be the first republic to secede from the Soviet Union.

Conclusion

Ranajit Guha (1989) in his study of English domination in India delineates how the old paradigm of Indian social organization was intended to "dissolve *ideally* into a hegemonic dominance" (Guha 1989, 228) of the English. Guha criticizes Gramsci's blending of hegemony and domination into a single notion of hegemony and argues that a coercive domination of the regime should not be erroneously mistaken for hegemony. The coercive dominance of the colonizers and a hegemonic consent of the subjected population are autonomous notions, argues Guha. Through his historiography, Guha demonstrates that the political and economic domination of the English in India had never become fully hegemonic in Gramsci's (1985) sense. In spite of overpowering technologies of domination, Indians maintained multiple sites of resistance and autonomy.

Similarly, as argued in this essay, an ultimate goal of the Soviet state was to spin a seamless web of hegemony over the local population in Lithuania. Through physical changes in the environment, the Soviet governmental institutions sought to control, manipulate, and impute their ideologies into the minds of its new citizens. The chemical plant was designed as a material agent that dictated its own organizational logic of time and space upon the local population. The chemicals were conceived as material and symbolic agents of collectivization and urbanization. Indeed, the foundation of the chemical plant in Kedainiai did modernize the geography of Lithuania and irreversibly changed the demographics of the country. The chemicals did enter the local grocery stores, homes, and the bodies of the Kedainees, making them vulnerable and pliable subjects of Soviet domination in the short-term.

Parallel to this profound anthropo-material transformation in the local ecology, however, the chemicals disrupted the traditional communal world, alienated the local populations from their homes, tools of labor, and neighbors, and fertilized capitalist mentalities of consumption and monetary market. The deepening schism between traditional know-how and expert knowledge was perhaps one of the most devastating losses for the culture, as it marked the emergence of new classlike hierarchies and destruction of the local traditions. Inserted in Kedainiai by alien institutions, the chemical plant and its products became a symbol of Soviet imperialism and a target for the nationalist resistance movements. So while the sulfuric acid of the Kedainiai plant produced the fertilizers that fed the growing cities and Soviet economy in the short-term, it slowly eroded the core of Soviet ideology by nourishing the capitalist mentalities of monetary exchange and consumerism in the long-term, and by feeding the Lithuanian nationalist movement that the Soviet leadership sought to starve out.

Does all this amount to saying that chemicals are inherently capitalist? Socialist? Nationalist? Imperialist? It would be naïve to insist that a technology as complex as the chemical industry has an inherent political or economic destiny. As a political tool, the chemical industry and its products seem to change hands through the course of this history. As an economic tool, the chemical industry was constitutive of the processes of socializing and capitalizing Lithuania. From the perspective of the 1960s, the Kedainiai chemical plant seemed to have become an ally of Soviet strategists by reorganizing the flows of trucks, food, building materials, money and humans according to the wishes of its socialist designers. Simultaneously, the chemicals escaped from the laboratories built by the Soviet politicians and acted as autonomous catalysts that fostered nationalism and capitalism. Independent of Soviet ideologies, ignorant of clever calculations and immune to ideological inscriptions, the chemicals permeated every sphere of life in Lithuania. Their molecules were freely moving from the mines to the furnaces, to the trucks, the ground and the human body. The chemicals were persecuted as "unhealthy," and the plant held up as an icon of Soviet imperialism by the nationalist movement they helped to foster. Yet it was the chemical industry that was to serve as the cornerstone to the new economy of the Lithuanian state, freed from Soviet imperialism by the nationalist movement that had scorned it.

13

Conclusion
Environmental Security in an Uncertain World

MONICA J. CASPER AND BARBARA A. BARNES

I think we ought to have high—high standards and set by—by agencies that rely upon science, not by what may feel good or what sound good [sic]. And I think it's important to give people time to say we're going to conform to standards, and if they don't, I think we ought to fine them. I mean, I think we ought to be tough when it comes to our environmental laws. But I don't—I don't believe that [the Clinton administration] has got it right when it comes to the environment. They try to sue our way to clean air and clean water or regulate our air—way to clean air and clean water [sic].
—George W. Bush, GOP Debate, Iowa, January 15, 2000

I also strongly believe that we can explore for natural gas in Alaska without damaging the economy—the environment. And I believe it's necessary to do that!
—George W. Bush, campaigning in Orlando, Florida, December 4, 2001

Within the pages of this book, we have traveled to Japan, Hungary, Lithuania, Vietnam, Cairo, the Persian Gulf, and various corners of the United States. Our journey has taken us into a wide range of environments—from deforested highlands, to urban streets, to not-so-pristine bays, to mauve deserts, to office buildings, to women's health conferences, to scientific laboratories, to hazardous waste sites, and beyond. We have explored the (usually) unwelcome intrusion of dangerous chemicals into bodies and communities, and we have seen varying levels of local and national interest in mediating this intrusion. But perhaps most striking when these chapters are taken as a whole is the utter relentlessness of the *global* nature of the issues at hand. That is, chemical toxins are indiscriminate and largely successful immigrants, crossing local and national borders, infiltrating communities, and vexing stakeholders. While the authors herein have offered sharp theoretical insights about these complex chemical maneuvers, in closing we want to spotlight policy. Or rather, we want to show how and why policy matters.

In the aftermath of 9/11, we have heard much dialogue and rhetoric about national security, and specifically about homeland security. In the United States, most political decisions appear to be made and defended in terms of protecting the country and its inhabitants. The current Republican administration of George W. Bush is intensely focused on these issues, with the United States being portrayed by its leaders as if it were the first nation ever to suffer at the hands of terrorists. (This, despite longstanding, violent conflicts that continue to rage in the Middle East, Africa, and elsewhere.) Many commentators have offered critiques of this myopic approach, which has prevented attention to other important issues and concerns, and we will not restate their cogent arguments here. What we offer instead is an appropriation of the language of security for a different purpose, one geared toward expanding rather than constricting borders. We contend that security should be construed as more than just protecting a privileged way of life, and instead should encompass the defense of human and ecosystem health in all its dimensions.

President Bush and his staff have emphatically, rabidly, and xenophobically pursued "homeland security" through a variety of policies, including the formation of an Office of Homeland Defense, which itself became embattled. These decisions have garnered the lion's share of media attention in the wake of the terrorist attacks. Yet behind the scenes another drama unfolds, one in which decisions are being made every day about issues that Americans care about but are seldom being informed about. We want to focus here, for obvious reasons, on environmental issues. Below, we offer a partial list of actions taken by the Bush Administration in the first two years of his tenure as President. While these policies reflect a small span of time, between 2001 and 2002, they will likely have serious consequences well into the future. Our list can thus be read as a harbinger of environmental health for the coming decades.

Note that our intention here is not to stress the actions of the United States to the exclusion of other nations. We could just as easily formulate a list of environmental policies for the U.K., Russia, South Africa, Vietnam, or any other country. Indeed, with very few exceptions, most industrial and developing nations have failed to adopt progressive environmental policies. We highlight the United States in part because it is convenient to do so; with just a little bit of digging, we have the information at our fingertips. Yet, at the risk of sounding like apologists for the "last remaining superpower," we do acknowledge that the United States maintains a position of importance in the world. The decisions made in Washington, D.C. extend far beyond the borders of that municipality, to the four corners of America and to other nations. Like dirty air, antienvironmental policies creep across political boundaries to affect bodies, ecosystems, communities, and nations at great distance from their origins.

The Bush Environmental Record: 2001–2002[1]

- Bush's energy plan, approved by the House of Representatives on August 1, 2001, focused on increasing the supply and continued use of fossil fuels. The centerpiece of the plan involves drilling in the Arctic National Wildlife Refuge (ANWR), a 19.5 million-acre area of which 1.5 million acres lies along the coastal plain of northeast Alaska. The ANWR was until this policy shift specifically protected from oil exploration and development; it is extremely fragile ecologically and is home to thirty-five mammal species and some one hundred and fifty bird species.

- The energy bill dedicates only $5.9 million in subsidies for energy efficiency and renewable energy, while setting aside about $27 billion for the coal, oil, and gas industries. In addition, the administration did not address Corporate Average Fuel Economy (CAFE) standards, leaving in place the "SUV loophole." This allows sport utility vehicles and minivans to be classified as light trucks (an exemption originally designed for the benefit of farmers), and thus to escape the 27.5 mile-per-gallon standard required of cars. Closing this loophole could save one million barrels of oil per day by 2015, more than the ANWR would be expected to produce in the same time frame.

- On March 20, 2001, Environmental Protection Agency (EPA) Administrator Christine Todd Whitman announced that she would delay a rule that would have restricted the amount of arsenic allowed in tap water. That rule was scheduled to take effect March 23. The National Academy of Sciences has argued that the standard for arsenic in drinking water needs to be improved "as promptly as possible."

- Riding the campaign trail in September 2000, Bush pledged to curb carbon dioxide pollution, promising that power plants would be required to meet clean air standards. On March 13, 2001, he reversed that pledge, stating that he did not believe the government should impose on power plants mandatory emissions for carbon dioxide.

- In March 2001, Bush criticized the Kyoto Protocol on global warming and reversed a campaign pledge that promised to reduce carbon dioxide emissions. Three months later, in June, he told reporters that by working cooperatively, the U.S. could help reduce greenhouse pollution from Third World countries. On July 6, the administration announced a plan that would reduce funding by $41 million for a program limiting greenhouse gases from developing countries, shifting more responsibility for pollution control to private industry. Bush eventually removed the United States completely from the Kyoto Treaty global warming accord, generating significant international criticism.

- Bush reversed the Clinton administration's actions setting aside environmentally sensitive areas as national parks or monuments, hoping instead to open them to oil and gas exploration. These areas include Grand Staircase-Escalante in Utah, Canyons of the Ancients in Colorado, the Upper Missouri Breaks in Montana, and the Coastal Monument in California.

- In February 2002, Bush endorsed a controversial plan to store 77,000 tons of high-level nuclear waste in an underground facility in Yucca Mountain, Nevada, despite evidence that the public will not be protected from radiation contamination.

- In May 2002, Bush decided against protecting more than 9 million acres of Alaska's Tongass National Forest, opening temperate rainforest to logging and other commercial activities.
- In June 2002, the Bush administration weakened air pollution rules that would allow some 17,000 of the country's biggest polluters to avoid installing pollution-controlled equipment when plants are expanded or modernized.
- In the second half of 2002, the Bush administration reversed decades-old foreign policy by instituting a "first strike" approach (in part to wage war against Iraq) and substantially increased military and defense funding.
- Bush cut $500 million from the EPA's 2002 budget, including $158 million that had been targeted to enforcement of laws to ensure clean air and water.
- Bush cut the U.S. Fish and Wildlife Service budget by $168 million, slashing money dedicated to protecting wildlife habitats, wetland restoration, and endangered species.
- At the Bureau of Land Management, the balance has shifted from conserving to exploiting public lands. The 2002 budget increased money for oil drilling and mining by roughly $15 million and made an equal cut in conservation funds.
- The Bush administration implemented deep cuts in the federal Superfund program, which will slow or halt cleanup efforts at thirty-three toxic waste sites in eighteen states. With the budget reduction and failure to reauthorize the program, revenue for the fund has shifted from industry to individual taxpayers, in the process freeing petrochemical industries from a heavy corporate tax.
- Bush abandoned a campaign pledge to invest $100 million in rainforest conservation.
- Bush rescinded a proposal to increase public access to information about the potential consequences resulting from chemical plant accidents.
- Bush eliminated funding for the Wetlands Reserve Program, which encourages farmers to maintain wetlands habitat on their property.
- Bush appointed Senator John Ashcroft as Attorney General. Ashcroft had an extremely poor environmental voting record in the Senate and is openly hostile to most environmental regulations. He voted against additional funding for environmental programs including the Clean Water Action Plan and toxic waste cleanup at Superfund sites. He voted for a bill to roll back clean water protections, to prevent the EPA from enforcing arsenic standards for public drinking water, and to allow mining companies to dump cyanide and other mining waste on large areas of public lands next to mining sites.

- Bush appointed Senator Spencer Abraham as Energy Secretary. While in the Senate, Abraham led efforts to prevent the Clinton administration from increasing fuel economy in cars and light trucks. He cosponsored two separate bills that would have allowed drilling in the fragile Arctic National Wildlife Refuge. He voted to kill an amendment that would have added $62 million to the Energy Department's solar and renewable energy programs, and he voted to delay reforming the way oil companies pay royalties for drilling public lands. Abraham also supported establishment of an aboveground "interim" nuclear waste dump near Yucca Mountain in Nevada. In 1999, Abraham sponsored legislation that would have abolished the Department of Energy.

- Bush appointed Christine Todd Whitman as Administrator of the EPA. As Governor of New Jersey, Whitman had a mixed record on the environment. On the one hand, she joined with other Northeastern governors to insist that Midwest utilities clean up coal-fired power plants and she advocated protecting 1 million acres of open space in her state. Yet she also cut New Jersey's environmental enforcement budget significantly, resulting in an 80 percent reduction in fines assessed to polluters, and she proposed watershed management rules that were so ineffective they were opposed by the New Jersey Assembly for failing to meet legislative intent. She weakened state oversight of pesticide use and failed to implement laws passed to protect farmworker health and safety; she tried to eliminate the Clean Water Enforcement Act; she eliminated a more protective state hazardous waste program in favor of a weaker federal program; and she failed to adequately monitor water pollution in the state, which led to EPA sanctions.

- Bush appointed former California Agriculture Secretary Ann Veneman as national Agriculture Secretary. Her record is a major cause for concern. In Veneman's private law practice, she represented clients whose positions run counter to the environmental protections that most Americans seem to want. For example, she represented a coalition of loggers, miners, and off-road vehicle enthusiasts in a case involving the Sierra Nevada Environmental Program. In California, she opposed efforts to ban methyl bromide, a toxic ozone-depleting pesticide. When campaigning for Bush in that state, she told farmers and ranchers they would no longer be subjected to "unnecessary and burdensome" environmental and safety regulations. Veneman also played a major role in promoting free trade agreements without adequate environmental, safety, labor, and human rights standards.

- Bush nominated David Lauriski, an ex-mining company executive, as Assistant Secretary of Labor for Mine Safety and Health; J. Steven

Giles, an oil and coal lobbyist, for Deputy Secretary of the Interior; and Linda Fisher, a Monsanto executive, for the number two job at the EPA.

And the list goes on and on.

Redefining Homeland Security

To borrow a "down-home" aphorism of the sort that Dubya is so fond of, the Bush environmental agenda looks like someone put the fox in charge of the hen house. (And somewhere in America, former Vice-President and environmental advocate Al Gore is likely shaking his head in bewilderment.) We can only speculate, nervously, on what the remaining years of this presidency have in store for the planet. What this list of repressive policies suggests is that, at least in terms of the environment and despite the patriotic rhetoric, homeland security is *not* at the top of President Bush's agenda. Indeed, one would guess from these policies and appointments that the Bush administration does not care if our home—the planet—goes to hell in a handbasket, as long as the interests of corporate America and a few wealthy individuals are protected. As the group Physicians for Social Responsibility phrased it in a recent mailing, "it seems the only environment President Bush cares about is the *business* environment."[2]

While the Bush administration has thus far exhibited an appalling lack of regard for ecosystem and human health, we would be remiss if we did not also mention that the Clinton administration generated its share of antienvironmental legislation. On a largely proenvironment platform, President Clinton and Vice-President Gore nonetheless succumbed to corporate interests in loosening domestic regulations, fostering global trade agreements unfriendly to environmental causes (such as NAFTA), and generally attempting to build a "centrist" or moderate position that placed market concerns before preservation of the planet. There are, of course, crucial differences between Republicans and Democrats—one need only compare the Reagan years, in which environmental programs were eviscerated, to the environmental gains made during the Clinton years. However, irregardless of party affiliation, environmental legislation and policy in the United States reflect the influence of corporate interests, creating a pervasive, bipartisan "business as usual" milieu. Capitalism wins, and more often than not, the environment loses.

This is unfortunate. As a number of commentators have argued, proenvironment legislation, much of it enacted since the 1960s, actually does make a positive difference in the quality of our air, water, and food. The National Environmental Policy Act (NEPA), the Clean Air Act (CAA), the Resource Conservation and Recovery Act (RCRA), the Comprehensive Environmental Response, Compensation, and Liability Act (CERCLA), the Clean Water Act (CWA), the Endangered Species Act, the Toxic Substances Control Act (TSCA), Food Quality Protection Act (FQPA), Emergency Planning and Community Right to Know Act (EPCRA), the Safe Water Drinking Act (SDWA)—this alphabet soup of policies has had important, measurable impacts on the lives of citizens, ecological health, and industrial practices (cf. Schettler et al.). As has the creation of government agencies such as the Occupational Safety and Health Administration (OSHA), the Environmental Protection Agency (EPA), the Food and Drug Administration (FDA), and the Consumer Product Safety Commission (CPSC).

To note one example, prior to the implementation of the Marine Protection, Research, and Sanctuaries Act of 1972, the U.S. Army used ocean dumping as its preferred method of chemical weapons disposal (Koplow 1997). Environmentalism has advanced to such a point that ocean dumping of any chemical waste now would horrify most people.

Into the linguistic political space created by 9/11, where notions of security dangle from the collective tongue, has crept a growing awareness that we, American citizens who are also citizens of the world, cannot afford to compromise our environment in the service of narrow-minded foreign and domestic policies. Consider these sardonic, apt words from commentator Bill Moyers, writing in *The Nation*:

> What else can America do to strike at the terrorists? Why, slip in a special tax break for poor General Electric, and slip inside the EPA while everyone's distracted and torpedo the recent order to clean the Hudson River of PCBs. Don't worry about NBC, CNBC or MSNBC reporting it; they're all in the GE family. It's time for Churchillian courage, we're told. So how would this crowd assure that future generations will look back and say "This was their finest hour?" That's easy. Give those coal producers freedom to pollute. And shovel generous tax breaks to those giant energy companies. And open the Alaska wilderness to drilling—that's something to remember the 11th of September for. And while the red, white and blue waves at half-mast over the land of the free and the home of the brave—why, give the President the power to discard democratic debate and the rule of law concerning controversial trade agreements, and set up secret tribunals to run roughshod over local communities trying to protect their environment and their health. (Moyers 2002, 286–87)

Moyers poses the question that many other Americans are wondering about in these postapocalyptic times and that many politicians are dancing around. How is the emphasis on "homeland security" obscuring other issues, while also making possible the passage of a conservative agenda that seems contrary to the desires of most Americans? It is not hard to fathom why many other nations are suspicious of the United States, when every decision made in the Capitol—from environmental legislation to foreign policy—appears to serve special interests in the guise of national security.

We want to suggest here that the quest for environmental security, which should by all measures be a global endeavor, not be confused with President Bush's parochial vision of homeland security. Surely, as the chapters in this book suggest, progressive environmental policy would recognize that bodies and communities matter, and that they matter across borders. It is not just the bodies of people who reside within the borders of the United States that we should care about, but the bodies of people all over the world, many of whom are at grave risk every day. While toxins may seep into and come to inhabit bodies and communities at local levels in the intimate spaces where we live, work, and play, it is in part global conditions that make this seepage possible. And it is progressive national policies, and the willingness of world leaders to engage in international cooperation, that might still foster a planet of healthy neighbors rather than one of cancerous terrorist cells.

People in the industrial world, and increasingly in the developing world, are thoroughly modernized, and it would be difficult if not impossible to turn back the clock. Nor would we necessarily want to. Chemicals saturate our existence, from the food we eat, to the detergents with which we scrub our toilets, to the drugs that may save our lives, to the materials that surround us when we drive in cars or fly in planes, to the dishes off of which we eat. That many of these same chemicals pose hazards to our health and well-being, however, is not something that we should ignore. That poor people the world over are far more likely to be victimized by toxic pollution than their richer, more resourceful neighbors is also something that should not be ignored. We cannot continue to produce, disseminate, and use potentially lethal chemicals without a sea change in public awareness and policy making.

The title of this book refers to the artificial or industrial nature of the chemicals discovered and applied in the twentieth century. We do indeed live on a synthetic planet, as each chapter in this book has shown in different ways. However, in closing, we want to draw out another meaning of the word "synthetic," that which refers to creating a whole from parts. We want to suggest that the insights contained in this book, focused on the origin and impact of synthetic chemicals, be used to envision a different form of environmental politics. Rather than emphasizing homeland security for the good of only one nation, a dubious and cynical undertaking at best, we want the ideas presented here to foster notions of global community. In following the molecule, we have learned that toxins respect no boundaries and obey no borders, be they corporeal or geographic. Perhaps there is a lesson here for the realm of politics, which is too often heavily Balkanized and partisan, creating different kinds of hazards as borders, boundaries, and bodies are violently maintained and rearranged. Synthetic organisms that we are, let us instead strive for worldly synthesis in the name of environmental and embodied security. For the good of the planet, and for our own good, policy matters.

Notes

Chapter 1

1. "Nature" has stood as a much-contested term in anthropology for decades. Interrogated aggressively in feminist anthropological debates in particular (MacCormack and Strathern 1980; Reiter 1975; Ortner and Whitehead 1981; Delaney and Yanagisako 1995), though prominent in a range of anthropological discussions, nature comprises a category often fundamentally opposed to culture. Yet nature is riddled with culture, not least the cultural interpretation of the natural realm—nature and culture are theoretical constructs that developed out of exegetical convenience and from a specific European intellectual tradition (Strathern 1980, 177). While understanding the problematic nuances of this term, I have used the word "nature" throughout this chapter in an attempt to engage with prevalent Japanese discourses on the natural milieu. In many respects, it is important to focus on conceptions of nature when thinking about toxic pollution, since nature is used to explain not only characteristics of the environment, but also the "normal" healthy state of the body and, not infrequently, attributes of nation as well. (Japanese, in my experience, bear strong conceptions of how "Japanese" nature *should* be that derive in part from traditional aesthetics and Japan's long history of constructing and improving upon the natural milieu [Berque 1997; Kalland and Asquith 1997; Kirby 1999a]. This tradition is reflected in Japan's artifice-laden, manicured gardens and miniature bonsai trees, and it also influences relations with nature at highly commercialized natural touristic sites, theme parks, artificial beaches and indoor ski areas in recent decades [Kirby 1999a; Kirby 1999b].)

2. While Foucault eloquently constructs a macro-social, macro-historical analysis of discipline, examination, and the "micro-physics of power" (Foucault 1991: 26), his panoptical treatment of bodies in institutional structures reveals little of the embodied social knowledge of disciplinarians and the disciplined that concerns embodiment scholars, less still the "weapons" that those in disciplinary apparatuses might have at hand (Scott 1985, 1990).

3. Paul Farmer (1993), though, finds ample transnational connections between marginalized settings and the "First World" from his vantage in Haiti.

4. Sometimes possibly psychosomatic, though the term retains little meaning in an embodied analysis.

5. "Environment" in common usage usually evokes an idealized notion of "nature," or ecology, separate from human contact. In this chapter, as I describe below, I attempt to use the term "environment" in such a way that it can acknowledge the interplay that environment has with ideas of nature, particularly in the Japanese context.

6. "Landscape," of course, is a highly cultural term that reflects a society's way of seeing (and representing) the environment around them (Bender 1995, 1998; Hirsch and O'Hanlon 1995). I use the term here with these nuances very much in mind.

7. This is not to say that most or all Japanese educators would steadfastly align themselves with *nihonjinron* writers; rather, these frequently left-wing professionals tend to carry around sometimes vague conceptions about Japanese distinctiveness that display a close similarity with *nihonjinron* tenets (Yoshino 1992, 131).

8. Though apparently a contradiction in terms, "native ethnology" reflects Yanagita's stated conviction that Japan, unlike other (Western) societies, boasted its own original culture embedded in the lives of the common people (jōmin) and did not need, as did Frazer, to go outside its borders to map out primitive origins and beliefs (Hashimoto 1998, 142; Harootunian 1998).

9. Of course, any characterization of the fickle, mercurial Japanese climate as benevolent seems clearly idealized and abstracted from the meteorological harshness of various seasons in the archipelago.

10. Of course, over many months of ethnographic research, one key realization I have had is that there is no such thing as an "ordinary" Japanese person. Even the most superficially

quotidian informant has revealed intriguing perspectives and, not infrequently, trenchant criticisms that have guided my research.

11. The pattern of this news synopsis in the paragraphs below derives from a close study of the *Asahi, Yomiuri, Mainichi,* and *Sankei Shimbun,* as well as the *Japan Times* and relatively less television news analysis, from early February 1999 on into the summer. There are too many individual sources to cite reasonably here. Despite some minor variation between different news organs at times, the basic pattern of the coverage is consistent with this synopsis.

12. Vegetables Take Fall (1999), Vegetables Under Fire (1999).

13. TV Asahi Admits Inappropriate (1999).

14. Because tea is typically steeped in hot water rather than directly ingested, the danger of dioxin intake is reportedly greatly diminished (Saitama Declared Safe [1999]).

15. Waste Reduction Comprehensive Planning Office 1995: 18–22.

16. The government's success at hitting this ambitious target is still unclear.

17. Japan boasts some of the world's strictest environmental laws in response to the pollution debacles of the 1950s, 1960s, and 1970s (Kalland and Persoon 1995; Broadbent 1998). As a direct result of these laws, Japan as a whole has, for example, seen an impressive reduction of sulfur dioxide emissions by international standards (OECD Environmental Data 1999; Broadbent 1998). However, partially due to the fact that Japanese industrial sites and car-exhaust emissions tend to be concentrated around urban agglomerations, major cities in Japan can be highly polluted (Broadbent 1998).

18. All names of communities and informants in this chapter are pseudonyms, due to the terms of my field interviews. I have also, occasionally, altered certain biographical or geographical details in an attempt to protect the identities of my interlocutors. However, I have endeavored to change as little as possible in order to preserve the richness of ethnographic detail in my research findings.

19. My informants in Horinouchi spanned socio-economic categories (recently developed areas of Western Tokyo often have long-term locals who might stay on and work as green-grocers or small-scale merchants in the area, providing some contrast to the more solidly middle-class arrivals who tend to commute to their jobs (cf. Robertson 1991; Bestor 1989) and ranged in age from mid-teens to those in their eighties.

20. Despite the government's lowering of dioxins' "tolerable daily intake," a report on dioxins in mother's milk exposed the fact that infants can take in up to twenty-six times the tolerable daily intake of dioxins even when assessed according to the erstwhile higher tolerable level (Mother's Milk Dioxins 1999; Dioxin in Mother's Milk 1999; cf. Ministry of Health and Welfare 1999).

21. An article I am currently writing presents these fascinating reproductive, gendered, and environmental elements of life in Japanese cities in greater scope and detail.

22. Below, I cite residents' descriptions of their symptoms, combining interview transcripts and questionnaire responses. Unfortunately I lack space here to describe aspects of these data-gathering methods in greater detail (cf. Kirby 2001, chapter 3).

23. This scientist also found that the agency in question had systematically distorted the negative information that his surveys had uncovered.

24. The new mayor had campaigned strongly on behalf of local environmental issues, partly due to the poignancy of dioxins and other toxic pollution in the ward and in the media at the time.

25. Though as we have seen, it is not infrequently the case that attempts to reign in toxic excesses in one sector merely transpose toxic defilement to another troubled site, as in the case of the Izawa waste facility and in toxin-ridden rural landfill sites.

Chapter 2

1. Policy makers both within and outside the EPA have contested the notion of comparative risk assessment and ranking of hazards as practiced in *Unfinished Business* and related studies in the 1980's. Critics argue that the "(r)anks did not take into account the feasibility of controlling risks, the economic benefits of activities posing risks, the limits of EPA's statutory authority, or the distribution of risks and benefits geographically, over time, or among people." (Schierow 1998, np) That said, the report is still widely cited and regarded as significant in calling attention to many critical but overlooked threats to environmental

health. Further, the inclusion of "economic benefit" in risk analysis is even more controversial than ranking of environmental threats.

2. It is interesting to note that many of the chemicals responsible for indoor air pollution also appear as the cause of other ranked problems such as worker exposure (ranked as the number 1 problem), hazardous waste sites, hazardous/toxic air pollutants, and groundwater contamination. In other words, although the problems are split into discrete categories in order to be ranked, many of the same substances pose problems to people or the environment in various stages of their "life cycles." It is also interesting to note that the category of "drinking water as it arrives at the tap" is ranked 9 of 29. This category is related to indoor air pollution in that it includes inhalation of VOCs, especially chloroform/ trihalomethanes, from heated tap water.

3. The situation here reminds me of vehicle airbags, which not only do not protect all people equally, but can actually kill people who aren't adult men. According to Allstate Insurance (1998) "Inflating air bags have caused a small number of deaths or serious injuries to children, smaller-stature adults, and pregnant women. As of July 1996, twenty-two infants and children and nineteen adults, mostly elderly and/or short women, have been killed in the United States by inflating airbags." While there are no specific height and weight parameters for greater risk of injury from airbags, the key factor is seat distance from the airbag. Since a "short" driver (most often short means an average size woman in the U.S.) is likely to have shorter legs than most adult white men, they will need to sit closer to the steering wheel to be able to drive—putting them at risk of airbag injury rather than protection.

4. The information for this section comes from EPA publications, or from publications by researchers affiliated with the EPA who work on indoor air quality issues. For the purposes of this chapter, the validity of this information will not be challenged. The intent here is to establish EPA beliefs of the risks posed by VOCs, in order to contrast those beliefs with the strategies they've adopted. The construction of risk is a highly interpretative and contested process that cannot be separated from power, however a full discussion of the construction of VOC risk is beyond the scope of this chapter.

5. The EPA publication *The Inside Story: A Guide to Indoor Air Quality* summarizes sources of indoor air pollution as follows: "There are many sources of indoor air pollution in any home. These include combustion sources such as oil, gas, kerosene, coal, wood, and tobacco products; building materials and furnishings as diverse as deteriorated, asbestos-containing insulation, wet or damp carpet, and cabinetry or furniture made of certain pressed wood products; products for household cleaning and maintenance, personal care or hobbies; central heating and cooling systems and humidification devices; and outdoor sources such as radon, pesticides, and outdoor air pollution" (US EPA and Commission 1995, 6).

6. Sick Building Syndrome (SBS) and Multiple Chemical Sensitivity (MCS) are two syndromes that can result from exposure to a combination of harmful substances. The medical establishment has only recently begun to research these illnesses, and knows very little about them.

7. S. 855, the "Children's Environmental Protection Act," introduced by Sen. Barbara Boxer in May of 2001, defined the term "vulnerable populations" as "children, pregnant women, the elderly, individuals with a history of serious illness, and other subpopulations identified by the Administrator as being likely to experience special health risks from environmental pollutants." (S. 855, 107th Cong., 2d Sess., §502 (2001)). This act was referred to the Senate Environment and Public Works Committee.

8. Section 503 of S. 855 contained language to address the inadequate data on health risk for children and vulnerable populations, and the need to reevaluate existing standards based on this biased data:

"(1) IN GENERAL-In establishing, modifying, or reevaluating any environmental or public health standard for an environmental pollutant under any law administered by the Administrator, the Administrator shall take into consideration available information concerning—

(A) all routes of children's exposure to that environmental pollutant;

(B) the special susceptibility of children to the environmental pollutant, including neurological differences between children and adults, the effect of in utero exposure to that environmental pollutant, and the cumulative effect on a child of exposure to that environmental pollutant and other substances having a common mechanism of toxicity.

(2) ADDITIONAL SAFETY MARGIN-If any of the data described in paragraph (1) are not available, the Administrator shall, in completing a risk assessment, risk characterization, or other assessment of risk underlying an environmental or public health standard,

adopt an additional margin of safety of at least 10-fold to take into account potential pre-natal and post-natal toxicity of an environmental pollutant, and the completeness of data concerning the exposure and toxicity of an environmental pollutant to children." (S. 855, 107th Cong., 2d Sess., §503 (2001))

9. The courts overturned CPSC's attempted ban of formaldehyde. See below for discussion of regulatory inadequacy.

10. In other words, there are no specific legislative requirements to reduce indoor air pollution. In contrast, outdoor air pollution is subject to legislated deadlines through the Clean Air Act—for example, national air quality standards must be met by a certain date (U.S. GAO 1991, 6). This means that in a "constrained budget process," indoor air pollution control measures can always be postponed, while those with mandates cannot (U.S. GAO 1991, 6). Hence, problems that pose a lesser risk to the public but which have legislative mandates are likely to receive greater attention than those that pose a greater risk but have no mandates.

11. Title IV of the Superfund Amendments and Reauthorization Act (SARA) of 1986 directed the EPA "to coordinate Federal indoor air quality activities" (U.S. EPA 1995a, i). Title IV further requires the EPA to ". . . develop an indoor air research program, disseminate the results of the research, establish an advisory committee comprised of federal agencies to assist the EPA in carrying out the program, and report to the Congress on federal indoor air activities" (U.S. GAO 1991, 3).

12. Besides having little or no data on most of the thousands of chemicals on the market, what data does exist is only on a chemical-by-chemical basis. Synergistic effects remain entirely unknown.

13. Scientists practicing Quantitative Risk Assessment (QRA) also have a wide margin of dis-cretion as to how they conduct and interpret the results of their studies. The EPA relies on QRA reports to determine the safety of a substance. For a concise discussion of the inter-pretative basis of QRA see Rosenthal, Gray, and Graham (1992).

14. Cost-benefit analysis is the practice where for any proposed regulation, economic costs are weighed against proposed benefits, such as lives saved or ecological protections. This prac-tice became standard during the Reagan/Bush presidencies.

15. Toxic Substances Control Act, Federal Insecticide, Fungicide, and Rodenticide Act, Federal Hazardous Substances Act.

16. BCIA membership includes manufacturers of chemicals, consumer products, building ma-terials, and building owners and/or tenants of commercial buildings (BCIA prepared state-ment in hearing on H.R. 2919, 103rd Cong., 1st Sess. (1993), 86).

17. CSMA "consists of more than 400 companies involved in the formulation, manufacture, and marketing of household and institutional chemical specialty products including, detergents, cleaning compounds, disinfectants and sanitizers, waxes, polishes, floor main-tenance products, home, lawn, and garden pesticides, and automotive specialty products" (Ralph Engel, President, Chemical Specialties Manufacturers Association, testimony in hearing on H.R. 2919, 103rd Cong., 1st Sess. (1993), 100).

18. The *EPA Journal* cautions that views expressed by the authors "do not necessarily reflect the views and policies of the EPA" (1993, 9). However, because the majority of contributing authors are EPA scientists or administrators, I believe these articles can reveal important information about the EPA's approach to indoor air quality.

19. Employees also must rely on the employer's willingness to follow voluntary EPA guidelines for building management: ventilation systems need to be kept in good working order, toxic building materials (such as new carpets) need to have time to outgass before employees are required to work in proximity to them, etc.

20. "In order of effectiveness."

21. Organizations listed as having "participated in the development of this brochure":
American Federation of State, County, and Municipal Employees, American Fiber Manufacturers Association, American Lung Association, American Textile Manufacturers Institute, Carpet and Rug Institute, Carpet Cushion Council, Floor Covering Installation Contractors Association, Floor Covering Adhesive Manufacturers Committee of the Na-tional Association of Floor Covering Distributors, Georgia Tech Research Institute, National Institute of Standards and Technology, Styrene Butadiene Latex Manufacturers Council, The Adhesives and Sealants Council, Inc., CPSC, EPA, U.S. General Services Administration.

22. According to Fagin, "Most experts on nontoxic building materials say, for example, that you can forget about going to the local hardware store or lumber yard for help. Such stores provide little information on product content and alternatives, and most products that are truly low in toxics are not produced by companies that have big distribution networks that ensure their presence on the shelves. Even products one might think are nontoxic—solid wood, for example—are often treated with such chemicals as preservatives, insecticides, or fungicides" (Fagin and Lavelle 1996, 202). And further, "Price, of course, is always an important issue. Toxic-free building materials generally are more expensive, not only because of the ingredients, but also because the companies producing them are so small that they do not realize economies of scale and because there are few distribution networks for such products" (Fagin and Lavelle 1996, 206).

23. For a comprehensive environmental inequality literature review see Szasz and Mueser (1997).

24. *Indoor Environment Connections*, an IAQ industry trade publication founded in 1999, demonstrates the fast growth of the IAQ industry, which has received great encouragement from the EPA. According to the *Indoor Environment Connections* website, "Indoor environments is (sic) not a flat market by any means. It's a marketplace full of individuals, businesses, and organizations that we know are strategically positioning themselves to do great things in the new millennium. . . ." (IE Connections Online 2002, website). It is interesting to note that the preferred EPA approach to solving the industrially produced IAQ problem is to support growth of a new industry to produce and market "solutions," rather than addressing the root causes of the problem itself.

Chapter 3

1. Not all countries have signed the CWC. Key exceptions include Iraq and North Korea, among others. However, only eight countries have declared possession of existing or former chemical weapons production facilities: China, Japan, France, India, United Kingdom, United States, Russia, and Canada. Only four have declared possession of a chemical weapons stockpile: India, United States, Russia, and South Korea. And seven nations have declared that chemical weapons were abandoned on their territory: Belgium, Germany, United Kingdom, China, Italy, France, and Japan.

2. For a report on chemical weapons activities on Johnston Island, see Casper 2002.

3. Endocrine disruption also impacts wildlife, and indeed, affected animals are often seen as harbingers of the human threat (Christensen and Casper 2000).

4. PMCD Fact Sheet, *FM_emissions—5/98*.

5. PMCD Fact Sheet, *standards.p65—12/97*.

Chapter 4

1. "Can the subaltern speak?" post-colonial critic Gayatri Spivak queries in a widely quoted article by that name (1988). "The subaltern is always speaking," Indonesian scholar Laurie Sears replies in *Shadows of Empire* (1996). "The problem for post-colonial intellectuals— whether they have inherited the subject position of the colonizer or the colonized—is how to listen when the subaltern speaks." This paper is intended as an attempt to listen. Underlying its approach are theoretical matters currently debated in languages particular to the social sciences: problematizations and deconstructions of the uses and languages of power, along with attention to social constructions of reality, to the power of discourse, to agency, and to engagement with issues of local and global, of bodies and nations. But since the goal of my work is to broaden discussion, not restrict it, I here heed the call from Edward Said's first address as head of the MLA, to avoid the elitism of terms with special meanings and speak in a common language, acknowledging as I do so the limitations of a seeming transparency. (For discussion, see, among others, Abu Lughod 1991, Trinh 1989, Patai 1991, Visweswaran 1994.)

2. The conference drew 280 scientists from Vietnam, and 120 from the U.S., Australia, Canada, the U.K., France, Germany, Italy, Japan, the Republic of Korea, Laos, New Zealand, the Netherlands, Norway, Russia, Singapore, Switzerland, Sweden, and Taiwan. Roughly

100 studies were presented. The conference was jointly coordinated by the U.S. National Institute of Environmental Health Studies and the Vietnamese Ministry of Science, Technology, and the Environment. The first officially recognized joint research between the U.S. and Vietnam, soil sampling near Da Nang, was begun.

3. See Gordon, who speaks of the need to "follow the ghosts and spells of power" in order to understand social life, "in order to tame [the] sorcerer and conjure otherwise" (1997, 7, 28).

4. See Kleinman, Das, and Lock (1997), *Social Suffering,* introduction and passim.

5. For a history of the development of the use of herbicides in war, and plans to use them in World War II, see Cecil (1986), Galston (1972), Neilands et al. (1977), Westing (1984). A definitive history tracing the interweavings of politics in science in the development and use of these chemicals has yet to be written. Testing of herbicides and defoliants began in 1961 in Vietnam, though their use in warfare did not begin until January, 1962. Agent Orange itself was in use from 1965–1971, accounting for roughly 61 percent of the 72,740,400 liters of defoliants and herbicides sprayed between 1961 and 1971. The U.S. stopped its own use of defoliants and herbicides in 1971; in 1972 it took the remaining barrels of Agent Orange to be stored on Johnston Island in the Pacific, where they were destroyed in 1977. However, the U.S. continued to supply other chemicals to the Saigon regime until the end of the war in 1975 (Young, 13; Dai, 22).

6. Based on statistics from a 1974 National Academy of Science review of a herbicide applications log kept by the U.S. Military Assistance Command, Vietnam, and on a 1985 review of Vietnam era records by a joint group of military records specialists (Young and Reggiani 1988, 13).

7. For a history of the evolution of this Air Force unit, see Cecil (1986). The motto of the group was "Only You Can Prevent Forests," the radio call signal was first "Cowboy," and then, "Hades."

8. The head of the Japan Science Council, Yoichi Fukushima, set the figure at half the arable land (Committee of Concerned Asian Scholars 1970, 113).

9. See, notably, the work of Dr. Jeanne Stellman, Professor of Clinical Public Health at Columbia University.

10. See Young and Reggiani (1988), Nielands et al. (1972), Cecil (1986), and Westing (1984) for the beginnings of fuller sketches.

11. Accounts vary.

12. Lewy (1978) 257–8. See Cecil (1986, 155) for reference to Kennedy's desire to experiment with the counterinsurgency potential of the chemicals. While Le Cao Dai (2000) speaks of the use of herbicides as a matter of U.S. initiative with South Vietnamese (Ngo Dinh Diem) assistance (12), Lewy says the American Military Assistance Advisory Group (MAAG) brought the proposal for herbicide use to Washington from the South Vietnamese (257), and Buckingham (1982) writes that Ngo Dinh Diem asked the U.S. to conduct the spraying (iii).

13. U.S. Department of the Air Force, cited by Lewy (1978, 259).

14. By subtracting the figures for Saigon, which was less affected by the spraying, the Army figures showed an increase in all three defects in the rest of the country, though it would be "totally incorrect," they said, to take this as proof of the effect of herbicides, since other factors might also be responsible. In heavily sprayed Tay Ninh province, the AAAS study, based on more complete hospital records than those used by the Army, also found evidence of a stillbirth rate more than double that for the country as a whole. The Saigon Children's Hospital showed a "disproportionate increase" in pure cleft palates and spina bifida for the years 1967–1968. Again, the team stressed that the affects could not safely be attributed to herbicides, and called for further study (Neilands et al. 1972, 282).

15. Lewy (1978) relates that the study was "accidentally found"; Uhl and Ensign claim it was leaked to Nader's Raiders by a source at the Food and Drug Administration (1980, 146). Regianni, observing merely that the results 'became known', sets the date the study became public knowledge as the birth date of Agent Orange as a matter of public concern, noting that later analysis revealed that the cause of the toxicity was a contaminant, not 2,4,5-T itself (Young and Reggiani 1988, 33–34).

16. The four listed as having sufficient evidence are Hodgkins disease, non-Hodgkins lymphoma, soft tissue sarcomas, and chloracne. The six listed with limited evidence are respiratory cancers (lung, larnyx, trachea, bronchial), prostate cancer, multiple myeloma, peripheral neuropathy, poryphyria cutanea tarda, and spina bifida.

17. Nineteen of the twenty blood samples taken in 1999 from this heavily exposed southern city showed elevated levels of TCDD dioxin (a marker for Agent Orange and other dioxin-contaminated herbicides), compared both to samples taken from the unsprayed north, and to World Health Organization standards for acceptable body burden (10 parts per trillion). The average in the north was 2.2 parts per trillion (ppt), while the samples in the south ranged up to 271 ppt, with 13 of the samples higher than 55 ppt, and five of the samples over 100 ppt.

18. A comparative study of the development of U.S. and Vietnamese scientific knowledge on this issue should yield insights both for the study of science and for the study of cultures.

19. See the work of the Canadian Hatfield group in general, and in particular, Dwernychuk. See also the work of Schecter, Dai, Constable, et al.

20. See Westing (1984), Schecter (1994), Cecil (1986), Young and Reggiani (1988), among others.

21. See Arthur Kleinman (1998), *The Illness Narratives.*

22. The question had been drawn to my attention by a whack on my shoulder from a shop-keeper in Hue. "Why hasn't your government done anything to help those people it hurt during the war?" she demanded. She was thinking especially about the people in surrounding villages "suffering from Agent Orange," she said. It was 1997. I was in my seventh year of half-time living in Vietnam, where I worked as a teacher and journalist; that year I was leading a small study-abroad pilot project, and writing occasional features for *Viet Nam News.*

23. By 2001, he was dean of the department and head of a center he had created, the "Office of Genetic Counseling and Disabled Children."

24. In 2000 and 2001, I conducted thirty-eight open-ended interviews in a dozen villages and three towns in the north, center, and south of Vietnam. The people interviewed came from many parts of the political spectrum: some fought for the revolution; some joined the Advanced Youth Brigades, some were wives or children of soldiers who fought for the Saigon regime, some cleared land in New Economic Zones, and some helped rebuild homes in towns and villages that were razed and abandoned for years during the war. Thirty-one now live in villages, and the other seven in provincial capitals.

    Thirty of the interviews were made possible by the Vietnamese and International Red Cross organizations, during preparations for a program to assist those the agency awkwardly but accurately labels "the disabled poor, including those thought to be affected by Agent Orange." The first eight interviews were conducted thanks to the help of the Committee for Protection and Care of Children (CPCC), in a northern province a few hours drive from Hanoi.

    Interviews included five open-ended topics, developed together with the CPCC and Red Cross over the course of the initial interviews: description of a family's current health and economic situation, exposure of a family member to chemicals during the war, help they have received, help that they would find useful, and comments they would like to have transmitted to a larger audience, including Americans. This last question grew out of a question posed by a Japanese visitor on yet another visit organized by the Vietnamese Red Cross. The man was a member of a citizens' delegation from Sapporo, investigating damage caused by the Japanese occupation during World War II, and by Japan's support for America during the Vietnam War. At a home for disabled veterans he asked a man who had lost both legs, "Is there anything you would like to ask America?" On a subsequent visit, the question was picked up by a representative of the Red Cross who had been present. It became a standard question, which was sometimes greeted with a sad shake of the head, or a gentle dismissal: "Oh, that was a long time ago . . ."; other times, it opened the doors to deep feeling. The length of our discussions depended on my reading of the family's eagerness to talk, and on time constraints.

    I was at first hesitant to do the work, not wanting to stir up painful memories or raise false hopes. The Vietnamese doctors and social workers I met told me most people would be eager to talk longer than we had time to listen. It turned out they were right: over and again I was thanked for my visits, and told, when I apologized for having only small gifts to share, that the recognition and attention I gave were "precious delicacies for the spirit." I came to think of my hesitation as misplaced, or even a tool that helped keep in place the distances between our worlds, helping to mask uncomfortable imbalances of power and privilege. The families lived with their situations every day; they were not forgetting. They were for the most part articulate, and grateful to be heard.

25. For that morning, "we" were my friend, a representative of the CPCC, a man I took to be from public security, and myself. The names used are pseudonyms, following American academic convention. However, a writer friend in Vietnam tells me it is more honest, and more respectful, to use the real name, especially since the stories were being told in a setting where many others observed and participated in the interviews, and since the families I have quoted asked that their words be conveyed.

26. The communities that have supported these families for decades are themselves struggling with the consequences of war, whether that be residual chemicals, bomb craters, unexploded ordnance and mines, or several of these at once, and more—to speak only of damage to the land. In Ha Nam, the provincial capital had been completely razed by bombing except for the skeleton of a church, a Red Cross doctor told me. In Thua Thien Hue, the village I visited had been a no man's land for four or five years; returning villagers were charged with filling in the bomb craters on their own land. How did they even know what land was theirs, I asked. The river was still there, I was told, and the stubble of clumps of bamboo, or sometimes the roots of trees. A grandfather spoke of returning from a "strategic hamlet" to find his shelter full of the bones of people he did not know. Large parts of Dong Nai were laid waste by defoliants, or contaminated by chemical runoff from the base; villagers moved from place to place "in circles," as a doctor from the Red Cross put it, looking for shelter from the bombs.

27. While this is not an exact description of a barrel of the dioxin-contaminated mix of 2,4,-D and 2,4,5-T that was, strictly speaking, code named Agent Orange, barrels of a variety of chemicals are still being uncovered today, and causing deaths. It is unlikely, however, that the barrel mentioned dioxin. Could it be a mis-reading of the English "Do not . . ." or "danger"?

28. "*Vung xa vung sau,*" an expression much in use at the time to indicate pockets of poverty in the distant hinterlands.

29. It is commonly held that trouble may be caused by neglect of the ancestors' graves.

Chapter 5

1. Both are Marxist categories. Use value refers to the concrete ability of a product to satisfy human needs, while exchange value refers to the value of a product, usually monetary, for which it could be exchanged on the market.

2. Vészi's novel *Géza Gazda's Forints* is about the Stalinist hero of material conservation and waste recycling, of whom more later.

3. The representation and deconstruction of this worker-hero that is perhaps best known to Western audiences is Polish film director Andrzej Wajda's *Man of Marble.*

4. Several authors notice this social contructivist attitude to nature in Marx's writings and explain it with Marx's need to distinguish his materialism from biological reductionism (O'Connor 1991).

5. This is Robert Blauner's term for largely automated industries constituted by flows, such as the chemical industry (1967).

6. The fact that production increased at a greater rate in the first half of the decade than in the second reflects the opening of many new chemical factories at the beginning of the 1960s.

7. I am borrowing Ann Anagnost's distinction between producing and consuming bodies (1995).

8. A major chemical plant started dumping toxic wastes in this small village in 1978. What made the case infamous was the public health scandals and the many years of litigation and public hearings on whether to clean the dump up by an incinerator that would also be built in Garé. As of 2002, the dump is still there.

9. Incinerators simply decrease the volume of waste but whether they actually reduce its toxicity is dependent on the composition of the burned wastes. Incineration itself has its waste products (e.g., bottom ash and fly ash) which are still considered toxic and which thus have to be screened from the air and landfilled. Incinerator emissions of dioxins and furans, the most toxic substances ever known, account for 80 percent of all such emissions in industrialized countries.

10. With charges of $1,500 for burning one ton of hazardous waste, a medium sized facility (50,000 t./yr.) can earn its investment (construction) costs (about $50–60 million) within one year.

11. Among the concerns and demands of MZP were racial purity, increasing male potency and fertility through improving environmental quality, banning the use of harmful salt produced by new-Zionists around the world to poison others, and forcing AIDS patients entering the country to wear yellow tags (note that the color of David Stars Jews had to wear in Nazi-ruled countries prior to and during World War II was also yellow).

Chapter 6

1. Resonates with Don, the railroad worker, from Nelkin and Brown, who believed that he brought home pesticides on his clothes (1984, 49).
2. Gathering information from a variety of articles is a common experience for patients. See for example, Nelkin and Brown (1984, 32).
3. Of course, we also have the counter example of gun control. Groups in favor of gun control try to use statistics on accidental children's deaths to move legislation for stricter gun control, but have thus far failed.

Chapter 7

1. The first large and highly visible protest in the environmental justice movement was in 1982 against the decision by then governor of North Carolina James Hunt to site in the predominantly African-American, rural community of Afton, North Carolina, a landfill for PCB-contaminated soil illegally dumped by a New York trucking company. For accounts of this and other protests in the environmental justice movement see, for example, Bullard (1990, 1993). The protest in Afton set off a round of investigation into disproportionate amounts of pollution in low-income communities of color. See, for example, U.S. GAO (1983), United Church of Christ Committee for Racial Justice (1987), Gelobter (1988), Lee (1992). These reports helped bring environmental discrimination into public awareness. Environmental justice advocates were equally critical of environmental organizations that had not been concerned with the social justice dimensions of environmental problems (Bryant et al. 1990; Moore et al. 1990).
2. In the larger ethnography of which this chapter is a part, I look at the marginal material and political conditions of pollution prevention activism in the United States at the turn of the twentieth century; how one organization built pollution prevention campaigns in the 1980s and 1990s; how in the early 1990s this group took heed of criticisms from the environmental justice movement and made a concerted effort to branch out into community organizing in predominantly low-income minority areas disproportionately impacted by pollution; what that effort took, how it went, and how the staff of the organization and the newcomers together formed an agenda; what resources they found in health and environmental agencies (discussed in this chapter); how the limited criteria for action I discuss in this chapter evolved and solidified in public health and regulatory agencies; and the issues of power, knowledge, and identity between and among newcomers and seasoned activists working in pollution prevention (Hoffman in progress).
3. My account is based on participant observation and ethnographic interviews I conducted between November 1999 and August 2001.
4. I have used pseudonyms for places, people, environmental groups, and local government agencies. I have called federal agencies by their actual names.
5. Involvement of residents of areas disproportionately impacted by pollution in health and regulatory politics through organizing by environmental groups is more of an exception than a rule. Many pollution prevention campaigns come directly from the affected community and from involvement with social justice and civil rights organizations. I chose this case not because it is the norm, but because collaboration between the Clean Air and Water Network and Springfield residents was relatively well-established and because I was successful at negotiating access to it. In addition to my role as participant observer, I worked as a volunteer assistant with the Clean Air and Water Network in support of their community organizing in Springfield.
6. Roughly fifty groups signed on to the alliance's statement. These include labor and religious organizations, in addition to environmental health and antitoxics groups. About five organizations, including the Clean Air and Water Network, were actively involved in building the alliance.

7. I began my fieldwork toward the end of the series of about fifty meetings and was able to attend only one of them. My account here is based on interviews with the community organizers.

8. One particularly egregious example of racism in medical science is the investigation by the United States Public Health Service of the natural history of untreated syphilis between 1932 and 1972. The PHS studied several hundred black men with syphilis, whom they did not tell about, nor treat for their conditions (Jones 1981). In another example, throughout the twentieth century, medical researchers have used the prevalence of sickle cell anemia in Blacks to assert race as a biological rather than ideological category (instead of accounting for the distribution of the disease in terms of genetics and politically influenced patterns of mating), and to claim the genetically based racial distinctiveness of "blacks" and "whites" (Tapper 1999).

9. In the political economy of high tech lab equipment, private industry is often better equipped, having the financial capacity to buy or develop it. Smaller government budgets are more prohibitive. Without a stronger ability of government to govern private industry, the question of whether or not knowledge about toxics will be produced and the quality of that knowledge comes under strong influence of an unregulated set of private interests.

10. I was present in meetings between the interested Springfield residents and those working on the dioxin prevention campaign at the Clean Air and Water Network. This account is based on my observations of these meetings.

11. There were differences to be worked out in the process of forming this agenda. For example, the more experienced pollution prevention activists knew that action rarely comes from testing and that, in fact, testing is often used as an excuse for a government agency or polluter to do nothing. Additionally, the Springfield residents supported the Clean Air and Water Network's tactics, but had little or no experience with it. For a discussion of the dynamics involved in forming this agenda, see Hoffman (in progress).

12. This meeting was small and by invitation only, not for the general public. I was not present and rely on participants' accounts here.

13. Pollution data has been made available through the Toxics Release Inventory since the late 1980s. Cancer incidence is available through the National Program of Cancer Registries, formally established by Congress only in 1992. Several states had established cancer registries earlier; for example Connecticut began collecting this information in 1941. While pollution causes many kinds of illness, cancer is one of the few kind of illness for which data has been collected. See Steingraber (1993).

14. In Love Canal in the mid-1950s, developers built a neighborhood on and adjacent to an abandoned dumpsite of Hooker Chemical Corporation, resulting in seepage of dioxin and other toxins dumped there into the homes. In the subsequent decades, exposure to these toxins caused high numbers of birth defects, miscarriages, cancers, and central nervous system problems. In Times Beach, as in other rural communities in Missouri, dioxin was sprayed in recycled waste oil on dirt roads for dust control throughout the 1970s. See Gibbs (1995).

15. For an analysis of the dynamics between and among newcomers and seasoned activists in the Dioxin Prevention Alliance, see Hoffman (in progress).

16. This part of my account is based on my observations and the Water Quality Bureau's transcript of the meeting.

17. Pete was referring to EPA's then recent decision to override the State and Regional Water Quality Bureau's list of toxic pollutants it planned to prioritize and address. The state and regional agencies did not include dioxin; EPA added dioxin to the list.

18. EPA published its first review of the scientific literature on the health effects of dioxin, which included an estimate of the cancer risk associated with it, in 1985. Industries that produce dioxin have kept the question of dioxin's health risks open in EPA over all these years, largely through inclusion on the EPA's Science Advisory Board, pushing the agency for more studies, even as each new study confirms and expands the bad news about dioxin. In 2000, EPA released a draft of its most recent, extremely comprehensive dioxin exposure and risk assessment but industry pressure thus far has prevented the release of the official report. It is through processes such as these that industry continues unduly to influence criteria for action in regulatory agencies, criteria that have severe consequences indefinitely. EPA does not have, after twenty-seven years and counting, a practical plan for compelling industries to stop producing dioxin. See Hertsgaard (2001) and Pianin (2001).

19. For a discussion of the evolution and solidification of limited criteria for action in health and regulatory agencies I discuss in this chapter see Hoffman (in progress).

Chapter 8

1. AIDS, which began making an impact on mortality rates during the 1980s, represents an obvious and important exception to this trend. Age-adjusted death rates for a variety of causes, going back to 1900, are available on-line from the National Center for Health Statistics at http://www.cdc.gov/nchs/datawh/statab/unpubd/mortabs/hist293.htm.

2. According to the National Cancer Advisory Board, although tobacco use accounts "for much of this alarming and wholly unacceptable increase . . . other contributing factors remain undiscovered and unconfirmed" (National Cancer Advisory Board 1994, 10).

3. Only recently (October 2002) did the National Cancer Institute release new figures indicating that the incidence rates of a number of cancers, including breast, have not decreased over the decade—as the NCI and the ACS have been claiming for the last few years—but have actually continued to climb. Delayed reporting and reporting errors were the reasons cited for the discrepancies.

4. All budgetary figures can be found in the NCI portion of the *NIH Almanac*, available on-line at http://www.nih.gov/about/almanac/organization/NCI.htm

5. Only the NCI, for example, among all the institutes of the NIH, submits its budget proposal directly to the Office of the President. The President's direct oversight of the NCI's budget was written into the National Cancer Act of 1971 to insure that the NCI would not be short-changed by the NIH. See Richard Rettig (1977) for a history of the National Cancer Act.

6. The chemotherapy screening program had two foci—plant-based compounds, most of which were gathered for the NCI by the U.S. Department of Agriculture, and synthetic chemicals, most of which were submitted by private industry, chemical companies in particular (Goodman and Walsh 2001).

7. For an analysis of breast cancer policy making in the U.S., see Carol S. Weisman (2001). The source for the disease-specific NCI budgetary figures for 1983 and 1987 is the National Cancer Institute Financial Management Branch (personal correspondence via fax, March 14, 2001). In response to my inquiry, Karen Colbart, an NCI staff member, put together a table entitled "National Cancer Institute Research Dollars by Various Cancers Fy1981–Fy1998." All figures are drawn from this table.

8. It is important to remember that the state is a complex maze of organized interests and bureaucratic fiefdoms more often working in ignorance of, or competition with, each other than in cooperation. The NIH is a case in point. In 1937 the NIH consisted of one institute, the NCI. In 1948 the National Institute of Mental Health was added. By 1952 there were seven separate institutes, today there are twenty-seven. Additionally, and importantly, in most instances the state neither acted alone nor initiated action. Rather, it responded to pressures from private industry, philanthropic foundations (major funders of medical research), the interests of organized medicine, cancer charities, patients groups, consumer rights organizations, and social movements. In fact, the definition and division of cancer research, regulation, treatment and prevention among various agencies within the state is, in large part, an outcome of pressures and demands that originated outside of it—but that discussion lies beyond the scope of this chapter. See James Patterson (1987) for a cultural history of cancer in the U.S. and see Robert N. Proctor (1995) for a political history of cancer research in the U.S.

9. A third model, equally important but beyond the scope of this chapter, is what I would call the behavioral, or public health, model. Since at least the 1970s the behavioral model is growing in importance by leaps and bounds. The primary places where it has been institutionalized within the state are the National Cancer Institute and the Centers for Disease Control and Prevention.

10. Taxol, which was approved for the treatment of ovarian cancer in 1992, was the first naturally occurring chemical substance to make it all the way from the NCI chemotherapy program to FDA-approval. The final step of this twenty-five year process was undertaken in 1989, when the federal government signed a CRADA with Bristol-Myers Squibb. The vast majority of chemotherapies, however, are synthetic chemicals (not naturally ocurring chemicals). Even Taxol is now produced semi-synthetically. See Goodman and Walsh (2001).

11. See Proctor (1995), especially pp. 36–48, for a fascinating discussion of Wilhelm Hueper.

12. These agencies were created, in large part, in response to Rachel Carson's *Silent Spring* (1962) and the environmental activism it catalyzed.

13. Even those funding niches within the NCI dedicated to the study of cancer prevention have pursued a largely biomedical agenda—focusing, for example, on pharmaceutical forms of prevention (called chemoprevention in the medical literature—literally, chemical prevention) while ignoring chemicals in the environment, or focusing on the effects of diet and nutrition while ignoring the use of growth hormones and pesticides used by agribusiness.

14. Ironically, the NBCC was founded, in 1991, by a group of women's cancer and breast cancer organizations, many of whom foregrounded industrial chemicals and environmental carcinogens in their political analyses and public statements. Although the story of feminist and lesbian cancer and breast cancer organizations in the late 1980s and early 1990s is an important one, and a missing piece of the puzzle, it is not the subject of this chapter. See Barbara Brenner (2000) for one of the few accounts of the U.S. breast cancer movement that discusses this early history. See Kelly Happe (forthcoming), especially chapter five ("Environmental Models of Disease in the Age of Genomics: The Case of Breast Cancer"), for an analysis of collective organizing around the environmental theory of breast cancer in Long Island. See Sabrina McCormick, Phil Brown, and Steven Zavestoski (2001) for a comparison of the environmental wing of the breast cancer movement in three of its principal locales: Long Island, Massachusetts, and the San Francisco Bay Area. And see Maren Klawiter (1999a, 1999b, 2000) for analyses of cancer organizing in the San Francisco Bay Area during the 1990s.

15. This chapter is based upon ethnographic research on cancer activism conducted in the San Francisco Bay Area between 1994 and 1999 and research on the pharmaceutical industry conducted between 1999 and 2002.

16. Feminist cancer activism includes the environmental wing of the breast cancer movement. In this chapter I move back and forth between different ways of referring to this field of activism because, although there is a great deal of overlap, there are differences that in certain circumstances become salient, but in many circumstances are not. The goals of the feminist cancer movement and the environmental wing of the breast cancer movement—at least in the San Francisco Bay Area—are very close to identical.

17. For example, although Greenpeace had produced a major report on breast cancer and dioxins entitled "Chlorine, Human Health, and the Environment: The Breast Cancer Warning," (Thornton 1993) and local Greenpeace organizers were active in various environmental justice campaigns in the San Francisco Bay Area, neither Breast Cancer Action (in San Francisco) nor the Women's Cancer Resource Center (in Berkeley) worked in coalition with Greenpeace during the early 1990s, or even, for that matter, with each other. The term "political fields" comes from Raka Ray (1998), who argues that the structure of a political field and a social movement organization's (SMO) position within it shapes the SMO's discourses and practices.

18. For a basic overview of the U.S. environmental movement and the development of movements around environmental justice and environmental racism, see Riley E. Dunlap and Angela G. Mertig (1992). For a thoughtful analysis of narratives of the environmental movement and their forms of inclusion and exclusion, see Marcy Darnovsky (1992).

19. The American Cancer Society has made high cancer rates the centerpiece of their public education materials and early detection campaigns since they were founded in 1913. Women's cancer and breast cancer organizations adopted a similar strategy in the 1990s, publicizing breast cancer statistics and framing them in terms as dramatic as possible.

20. The Northern California Cancer Center is the organization contracted by the National Cancer Institute to manage the Tumor Registry for the San Francisco Bay Area, as part of the Bay Area's participation in SEER (Surveillance, Epidemiology and End Results). SEER is the largest cancer database in the country and has, since 1972, been collecting population based data on cancer incidence, treatment and survival. SEER data covers 14 percent of the U.S. population and is the best source of data from which to make estimates about the U.S. population, since there is no nationwide, population-based cancer surveillance in the U.S.

21. The dominant narrative about black women within the epidemiological discourse on breast cancer emphasizes the disproportionately high rate of breast cancer *mortality* among black women by contrasting it to their relatively low rate of *incidence*. In both cases, the implicit comparison group embedded in this discourse is white women, and the discourse has

the effect of minimizing the incidence of breast cancer among black women in the United States. The data published in the report of the Northern California Cancer Center demonstrated that, although black women in the Bay Area have lower incidence rates than white women in the Bay Area, they have higher rates than almost every other group of women in the world. Only women living in Hawaii and white women in Atlanta, Georgia had higher rates than black women in the Bay Area.

22. I began doing participant-observation of the TLC in October 1994, shortly after its formation. The information about the first two meetings of the Toxic Links Coalition (TLC) is based upon interviews with cancer activist Judy Brady, and the public recounting of this history at various events.

23. Quote taken from AstraZeneca International, "Community and Company Projects: US National Breast Cancer Awareness Month," www.astrazeneca.com

24. Although the NBCAM's genealogy can indeed be traced to 1985, there was no "breast cancer awareness month" that year, but rather a week of activities designed around the promotion of breast cancer early detection practices. See Johns Hopkins Health Information, "How It All Began," included as part of a special feature called "Pink October: Breast Cancer Awareness Month," http://www.intelihealth.com (accessed October 2001).

25. Betty Ford, wife of former U.S. President Gerald Ford, created a furor in 1974 when she publicly revealed her recent breast cancer diagnosis and mastectomy and pointedly attributed her survival to early detection. This occurred during the Breast Cancer Detection Demonstration Project (discussed earlier in this article) and, because Ford's disclosure was so dramatic and so well-covered by the media, the BCDDP was flooded with new recruits and, throughout the country, requests for mammograms peaked. The consequences of Ford's disclosure can be seen in the breast cancer statistics. The breast cancer incidence rate spikes during this period of time, then falls back to a much more gradual rate of increase

26. Information on Zeneca comes from Scrip Reports (1996: 412). Salick Health Care was founded in 1983 by an entrepreneurial physician and it was the first company to open for-profit cancer treatment centers in the U.S. (Tanenbaum 2000, 52).

27. In 1997, the review panel of the United States National Toxicology Program recommended listing tamoxifen as a "known" human carcinogen. This recommendation followed on the heels of a similar action by the International Agency for Research on Cancer (IARC), of the World Health Organization, who, in February of 1996, classified tamoxifen as a Group 1 human carcinogen—the strongest possible classification. Interestingly, as far back as 1995, the Carcinogen Identification Committee of the California Environmental Protection Agency Office of Environmental Health Hazard Assessment (OEHHA) unanimously concluded that tamoxifen was carcinogenic to humans and recommended adding it to the state's list of cancer-causing chemicals, a public document that the Governor, under Proposition 65 (the antitoxics initiative approved by California voters in 1986) is required to maintain. Following the recommendations of the advisory panel, Zeneca launched an extensive campaign to keep the drug off the Proposition 65 list, and days before the deadline for listing tamoxifen, Governor Wilson stepped in and delayed the addition by calling for additional study and public hearings. Alan Bilbauer, a spokesman at Zeneca's U.S. headquarters in Wilmington, Delaware, rejected the claim that tamoxifen is a uterine carcinogen, arguing (in language reminiscent of the tobacco industry) that "there is a difference between association and causation." See *The Cancer Letter* (November 7, 1997) for a discussion of the US National Toxicology Program's recommendation; the WHO's classification of tamoxifen as a Class I carcinogen is from the "Official Press Release" of the International Agency for Research on Cancer of the World Health Organization, February 22, 1996; events related to the California EPA are in Paul Jacobs, "State Delays Putting Drug on Carcinogen List," *Los Angeles Times*, November 8, 1995. Bilbauer quote from Sabin Russell, "Wilson Intervened on Carcinogen List," *San Francisco Chronicle*, Thursday November 9, 1995.

28. See Klawiter (1999a) for a comparative analysis of Race for the Cure, the Women & Cancer Walk, and the Toxic Tour of the Cancer Industry—cancer events held on an annual basis in San Francisco.

29. WEDO is based in New York City and was founded in 1990, and was led by former U.S. Congresswoman and "cancer fighter" Bella Abzug (until her death in 1998). WEDO describes itself as "a global activist, advocacy and information organization that networks with some 20,000 women and men from groups in every region of the world. . . . WEDO is a highly

effective global network of women activists and leaders concerned with the environment, development, social and economic justice." WEDO was a major sponsor and organizer of the first World Conference on Breast Cancer, held in Kingston, Canada in July of 1997 and the second World Conference on Breast Cancer, held in July of 1999 in Ottawa, Canada.

30. In 1997, the West County Toxics Coalition was finally successful in getting Chevron to shut down their hazardous waste incinerator.

31. In addition to the local campaigns described in the body of this chapter, there were a number of campaigns and coalitions operating on a grander scale. For example, California Zero Dioxin Exposure Alliance formed to help coordinate and provide resources for anti-dioxin organizing activities throughout the state. As a result of their efforts and the growing recognition of the dangers of dioxin, three city councils in the Bay Area, Berkeley, Oakland and San Francisco, approved resolutions to create a dioxin-free environment. Californians for Pesticide Reform worked on a number of issues at the state level: improving access to information on pesticides through public right-to-know legislation; banning the use of the most harmful pesticides; and reducing the use of less toxic pesticides. Another national campaign with local roots was created in September 1996 when Commonweal (a retreat center for people with cancer and cancer survivors) invited representatives from organizations around the country to attend an organizing meeting that resulted in the formation of Health Care Without Harm. HCWH built upon local anti-dioxin oganizing but directed its focus to the elimination of hospital-generated dioxins and mercuries (one of the major sources of dioxins) by helping hospitals redesign their waste management systems in order to minimize the production of PVC waste. At a broader level, HCWH marked the development of "environmentally responsible health care." Breast Cancer Action was a charter member of Health Care Without Harm, and other feminist cancer organizations contributed to HCWH. See http://www.noharm.org/ for additional information.

32. Dioxin is the common name for a class of seventy-five chemicals. It has no commercial use but is a toxic waste product formed when waste containing chlorine is burned or when products containing chlorine are manufactured. PVC (polyvinyl chloride) plastic is a major source of the chlorine in medical waste. See *Health Care Without Harm: The Campaign For Environmentally Responsible Health Care*. Dioxin is one of the most toxic chemicals in the world and has been linked to cancer, diabetes, birth defects, endometriosis, and many other health problems. In February of 1997, a panel of scientists convened by the International Agency for Research on Cancer (IARC), a body of the World Health Organization, voted to classify a form of dioxin known as 2,3,7,8, TCDD as a proven human carcinogen. TCDD is 300,000 times more potent than DDT, which was banned by the U.S. in 1972. Dioxins are formed as unintended by-products of certain chemical reactions, especially those involving chlorine. They are exceptionally stable compounds, and therefore persist for long periods in the environment and in tissues of exposed individuals. See Health Care Without Harm's website http://www.noharm.org for additional information on dioxins and other toxic chemicals.

33. For an analysis of environmental activism and the politics of breast cancer and risk assessment science in Bayview-Hunters Point, see Fishman (2000).

34. Francine Levien died from breast cancer in 2001.

35. The Mission Statement eventually developed by MBCW reads as follows: "Marin Breast Cancer Watch is a grassroots organization dedicated to finding the causes and stopping the epidemic of breast cancer. We accomplish our mission through community-based participatory research, education, and public policy advocacy with a focus on creating a healthy environment."

36. In August of 2002, the long-awaited and much-anticipated results from the main component of the federally funded Long Island studies on possible links between pollution and high rates of breast cancer were finally announced. The findings did not show any relationship between breast cancer and the types of chemicals tested, though critics argued that the design of the study was flawed and the most important chemicals weren't tested. Researchers took blood and urine samples from more than three thousand Long Island women, as well as samples of carpet dust, tap water and yard soil to try and determine to what extent the women had been exposed to specific pollutants. The study found "no increased rate of breast cancer among women exposed to pesticides, but found that exposure to chemicals like car exhaust and cigarette smoke appeared to elevate a women's risk of

breast cancer by 50 percent" (Toy 2002). See Kolata (2002), Lerner (2002), Brody (2002), BCA (2002), and Fagin (2002a, 2002b, 2002c) for responses to the study's findings.

37. I was a participant observer with Marin Breast Cancer Watch for about three years, beginning in the fall of 1995, when the group first began meeting in Francine Levien's living room to discuss environmental issues and their relationship to breast cancer. Marin Breast Cancer Watch was mentored in their development and direction by Nancy Evans, then the president of Breast Cancer Action, Andrea Martin, founder of the Breast Cancer Fund, and Lorraine Pace, a breast cancer activist from Long Island, NY and the founder of two organizations: the West Islip Breast Cancer Mapping Project and Healthy Environment for a Living Planet (HELP).

38. MBCW is currently involved in five environmental research projects: (1) Adolescent Risk Factors Study; (2) Marin Breast Cancer Research Collaborative; (3) Marin Environmental Data Study; (4) Nipple Aspirate Fluid Collection Pilot Study; (5) Personal Environmental Risk Factor Study. Funders include the Marin County Health Department, the California Department of Health Services Cancer Research Program (CRP), the Centers for Disease Control and Prevention, and the Susan Love Breast Cancer Foundation

39. In "The Mindful Body" (1987), Nancy Scheper-Hughes and Margaret Lock conceptualize three different kinds of bodies: the individual body, the social body, and the body politic. My use of the terms "suffering body" and "political body" is indebted to their analysis and to the work of Arthur Frank (1991), who uses Bryan Turner's theory of bodily order (1984) to develop a typology of four bodies: the disciplined body, the mirroring body, the dominating body, and the communicative body."

40. MBCW eventually wore out their welcome at Marin Hospital, though it was never clear to me that this had anything to do with their environmental activism. My sense at the time was that it was more closely connected to criticisms of mainstream medicine and the pharmaceutical industry that were articulated not from an environmental perspective but from an alternative medicine perspective. Further supporting this interpretation is the fact that Francine Levien, the founder and President of MBCW (until her death in 2001), refused adjuvant radiation and chemotherapy in favor of nontoxic alternative therapies.

41. See Linda Hogle (2000) for a thoughtful analysis of AstraZeneca's advertising campaign (of tamoxifen to high risk women). Hogle's analysis draws upon data gathered by conducting a series of focus groups with healthy women. For an analysis of STAR (Study of Tamoxifen and Raloxifene), the follow-up trial to the Breast Cancer Prevention Trial, see Fosket (2002). STAR is an on-going trial designed to compare tamoxifen to raloxifene (an anti-osteoporosis drug manufactured by Eli Lilly) on healthy women.

42. Consistent with the eligibility criterion for the clinical trial testing tamoxifen, "high risk" has been defined as having a 1.7 percent chance of being diagnosed with breast cancer in the next five years.

43. The name "Prevention First" evolved in late 2001, although the member organizations had been meeting via conference call, and clearly working on the issues together, since early 2000. Prevention First applied for and received a two-year, $300,000 grant from the San Francisco-based Richard and Rhoda Goldman Fund, a foundation with a history of funding projects connected to breast cancer and the environment. They began drafting the grant proposal in early 2000 and funding commenced in April 2001. Personal correspondence with Barbara Brenner, Executive Director of Breast Cancer Action, San Francisco (May 6–7, 2002). Prevention First founding members include: Boston Women's Health Book Collective, Breast Cancer Action (San Francisco), Center for Medical Consumers (New York), DES Action (Oakland), Massachusetts Breast Cancer Coalition, National Women's Health Network (Washington D.C.), Women's Community Cancer Project (Cambridge, MA), Women and Health Protection (Canada), represented by Breast Cancer Action Montreal, and the Elizabeth May Chair in Women's Health and the Environment (Dalhousie University, Halifax). The Boston Women's Health Group is the radical feminist collective that created the *Our Bodies/Our Selves* series of manuals/books that are most often identified with the women's health movement of the 1960s and 1970s. The National Women's Health Network is one of the most important women's health activist organizations in the country. NWHN is very active in lobbying and legislation. Breast Cancer Action and the Women's Community Cancer Project are two of the most radical, feminist organizations of the U.S. breast cancer movement of the 1990s.

Chapter 9

1. This research was supported in part by NSF grants #SBR-9811962 (Science and Technology Studies Program), and 0080400 (Societal Dimensions of Engineering, Science, and Technology Program). I presented earlier versions of the paper at the Society for Social Studies of Science, Halifax, October 1998, and at CHEMRAWN XIV International Conference on Green Chemistry, Boulder, Colorado, June 2001.

2. The concept of Governing Mentalities is developed in Campbell, 2000. See especially chapter 2, "Governing Mentalities: Reading Political Culture," pp. 33–54.

3. On the social *re*construction of technologies, see Woodhouse et al. (2002).

4. For helping a nonchemist to grasp some of the technical details, my thanks to participants in the 2nd Annual Green Chemistry and Engineering Conference: Global Perspectives, National Academy of Sciences, Washington DC, June 30–July 2, 1998; the OECD Workshop on Sustainable Chemistry, Fondazione Cini, Venice, Italy, October 15–17, 1998; and especially members of the planning committee for CHEMRAWN XIV, held July 2001 at Boulder, Colorado, sponsored by the International Union of Pure and Applied Chemistry's Chemical Research Applied to World Needs. My thanks as well to Doryen Bubeck for excellent research assistance and to Nancy Campbell, Monica Casper, Kim Fortun, and Linda Layne for discussions of anthropological literature concerning bodies and nations.

5. Except where otherwise noted, all quoted material is drawn from interviews conducted by the author during 1998–2002 with government officials, university researchers, chemistry students, corporate executives, and interest group representatives—primarily from the U.S., but also from Britain, Denmark, Germany, Italy, Japan, Sweden, and The Netherlands.

6. For typical examples of the explication of brown chemistry as if it were the only way to do chemistry, see Wade (1987) and Masterton et al. (1985).

7. A small minority of chemists did continue to conduct research outside the mainstream, and their efforts have gained a bit of momentum in the past several decades. The work has tended to focus more on pharmaceutical and nutritional rather than industrial chemistry, as the main journals reveal: *Advances in Carbohydrate Chemistry and Biochemistry, Journal of Carbohydrate Chemistry*, and *Carbohydrate Chemistry*. Also see texts in the field including Pigman and Goepp (1948), McIlroy (1967), and Hecht (1999). The work on lipids is published in a single main journal, *Progress in Lipid Research,* published by Pergamon. Also see Gunstone (1970).

8. Nominations come from diverse sources, including self-nomination, and finalists are selected by panels of technical experts convened by the American Chemical Society. EPA makes the final selection, after attempting to make sure that the organization ranked first by ACS is not about to make headlines for some environmentally despicable act that would bring the agency into disrepute.

9. A key intermediate in the process is DSIDA (disodium iminodiacetate), traditionally manufactured via the Strecker process using ammonia, formaldehyde, hydrogen cyanide, and hydrochloric acid. Hydrogen cyanide is the worst of these, for its extreme acute toxicity means great care must be taken to protect workers, those living near chemical plants, and the environment.

10. The Gordon Conferences are prestigious scientific gatherings that operate largely via invitation. Conferences cover several dozen subjects ranging among many different facets of the natural sciences.

11. The concept of enunciatory community is developed in Fortun (2001).

Chapter 10

1. Versions of this chapter were presented at "Formations of Medical Techniques: Between Laboratories, Hospitals, and Public Space" (December 1–4, 1999, Paris, France), and "Social Change and the Politics of Sexual Health," (April 20, 2001, Baltimore, MD); an earlier slightly different version of this article appeared as "Acceder au pouvoir par les technologies: femmes et science dans la recherche sur les microbicides," published in *Sciences Sociales et Sante*, v. 18, n. 2, Juin 2000: 121–40. I would like to thank Lauren Wise, Adele Clarke, Lori Heise, Jennifer Hirsch, Judy Norsigian, Volona Rabeharisoa, Susan Reverby, and Kevin Whaley for their valuable critiques of drafts of this essay, and to Bowdoin College for research support through a Kenan Fellowship for Faculty Development.

2. *Our Bodies, Ourselves for the New Century* is the most recent version of the book, *Our Bodies, Ourselves*, edited by the Boston Women's Health Book Collective, which has been called "the bible of women's health" (Anstett, 1992, HE, 2E). First published in 1970, the book has been revised and expanded seven times over the years, and translated and/or adapted into nineteen languages. More than 6 million copies of it have been sold (http://www.ourbodies ourselves.org/adapt.htm).

3. As Judith Auerbach and Anne Figert (1995, 115) remind us, even in the United States "there have been many women's health movements . . . which overlap but have also been some-what distinct historically from feminism and from different feminist movements." Since the 1970s, there have been tensions within feminism generally, and women's health move-ments specifically, about which women participated in it and which (whose) problems were most urgent. The most visible and vocal feminist health activists in the 1970s assumed that unity among women derived from a potential identity between women. This identity, in turn, was based on the idea that women share the same experiences. For example, women are economically oppressed, commercially exploited, and legally discriminated against. In addition, women feel inadequate and attribute these experiences to personal flaws. These external and internal similarities create the basis for common feelings between women. The expression of this community of feeling and experience is women's politics and women's organizing (Delmar 1986). Critics of this perspective argue that this assumption is made by white, middle-class, heterosexual women—women who are relatively privileged in com-parison to other groups of women. According to these critics, women are situated differ-ently from one another and thus their experiences and feelings vary; the meaning of "woman" or "feminism" is not universal. The universalizing claims of feminism marginalize or exclude the lives of many women, such as women of color and working class women. For more on this paradox, see Davis and Fisher (1993) and Herrmann and Stewart (1994). For its discussion in the context of the international politics of women's health see Doyal (1996).

4. The eleven women's health advocates were Vicki Alexander (Community Family Planning Council), Rani Bang (Society for Education, Action and Research in Community Health), Liz Cameron (Empower), Muriel J. Harris (Society for Women and AIDS in Africa), Am-paro Claro (Latin American and Caribbean Women's Health Network/ISIS International), Lori Heise (Pacific Institute for Women's Health), Vicki Legion (Community Health Worker Program, Health Education Department San Francisco State University), Florence Manguyu (Medical Women's International Association), Nicolien Wieringa (Women's Health Action foundation), Maria Betania Avila (Brazilian Feminist Health Network), and Adrienne Germain (International Women's Health Coalition).

5. Adele Clarke (1998, 169–70) argues that between 1925 and 1963 birth control research shifted from the development of "simple" to "scientific" technologies. "Simple" technolo-gies are relatively simple to use, controlled by users, capable of being discontinued at any time, and used or not used at the time of a given intercourse. Examples of simple technolo-gies are "barrier methods" of birth control, spermicides, and "natural" birth control. They are low technology, although they require some science to formulate, test, and produce them. Their effects are localized to the reproductive system, and most are considered safe enough to be distributed over the counter. Reproductive scientists typically view simple technologies as nonscientific, and hence not interesting or worth attending to, derived from clinical practice and applied research instead of from basic science. "Scientific" tech-nologies are high technology methods of contraception resulting from basic science and in the United States all of them are mediated by the medical profession for initiation, moni-toring, and often for removal. Their effects are systemic, permanent, and sometimes in-volve surgery. Examples of scientific technologies are hormonal methods, sterilization, and IUDs.

6. A notable exception to this was in 1951, when feminist health advocate Margaret Sanger approached reproductive biologist Gregory Pincus and persuaded him to begin research on a "'universal contraceptive' that could be used by all women, regardless of colour, class, age, or educational background" (Oudshoorn 1996, 157). Even in that famous instance, the production of the birth control pill by Gregory Pincus and M. C. Chang proceeded without the benefit of Sanger's active engagement in the reproductive science.

7. Behind the publication of the birth control chapter was communication between me and a reproductive scientist from Johns Hopkins and a member of WHAM because I wanted to ensure the accuracy of translating science to women. Alongside of the publication was the

participation of a member of the Boston Women's Health Book Collective on the Committee responsible for publishing *Contraceptive Research and Development* (Harrison and Rosenfield 1996).

8.   The International Women's Health Coalition is a nonprofit organization that works collaboratively with feminists, women's organizations, health professionals, and officials in the North and South to promote women's reproductive health and rights. The Pacific Institute for Women's Health is a nonprofit research and advocacy organization dedicated to improving women's health status worldwide. It works with women's organizations, health professionals, and researchers in the North and South to develop high-quality, research-based activism.

9.   Germain and Heise belonged to different women's health advocate networks. Heise's focus was on advocacy in the areas of HIV/AIDS and violence against women. Germain's focus was on reproductive rights projects, and she identified women's health advocates from this area of women's health politics to invite to the meeting (Heise personal communication, October 4, 1999).

10. The next three paragraphs draw heavily on Bell and Wise (1998, 288 and footnote 2, 336).

11. Letter, Carolyn Caddle-Steele, International Women's Health Colaition, to Susan E. Bell September 1, 1999.

Chapter 11

1.   This research is supported by grants to the first author from the Robert Wood Johnson Foundation's Investigator Awards in Health Policy Research Program (Grant # 036273) and the National Science Foundation Program in Social Dimensions of Engineering, Science, and Technology (Grant # SES-9975518). We thank Theo Luebke and Joshua Mandelbaum for many discussions and comments on earlier material that has informed this paper. We thank Lundy Braun, Monica Casper, Adele Clarke, and Charles Engel for helpful discussions on the conceptual framework and readings of the manuscript. We are grateful to the scientists of the Boston Environmental Hazards Center for permitting us access to their work.

2.   This is a more inclusive definition of environmental causes than we employ in our examination of asthma and breast cancer, two other illnesses we are examining as part of a larger research project. This is due in part to the possible interactive effects of toxins and medical treatments that we mention in the text. Also, in breast cancer, there is general acceptance that estrogen in medical treatments (e.g., hormone replacement therapy) is a potential carcinogen, whereas environmental estrogens are not generally seen as risk factors. For asthma, there are no suspected treatment-related causes.

3.   We do not intend to view all government agencies as identical. Many different government agencies became involved in the effort to understand GWRIs, especially the Department of Defense, the Department of Veterans Affairs, the Centers for Disease Control, the Institute of Medicine, and the National Institute of Health. Because of questionable efforts by some of these agencies, the president formed a Presidential Advisory Committee to investigate further GWRIs. We make clear when appropriate the differences among agencies. From the point of view of veterans, the DOD, and to a lesser extent the VA, have been most problematic.

4.   The lack of interest in GWRI research among public health professionals is evidenced in the fact that the only presentation at the 2000 American Public Health Association Annual Meeting was by the lead author of this paper.

Chapter 12

1.   An idea to build a chemical plant in Lithuania was first introduced by the GIPROKHIM, the central governmental planning agency for the chemical industry, and had to undergo some cumbersome procedures before it was actually materialized in 1963. It first appeared under the category of the "chemicalization" of the Baltic region that covered Estonia, Latvia, Lithuania, and Kaliningrad region in the GIPROKHIM's proposition to the USSR Ministry of Finances. When the final version of the plan of the regional chemicalization was approved by the ministry in only four months, the plant was already marked on the map. It came up as a dot near the major railroad artery connecting the Kola peninsula with

the Ukraine, in the center of Lithuania, on the banks of the river Nevezis. This approved document still had to be reviewed and confirmed by the Soviet Politburo and presented to the Lithuanian Ministry of Finances and the Lithuanian Board of Ministers for further specifications. The actual design and calculations regarding the installation of technologies were completed in January 1958. In March 1958, the Institute assigned the construction of the Kedainiai chemical plant to the Lithuanian Ministry of Construction which, in its turn, chose twenty Soviet construction subcontractors to carry out the project.

2. Among a number of studies that investigate the connection between scientific-technological progress and the formation of the modern nation-states. Bruce Bruan's work is particularly concerned with how modern science is woven into the new governmental regime. He builds on Bruno Latour's "anthropo-materialism" and argues that the nation state is not a purely social institution but an assemblage of social, industrial, geographical, historical, scientific, and cultural components. For Braun, modern science, technology, and industry in Victorian Canada were the instruments for the "the management of 'life' both at the level of the individual body (through ordering of space, medical and psychological exams, and so on) and the level of the social body (in response to comprehensive measurements like censuses, statistical assessments, and so on)" (Braun 2000, 27).

3. Heidegger's concept of "standing reserve" was introduced and developed in his two lectures at the Bavarian Academy of Arts (1950, 1955), "The Question Concerning Technology" and "Turning." In these lectures, Heidegger explains that the notion of "standing reserve" reveals the instrumental nature of technology that structures human existence by acting upon and organizing the world so as to make it available as a resource. In his reading, both humans and nature are ordered according to technology's instrumental mentality, and the lifeworld is rendered as a standing reserve available and ready for consumption. For example, a modern power-generating technology is conceptually different from old wind and water driven mills, as it no longer depends upon such contingent sources of energy as wind, water level in the basin or human physical strength. The coal-fired power requires consistent supply of coal and, by doing so, proceeds to exploit earth's natural resources, local communication infrastructures, transportation and human labor in a much more systemic and demanding manner than ever before. Through this system of exploitation, the earth loses its state of being and is turned into a "coal mining district" and "a mineral deposit" (Heidegger 1977, 14).

4. The notion of a scientific-technological revolution was introduced in the mid-1950s by Khrushchev's administration and denoted a qualitatively new stage in the development of human civilization. Arguably, the scientific-technological revolution was preceded by (1) the neolithic revolution that featured the creation of the first labor tools and the emergence of the antagonistic class society and (2) the industrial revolution that entailed the development of machines and the formation of the capitalist mode of production. The aftermath of the scientific-technological revolution would engage a closer collaboration between science and industry ensuring a more immediate implementation of the scientific achievements into practice and the foundation of socialist society. It is interesting to note that the Soviet effort to integrate science and technology into the economic and social relations remotely resonates with a cybernetic approach. Indeed, one of the predecessors of the scientific-technological revolution was a Ukrainian cybernetician, K. Dobrov. Unfortunately, the Soviet Politburo was not ready for the implementation of his radically democratic program and fell back to its common politics of the "iron hand."

5. The proposition that the minds of the Soviet citizens can be manipulated through industrialization was fully articulated and implemented by the Khrushchevian Politburo. Herbert Blumer (1990) in *Industrialization as an Agent of Social Change: A Critical Analysis* argues against this proposition. Blumer suggests that the causal explanation of the social change by industrialization ignores a massive number of other important actors and networks that composite social transformation. Blumer points out that industrialization and social change are mutually constitutive. Interestingly, Blumer arrived at this conclusion in the 1950s at the same time as the Soviet government launched the project of scientific-technological revolution as the means for taming its citizens.

6. For the Bolsheviks and, thus, the Soviet state, it is Karl Marx whose work on the issue of technology was of primary importance. In *Capital* Marx places a strong emphasis on modern technology as a necessary material condition in the transformation of social modes

from feudalism to capitalism. His position is, however, ambiguous. On the one hand, Marx argues that socialism, by definition, requires the development of ultimately different technologies than those of the repressive capitalist mode. On the other hand, Marx suggests that technology is historically contingent, or at least that there is nothing inherently repressive within modern sciences and technology. This optimistic theory of technology "enables us to envision the development of liberatory technologies in the context of a capitalist society" (Balbus 1994, 153). Obviously, the Bolsheviks adopted the second, more instrumental of the two positions by placing transformative agency onto industrialization. In the same way as Prakish's British colonizers, the Soviet imperialists assumed that scientific-technologies progress would automatically hegemonize the population.

7. Methodologically, this essay is based on my two-year intensive research on the development of the chemical industry in Lithuania and the Kedainiai chemical plant, in particular. I conducted twenty-five interviews with former workers, administrators, and the Communist Party leaders who were affiliated with the plant in the 1960s. I also researched the Kedainiai area local archives that inform this essay about the ways that the Kedainiai chemical plant affected economic, political, and social spheres and everyday practices of the local inhabitants.

8. According to the official reports in 1966 there were also 500 (6.9 percent) construction workers, 380 (5.3 percent) transportation employees, 170 (2.3 percent) men and women employed in the food and service industry, and 246 (3.4 percent) hired by the education and cultural institutions.

9. This transformation had even more profound impact in the rural areas where the farmers were ordered to be paid in money, not agricultural products as was customary in the past. They lost a direct connection to the land, even as they continued to labor over it.

10. It would be interesting to trace how these chemicals affected the bodies and the environment of the local inhabitants. However it is difficult to get an accurate view of this. The official statistics strategically avoid the subject of "harm" and "risk" posed by the chemicals to the human body. The Soviet medical records celebrate "magnificent amelioration of the health conditions" in Kedainiai due to industrialization, but do not mention any of the potential diseases or hazards resulting from working and living around the chemical plant.

11. The schools for the humanities and social sciences suffered even more severely from the new regime. The old programs and departments were dismantled, and the new ones became the primary educators in material empiricism and Marxism-Leninism. Four fifths of all education institutions in Lithuania were turned into technology, engineering, and science schools.

12. The "chemical" students constituted approximately 17 percent of all Lithuanian students in the institutions of higher education in 1966.

13. These were purely self-sustaining groups that received hardly any substantial financial or military support from foreign sources.

Chapter 13

1. Material for this list was gathered from a variety of sources including the websites of environmental groups such as the Natural Resources Defense Council, Sierra Club, Rocky Mountain Institute, Environmental Defense Fund, Audobon Society and several others. Government websites such as those of the Environmental Protection Agency and the Office of Homeland Security were also analyzed, as were two years' worth of newspaper articles. For an account of the Bush environmental record as Governor of Texas, see Abraham (2000) and Miller (2001).

2. Mark Crispin Miller (2001, 167–69) writes, "Of all the blots on Bush's record . . . none is quite as large, or evil-smelling, as his six years of environmental work in Texas. A man of oil and gas, the governor was—as it were by nature—always sympathetic to the planet's dirtiest polluters: the big oil, petrochemical, and automobile industries. . . . Under Bush, Texas had the nation's highest volume of air pollution, with the highest ozone levels of any state—while ranking forty-sixth in spending on environmental problems. Moreover, after 1994 Texas was the nation's leading source of greenhouse gases, accounting for 14 percent of the annual U.S. total. . . . However shocking, such statistics cannot quite convey the ugliness

of Bush's legacy as steward of the environment in Texas—a story not just of poor numbers but of townships darkened by thick toxic fogs, of schools shut down because of airborne poisons, of children suffering from damaged lungs as if they were heavy smokers. . . . While Bush's grim environmental record is his worst offense, it is also one that could have hurt him badly as a national candidate if it had ever been reported with due clarity. Most Americans are flaming liberals on environmental issues. . . . If the viewers had known more about the Texas governor's hard-nosed let-them-eat-smog approach to the environment . . . his canned assurances about the perfect sweetness of his 'heart' would not have helped him much."

References

2020 Workshop on the Role of Polymer Research in Green Chemistry and Engineering. 1998. Press Release. Amherst, MA: University of Massachusetts.

AICR. 2002. *Simple Steps to Prevent Cancer*. Washington D.C.: American Institute for Cancer Research.

Abraham, Rick. 2000. *The Dirty Truth: The Oil and Chemical Dependency of George W. Bush*. Houston: Mainstream Publishers.

Abu-Lughod, Lila. 1991. "Writing Against Culture." In *Recapturing Anthropology*, edited by Richard G. Fox. Santa Fe: School of American Research Press.

Accreditation Board for Engineering and Technology. 1991. *ABET Accreditation Yearbook*. New York: Accreditation Board for Engineering and Technology.

Aftalion, Fred. 1991. *A History of the International Chemical Industry*. Philadelphia: University of Pennsylvania Press.

Agency for Toxic Substances and Disease Registry (ATSDR). 2000. Annual Report. http://www.atsdr.cdc.gov.

Ahlborg, U. G., L. Lipworth, L. Titusernstoff, and C. C. Hsieh. 1995. Organochlorine compounds in relation to breast cancer, endometrial cancer, and endometriosis—an assessment of the biological and epidemiological evidence. *Critical Reviews in Toxicology* 25:463–531.

Akrich, Madeline. 1995. User representations: Practices, methods and sociology. In *Managing Technology in Society*, edited by Arie Rip, T. J. Misa, and J. Schot, 167–84. London and New York: Pinter/St. Martin's.

Alexander, Nancy J. 1996. Sexual spread of HIV infection. *Human Reproduction* 11(7): 111–20.

Allan, Stuart, Barbara Adam, and Cynthia Carter, eds. 2000. *Environmental Risks and the Media*. London: Routledge.

Allison, A. 1994. *Nightwork: Sexuality, Pleasure, and Corporate Masculinity in a Tokyo Hostess Club*. Chicago: University of Chicago Press.

Allstate Insurance Company. 1998. Airbag safety. Online at http://www.autotrader.com/research/shared/article.jtmpl?article_id=15481&make=&model=&year=&category_search=&refpage=insurance&restype=&ac_afflt-one

American Academy of Environmental Engineers. 1999. *Guide for Administrators and Faculty to ABET Accreditation in Environmental Engineering*. 2d ed. Annapolis, MD: American Academy of Environmental Engineers.

American Academy of Pediatrics. 2002. Reducing the Number of Deaths and Injuries From Residential Fires (RE9952). *Pediatrics* 105 (6): 1355–57.

American Cancer Society. 2002. *Cancer Facts and Figures–2002*. Atlanta, Georgia: American Cancer Society.

Anagnost, Ann. 1995. A Surfeit of Bodies: Population and the Rationality of the State in Post-Mao China. In *Conceiving the New World Order: The Global Politics of Reproduction*, edited by F. D. Ginsburg and R. Rapp, 22–41. Berkeley: University of California Press.

Anastas, Paul T., and Carol A. Farris, eds. 1994. *Benign by Design: Alternative Synthetic Design for Pollution Prevention*. Washington, D.C.: American Chemical Society.

Anastas, Paul T., and Tracy C. Williamson, eds. 1996. *Green Chemistry: Designing Chemistry for the Environment*. Washington, D.C.: American Chemical Society.

Anastas, Paul T., and John C. Warner. 1998. *Green Chemistry: Theory and Practice*. Oxford: Oxford University Press.

Anderson, Benedict. 1983. *Imagined Communities*. London: Verso.

Anderson, Deborah J., and Alison J. Quayle. 1996. Mucosal immunologic approaches. In *Contraceptive Research and Development*, edited by Polly Harrison and Allen Rosenfield, 446–73. Washington, D.C.: National Academy of Sciences.

Anstett, Patricia. 1992. Our bodies, our book. *Detroit Free Press*, September 21.

Antonetta, Susanne. 2001. *Body Toxic: An Environmental Memoir*. Washington, D.C.: Counterpoint.

Asad, Talal. 1986. "The concept of cultural translation in British social anthropology" in James Clifford and George E. Marcus, *Writing Culture*. Berkeley: University of California Press.

Associated Press. 1998. Agent Orange reports withheld, altered, paper says. Report on six-month study by *San Diego Union-Tribune*. November 1.

Auerbach, Judith D. and Anne E. Figert. 1995. Women's health research: Public policy and sociology. *Journal of Health and Social Behavior* (extra issue): 115–31.

Auerbach, Judith D. and Coates, Thomas J. 2000. HIV prevention research: Accomplishments and challenges for the third decade of AIDS. *American Journal of Public Health* 90(7):1029–32.

Axelrad, Bob. 1993. "Improving IAQ: EPA's program—pollution prevention must become routine." *EPA Journal* 19:14–7.

B.Sz. 1985. Szemétimport. Garbage Import. *Népszava*. July 20.

Baker, Carl G. 1977. Cancer Research Program Strategy and Planning—the Use of Contracts for Program Implementation. *Journal of the National Cancer Institute* 59, 2 (Supplement): 651–69.

Balbus, Isaak. 1994. *Marxism and Domination: A Neo-Hegelian, Feminist, Psychoanalytic Theory of Sexual, Political, and Technological Liberation*. Princeton: Princeton University Press.

Baughman, Robert W. 1977. TCDD and industrial accidents. Appendix in *The Pendulum and the Toxic Cloud: The Course of Dioxin Contamination*, by Thomas Whiteside. New Haven: Yale University Press. First published in Tetrachlorodibenzo-*p*-dioxins in the environment: High resolution mass spectrometry at the picogram level. Ph.D. diss., Harvard (1974).

Beck, Ulrick. 1992. *Risk Society: Towards a New Modernity*. Translated by M. Ritter. Thousand Oaks: Sage.

Begley, Sharon. 2002. "New Statistics show increase in cancer rates." *The Wall Street Journal*, October 16. http://www.sfgate.com/cgi-bin/article.cgi?file=/news/archive/2002/10/16/financial1029EDT0056.DTL

Bell, Robert. 1992. *Impure Science: Fraud, Compromise, and Political Influence in Scientific Research*. New York: Wiley.

Bell, Susan E. 1979. Political gynecology: Gynecological imperialism and the politics of self-help. *Science for the People* 11(5):8–14.

———. 1984. Birth control. In *The New Our Bodies, Ourselves*, ed. Boston Women's Health Book Collective, 220–62. New York: Simon and Schuster.

———. 1986. A new model of medical technology development: A case study of DES. In *Research in the Sociology of Health Care*, vol. 4, ed. J. Roth and S. Ruzek,1–32. Greenwich CT: JAI Press.

———. 1992. Birth control. In *The New Our Bodies, Ourselves*, revised ed. Boston Women's Health Book Collective, 259–307. New York: Simon and Schuster.

———. 1994. Translating science to the people: Updating *The new our bodies, ourselves*. *Women's Studies International Forum* 17: 9–18.

———. 1999. Narratives and lives: Women's health politics and the diagnosis of cancer for DES daughters. *Narrative Inquiry* 9(2):347–89.

Bell, Susan E., and Lauren Wise, with Suzannah Cooper-Doyle and Judy Norsigian. 1998. Birth control. In *Our Bodies, Ourselves for the New Century*, ed. Boston Women's Health Book Collective, 288–340. New York: Simon and Schuster.

Bender, B., ed. 1995. *Landscape: Politics and Perspectives*. Oxford: Berg.

———. 1998. *Stonehenge: Making Space*. Oxford: Berg.

Berer, Marge. 1993. Population and family planning policies: women-centred perspectives. *Reproductive Health Matters* 1: 4–12.

Berglund, Eeva. 1998. *Knowing Nature, Knowing Science: An Ethnography of Local Environmental Activism*. Cambridge: White Horse Press.

Bernauer, Thomas. 1993. *The Chemistry of Regime Formation: Explaining International Cooperation for a Comprehensive Ban on Chemical Weapons*. Geneva: United Nations Institute for Disarmament Research.

Berque, A. 1997 [1993]. *Japan: Nature, Artifice and Japanese Culture*. Yelvertoft Manor, Northamptonshire: Pilkington Press.

Best, Joel, ed. 1989. *Images of Issues: Typifying Contemporary Social Problems*. New York: Aldine.

Bestor, T. C. 1989. *Neighborhood Tokyo*. Stanford: Stanford University Press.

Biagioli, Mario, ed. 1999. *The Science Studies Reader*. New York: Routledge.

Birnbaum, Linda S. 2002. Health and environmental effects of dioxins. Paper prepared for presentation to the Yale Vietnam Conference 2002: The Ecological and Health Effects of the Vietnam War. New Haven, CT. September 13–15.

Blauner, Robert. 1967. *Alienation and Freedom: The Factory Worker and His Industry.* Chicago: University of Chicago Press.

Blaxter, Mildred. 1983.The causes of disease: women talking. *Social Science and Medicine,* 17: 59–69.

Blumer, Herbert. 1990. *Industrialization as an Agent of Social Change: A Critical Analysis.* New York: Aldine de Gruyter.

Bombeck, Erma. 1989. *I Want to Grow Hair, I Want to Grow Up, I Want to Go to Boise.* New York: Harper and Row.

Bosk, Charles L. 1992. *All God's Mistakes.* Chicago: The University of Chicago Press.

Boston Women's Health Book Collective. 1991. *History of the Boston Women's Health Book Collective.* Available from the BWHBC, 34 Plympton Street, Boston, MA 02118, U.S.A.

Bourdieu, P. 1977. *Outline of a Theory of Practice.* Cambridge: Cambridge University Press.

Bourdieu, Pierre. 1990. Structures, *Habitus,* Practices. In *The Logic of Practice.* Stanford University Press.

Brady, Judy, ed. 1991. *1 in 3: Women with Cancer Confront an Epidemic.* San Francisco: Cleis Press.

Bragg, Rick. 2002. Burning of Chemical Arms Puts Fear in Wind. *New York Times.* September 15.

Braun, Bruce. 2000. Producing vertical territory: Geology and governmentality in late Victorian Canada. *Ecumene* 7(1). 7–46.

Breast Cancer Action. 2002. "Activists Respond to First Findings from Controversial Ten-Year Project on Pollution and Breast Cancer Risk." Breast Cancer Action, June 5, 2002 Press Release. http://www.bcacation.org/Pages/GetInformed/PressReleases.html.

Brenner, Barbara A. 2000. Sister support: Women create a breast cancer movement. In *Breast Cancer: Social Construction of an Illness,* edited by Anne S. Kasper and Susan J. Ferguson, New York: St. Martins Press.

Brody, Jane. 2002. "Risks and Realities: In a World of Hazards, Worries Are Often Misplaced." *New York Times.* August 20, 2002. On-line version accessed.

Brown, Mark A., and Peter A. Johnson. 1994. Public distrust slows weapons destruction. *Forum for Applied Research and Public Policy* 9(2):126–131.

Brown, Michael. 1985.Disputed knowledge: Worker access to hazard information. In *The Language of Risk: Conflicting Perspectives in Occupational Health,* edited by Dorothy Nelkin. Beverly Hills: Sage Publications.

Brown, Phil. 1992. Popular epidemiology and toxic waste contamination: lay and professional ways of knowing. *Journal of Health and Social Behavior* 33:267–81.

———. 1995. Naming and framing: The social construction of diagnosis and illness. *Journal of Health and Social Behavior* (Extra issue):34–52.

Brown, Phil, and Edwin Mikkelsen, J. 1990. *No Safe Place: Toxic Waste, Leukemia, and Community Action.* Berkeley: University of California Press.

Bruce, Judith. 1987. Users' perspectives on contraceptive technology and delivery systems: Highlighting some feminist issues. *Technology in Society* 9: 359–83.

Brunnstrom, David. 2002. Vets Say Vietnam dioxin victims should be helped. *Reuters.* March 4.

———. 2002. Vietnam insists on Agent Orange damage repair plan. *Reuters.* March 6.

———. 2002. U.S., Hanoi don't finalize dioxin plan, to talk more. *Reuters.* March 9.

Bryant, P., C. T. Vivian, B. Chavis, A. Favorite, Sr., D. Malek-Wiley, F. Shuttlesworth, A. Braden, R. M. Smith, M. Henderson, S. Lewis, A. C. Alexander, B. Ewing, J. Dickerson, and R. Moore. *Letter to Group of Ten Environmental Organizations.* Reprinted in *Not Man Apart: The News-magazine of Friends of the Earth, USA,* 20, no. 2:16.

Buckingham, William A., Jr. 1982. *Operation Ranch Hand: The Air Force and Herbicides in Southeast Asia 1961–1971.* Washington, D.C.: Office of Air Force History, United States Air Force.

Bullard, Robert D. 1990. *Dumping in Dixie: Race, Class, and Environmental Quality.* Boulder: Westview Press.

———, ed. 1993. *Confronting Environmental Racism: Voices from the Grassroots.* Boston: South End Press.

Burawoy, Michael. 1985. *The Politics of Production.* London: Verso.

Burck, Gordon M., and Charles C. Flowerree. 1991. *International Handbook on Chemical Weapons Proliferation.* New York: Greenwood Press.

Burkett, B. G., and Glenna Whitely. 1998. *Stolen Valor: How the Vietnam Generation Was Robbed of Its Heroes and Its History.* Dallas: Verity Press.

Burleson, G. R., H. Lebrec, Y. G. Tang, J. D. Ibanes, K. N. Pennington, and L. S. Birnbaum, 1996. Effects of 2,3,7,8-tetrachlorodibenzo-p-dioxin (TCDD) on influenza virus host resistance in mice. *Fundamentals of Applied Toxicology* 29:40–7.

Callon, Michel. 1985. Some elements of a sociology of translation: Domestication of the scallops and the fishermen of St. Brieuc Bay. In *Power, Action, Belief: A New Sociology of Knowledge?*, edited by John Law. London: Routledge and Kegan Paul.

Campbell, Nancy D. 2000. *Using Women: Gender, Drug Policy, and Social Justice*, New York: Routledge.

Carson, Rachel. 1962. *Silent Spring*. Greenwich, CT: Fawcett Crest.

Casey, E. S. 1987. *Remembering: A Phenomenological Study*. Bloomington and Indianapolis: Indiana University Press.

Casper, Monica. 1998. *The Making of the Unborn Patient: A Social Anatomy of Fetal Surgery*. New Brunswick: Rutgers University Press.

————. 2002. Chemical weapons: Incineration island. *Bulletin of Atomic Scientists*. 58 (2), March/April: 17–9.

Casper, Monica J., and Adele E. Clarke. 1998. "Making the pap smear into the "Right Tool" for the Job: Cervical cancer screening in the USA, circa 1940–95." *Social Studies of Science* 28:255–90.

Cecil, Paul Frederick. 1986. *Herbicidal Warfare: The Ranch Hand Project in Viet Nam*. New York, London, Westport, CT: Praeger.

Centers for Disease Control and Prevention. 1994. "Deaths from Breast Cancer—United States, 1991." *Morbidity and Mortality Weekly Report*, April 22, 1994, v43, n15, pp. 273, 279–281. http://www.cdc.gov/mmwr/preview/mmwrhtml/00026281.htm.

Centers for Disease Control and Prevention, National Center for Environmental Health. 2001. National Report on Human Exposure to Environmental Chemicals. NCEH Pub. No. 01–0164.

Chemical Weapons Working Group. 1997. Dioxin and Agriculture. Brea, KY: Kentucky Environmental Foundation.

————. 1998. Chemical Weapons Incineration: Haz Waste Disposal or Dispersal? In *Common Sense*. Brea, KY: Kentucky Environmental Foundation.

Christensen, Vivian A. 1999. *Contested Knowledge in the Environmental Health and Toxic Waste Arenas*. Santa Cruz: University of California.

Christensen, Vivian A., and Monica J. Casper. 2000. Hormone mimics and disrupted bodies: A social worlds analysis of a scientific controversy. *Sociological Perspectives* 43:S93–S120.

Clarke, Adele E. 1998. *Disciplining Reproduction*. Modernity, American Life Sciences, and the Problems of Sex. Berkeley: University of California.

————. 2000. Maverick reproductive scientists and the production of contraceptives, c1915–2000+. To appear in *Bodies of Technology: Women's Involvement with Reproductive Medicine*, edited by Ann Saetnan, Nelly Oudshoorn, and Marta Kirejczk. Columbus, OH: Ohio State University Press.

————. 2000. Personal communication.

Clarke, Adele, and Virginia Olesen. 1999. Revising, diffracting, acting. In *Revisioning Women, Health, and Healing*, edited by A. E. Clarke and V. L. Olesen, 3–48. New York: Routledge.

Colborn, Theo, Dianne Dumanoski, and John Peterson Myers. 1996. *Our Stolen Future: Are We Threatening Our Fertility, Intelligence, and Survival?—A Scientific Detective Story*. New York: Dutton.

Comaroff, Jean, and P. Maguire. 1981. Ambiguity and the Search for Meaning: Childhood Leukemia in the Modern Clinical Context. *Social Science and Medicine*, 15B: 115–23.

Committee for Concerned Asian Scholars. 1970. *The Indochina Story: A Fully Documented Account*. Pantheon.

Congressional Quarterly Inc. 1998. *Congress and the Nation: A Review of Government and Politics*. Volume IX, 1993–1996. Washington, D.C.: Congressional Quarterly Inc.

Constable, John. 2002. Personal communication at the Stockholm Conference on the Long-Term Environmental Consequences of War.

Cozzens, Susan E., and Edward J. Woodhouse. 1995. Science, Government, and the Politics of Knowledge. In Sheila Jasanoff et al., *Handbook of Science and Technology Studies*. Beverly Hills: Sage.

CPSC and U.S. EPA. 1998. "What You Should Know About Using Paint Strippers—If not properly used, paint strippers are hazardous to your health and safety." CPSC Document #4423. EPA 747-F-95–002. Accessed online, July 1998: gopher://www.cpsc.gov:70/00/CPSCPubs/iaq/4423.txt.

CRJ/UCC. 1987. Toxic Wastes and Race in the United States: A National Report on the Racial and Socioeconomic Characteristics of Communities with Hazardous Waste Sites. Commission for Racial Justice, United Church of Christ, New York: Public Data Access.

Crawford, Robert. 1981. "Individual Responsibility and Health Politics." In *The Sociology of Health and Illness*, edited by Peter Conrad and Rochelle Kern. New York: St. Martin's Press.

Crawford-Brown, Douglas J. 1996. *Comparative Risk Assessment of Alternative Management and Treatment Options for the Army Chemical Weapon Incineration Program*. Chapel Hill: Institute for Environmental Studies.

Croissant, Jennifer, and Sal P. Restivo, eds. 2001. *Degrees of Compromise: Industrial Interests and Academic Values*. Albany, NY: State University of New York Press.

———. 1992. *Banning Chemical Weapons: The Scientific Background*. Cambridge: Cambridge University Press.

Crone, Hugh D. 1986. *Chemicals and Society: A Guide to the New Chemical Age*. Cambridge: Cambridge University Press.

Cronon, William. 1996. *Uncommon Ground: Rethinking the Human Place in Nature*. New York: W.W. Norton and Company.

Csordas, T. J. 1993. Somatic modes of attention. *Cultural Anthropology* 8(2): 135–56.

———. 1994. *Embodiment and Experience: The Existential Ground of Culture and Self*. Cambridge: Cambridge University Press.

Cummings, A. M., J. L. Metcalf, and L. S. Birnbaum. 1996. Promotion of endometriosis by 2,3,7,8-tetrachlorodibenzo-p-dioxin in rats and mice: time-dose dependence and species comparison. *Toxicology and Applied Pharmacology* 138:131–39.

DHHS (Dept. of Health and Human Services). Sept. 1987a. Everything doesn't cause cancer. Bethesda: National Institute of Health (NIH).

———. 1987b. Good news, better news, best news. Bethesda: National Institute of Health (NIH).

Dahl, Robert A. 1998. *On Democracy*. New Haven, CT: Yale University Press.

Dale, P. 1986. *The Myth of Japanese Uniqueness*. New York: St. Martin's Press.

Daniels, S. 1993. *Fields of Vision: Landscape Imagery and National Identity in England and the United States*. Cambridge: Polity Press.

Darnovsky, Marcy. 1992. Stories less told: Histories of U.S. environmentalism. *Socialist Review* 22:11–54.

Dauvergne, P. 1997. *Shadows in the Forest: Japan and the Politics of Timber in Southeast Asia*. Cambridge, MA, and London: MIT Press.

Davis, Derra Lee. 2002. *When Smoke Ran Like Water: Tales of Environmental Deception and the Battle against Pollution*. New York: Basic Books.

Davis, Fred. 1963. *Passage through Crisis: Polio Victims and Their Families*. New York: Bobbs Merrill.

Davis, Kathy, and Sue Fisher. 1993. Power and the female subject. In *Negotiating at the Margins*, edited by S. Fisher and K. Davis. New Brunswick, NJ: Rutgers.

Delaney, C., and S. Yanagisako, eds. 1995. *Naturalizing Power: Essays in Feminist Cultural Analysis*. New York and London: Routledge.

Delmar, R. 1986. What is feminism? In *What Is Feminism?*, edited by J. Mitchell and A. Oakley. New York: Pantheon.

Desjarlais, R. 1993. *Body and Emotion: The Aesthetics of Illness and Healing in the Nepal Himalayas*. Philadelphia: University of Pennsylvania Press.

Devesa S. S., D. G. Grauman, W. J. Blot, G. Pennello, R. N. Hoover, and J. F. Fraumeni, Jr. 1999. *Atlas of Cancer Mortality in the United States, 1950–94*. Washington, DC: U.S. Govt. Printing Office, [NIH Publ No. (NIH) 99–4564].

DeVito, Stephen C., and Roger L. Garrett. 1996. *Designing Safer Chemicals: Green Chemistry for Pollution Prevention*. American Chemical Society, Washington, D.C.

Dickson, R. Bruce. 1994. Regulation of indoor air: The last frontier of environmental regulation. *Natural Resources & Environment* 9:20–2, 55–7.

Dingwall, Robert. 1973. *Aspects of Illness*. New York: St. Martin's Press.

Dioxin in Mother's Milk. 1999. Asahi Evening News, August 3.

Dioxin: Levels High in Incinerator-Happy Japan. 1999. *Japan Times*, May 7.

Dioxins Highest in Japan, but Traces Found Everywhere. 1999. *Japan Times*, August 16.

Downs, Andrew. 1972. Up and down with ecology—The "Issue-attention Cycle." *The Public Interest* 28:38–51.

Doyal, Lesley. 1996. The politics of women's health: Setting a global agenda. *International Journal of Health Services*. 26(1): 47–65.

Dunlap, Riley E. and Angela G. Mertig, eds. 1992. *American Environmentalism: The U.S. Environmental Movement, 1970–1990.* Philadelphia, PA: Taylor and Francis.

Duus, P. 1976. *Feudalism in Japan.* New York: Knopf.

Dwernychuk, Wayne, Hoang Dinh Cau, et al. 2002. Dioxin reservoirs in southern Viet Nam—A legacy of Agent Orange. *Chemosphere* 47: 117–37.

Eades, J. S. 1998. Cities of sludge: The politics of waste disposal in New York and Tokyo. In *Towards Sustainable Cities: Readings in the Anthropology of Urban Environments,* edited by K. Aoyagi et al. Leiden: Institute of Cultural and Social Studies.

Edelman, Murray. 1971. *Politics as Symbolic Action: Mass Arousal and Quiescence.* Chicago: Markham.

Edelstein, Michael R.1988.*Contaminated Communities: The Social and Psychological Impacts of Residential Toxic Exposure.* Boulder: Westview.

Elias, Christopher J., and L. L. Heise. 1994. Challenges for the development of female controlled vaginal microbicides. *AIDS* 8: 1–9.

Endicott, Kenneth M. 1957. The chemotherapy program. *Journal of the National Cancer Institute* 19 (2): 275–303.

Engel, C. C., X. Liu, R. Clymer, R. F. Miller, T. Sjoberg, and J. R. Shapiro. 2000. Rehabilitative Care of War-related Health Concerns. *Journal of Occupational and Environmental Medicine* 42:385–90.

Epstein, Samuel S. 1979. *The Politics of Cancer.* San Francisco: Sierra Club Books, 1978; rev. ed. Garden City, N.Y.: Anchor Press/Doubleday.

Epstein, Steven. 1996. *Impure Science.* Berkeley: University of California.

———. 2000. Democracy, expertise, and AIDS treatment activism. In *Perspectives in Medical Sociology.* 3d ed. edited by P. Brown. Prospect Heights, IL: Waveland Press.

Erickson, J. David et al. 1984. Vietnam Veterans' Risk for Fathering Babies with Birth Defects. Atlanta: U.S. Dept. of Health and Human Services (CDC) Center for Environmental Health.

Evans, Nancy, ed. 2002. State of the evidence: What is the connection between chemicals and breast cancer? San Francisco: The Breast Cancer Fund and Breast Cancer Action. Report available at http://www.breastcacerfund.org and http://bcaction.org.

Fagin, Dan. 2002a. "Tattered Hopes: A $30-Million Federal Studey of Breast Cancer and Pollution On L.I. Has Disappointed Activists and Scientists." Newsday.com. July 28, 2002. http://www.newsday.com/news/local/longisland/nylicanc0728.story.

———. 2002b. "So Many Things Went Wrong: Costly search for links between pollution and breast cancer was hobbled from the start, critics say." Newsday.com. July 29, 2002. http://www.newsday.com/news/local/longisland/nylicanc0729.story.

———. 2002c. "Still Searching: A computer mapping system was supposed to help unearth information about breast cancer and the environment." Newsday.com. July 30, 2002. http://www.newsday.com/news/local/longisland/nylicanc0730.story.

Fagin, Dan, Marianne Lavelle, and Center for Public Integrity. 1996. *Toxic Deception: How the Chemical Industry Manipulates Science, Bends the Law, and Endangers Your Health.* Seacaucus, NJ: Birch Lane Press.

Farmer, P. 1992. *AIDS and Accusation: Haiti and the Geography of Blame.* Berkeley: University of California Press.

———. 1997. On Suffering and Structural Violence: A View from Below. In *Social Suffering,* edited by Kleinman et al. Berkeley: University of California Press.

———. 1999. *Infections and Inequalities.* Berkeley: University of California.

Fathalla, M. F. 1999. Contraception-21. *International Journal of Gynecology and Obstetrics.* 67: S5–S12.

Ferenczi, József. 1985. Szemét a Szomszédból: Kényszerből—Kísérletként. Garbage from the Neighborhood: Of Necessity—As an Experiment. *Kisalföld.* September 10.

Ferraro, Susan. 1993. "You can't look away anymore": The anguished politics of breast cancer. *New York Times Magazine,* August 15.

Fishman, Jennifer. 1999. Assessing breast cancer: Risk, science, and environmental activism in an "at risk" community. In *Feminist Ideologies of Breast Cancer,* edited by Laura Potts. London: MacMillan Press.

Florida Chemical Company Inc. website http://www.floridachemical.com/datasheets/ezmulse.html.

Florida, Nancy. 1995. *Writing the Past, Inscribing the Future: History as Prophecy in Colonial Java.* Durham and London: Duke University Press.

Fortescue, Stephen. 1986. *The Communist Party and Soviet Science.* Baltimore: John Hopkins University Press.

Fortun, Kim. 2001. *Advocacy after Bhopal: Environmentalism, Disaster, New Global Orders.* Chicago: University of Chicago Press.

Fosket, Jennifer Ruth. 2002. Breast Cancer Risk and the Politics of Prevention: Analysis of a Clinical Trial. Ph.D. dissertation, Department of Social and Behavioral Sciences, University of California, San Francisco, San Francisco, CA.

Foucault, Michel. 1970. The Order of Discourse. Inaugural lecture at the College de France.

———. 1991 [1975]. *Discipline and Punish: The Birth of the Prison.* London: Penguin.

———. 1977. *Discipline and Punish: The Birth of the Prison.* New York: Vintage Books.

———. 1978. *The History of Sexuality, Vol. I.* New York: Vintage Press.

———. 1994. *The Birth of the Clinic: An Archaeology of Medical Perception.* New York: Vintage.

Frank, Arthur W. 1991. *At the Will of the Body.* Boston: Houghton Mifflin.

Franklin, Jon. September 10, 2000. Personal correspondence via e-mail.

Franklin, S. 1997. *Embodied Progress: A Cultural Account of Assisted Conception.* New York: Routledge.

Freeman, C. 1977. In *Science, Technology, and Society: A Cross-Disciplinary Perspective,* edited by Ina Spiegel-Rosing and Derek de. Solla Price. Beverly Hills: Sage.

Fukuda K., R. Nisenbaum, G. Stewart, W. W. Thompson, L. Robin, R. M. Washko, D. L. Noah, D. H. Barrett, B. Randall, B. L. Herwaldt, A. C. Mawle, and W. C. Reeves. 1998. Chronic multisymptom illness affecting Air Force veterans of the Gulf War. *Journal of the American Medical Association,* 280:981–88.

Fuller, Steve. 2000. *The Governance of Science: Ideology and the Future of the Open Society.* Buckingham, UK: Open University Press.

Galston, Arthur W. 1972. Science and social responsibility: A case history. *Annals of the New York Academy of Sciences.* Vol. 196, Article 4: 223–235.

Gamson, William, Bruce Fireman, and Steven Rytina. 1982. *Encounters with Unjust Authority.* Homewood, IL: Dorsey.

Gazda, Géza. 1951. "Használjunk fed minden gramm hulladékot (Let's use every gram of waste!) *Szabad Nép. (Free People.)* August 14, p. 1.

GEAD documents. 1999.

Gehrs, B. C., M. M. Riddle, W. C. Williams, and R. J. Smialowicz. 1997. Alterations in the developing immune system of the F344 rat after perinatal exposure to 2,3,7,8-tetrachlorodibenzo-p-dioxin. II. Effects on the pup and the adult. *Toxicology* 122:229–40.

Gelobter, Michael. 1993. Race, class, and outdoor air pollution: The dynamics of environmental discrimination from 1970 to 1990. Ph.D. dissertation, Energy and Resources Group, University of California, Berkeley.

Gibbs, Lois Marie. 1995. *Dying from Dioxin: A Citizen's Guide to Reclaiming Our Health and Rebuilding Democracy.* Boston: South End Press.

Gill, Graeme. 1987. Khruschchev and Systematic Development. In *Khrushchev and Khrushchevism,* edited by Martin McCauley. London: Macmillan Press. 30–46.

Girard, Francoise. 1999. Cairo + five: Reviewing progress for women five years after the International Conference on Population and Development. *Journal of Women's Health and Law* 1(1): 1–14.

Giuiuzza, Paolo. 1998. Italian chemical industry and environmental issues. Presented at the OECD Workshop on Sustainable Chemistry. Venice. October 15.

Global Campaign for Microbicides. 2001. Legislative Message. http://www.global-campaign.org/dom/hotflash3dom.html.

———. 2001. Looking for Mrs. McCormick: Accomplishments to date.http://www.global-campaign.org/dom/accdom.html.

Global Campaign for Prevention Options for Women. 2001. http://www.global-campaign.org/inter/abouti.html.

Global Microbicide Project. 2001. http://www.gmp.org/.

Gluck, S. 1985. *Japan's Modern Myths: Ideology in the Late Meiji Period.* Princeton: Princeton University Press.

———. 1998. The Invention of Edo. In *Mirror of Modernity: Invented Traditions of Modern Japan* edited by S. Vlastos. Berkeley: University of California Press.

Goodman, John, and Vivien Walsh. 2001. *The Story of Taxol: Nature and Politics in the Pursuit of an Anti-Cancer Drug.* Cambridge: Cambridge University Press.

Gordon, Avery F. 1997. *Ghostly Matters: Haunting and the Sociological Imagination.* Minneapolis and London: University of Minnesota Press.

Gore, Albert. 1996. *The Best Kept Secrets in Government: How the Clinton Administration Is Reinventing the Way Washington Works.* New York: Random House.

Gottemoeller, Megan. 2000. Empowering women to prevent HIV: the microbicide advocacy agenda. *Agenda Magazine.* http://www.agenda.org.za/megan.htm.

Gramsci, Antonio. 1985. *Selections in Cultural Writings.* London: Routledge.

Gray G. C., J. D. Knoke, S. W. Berg, F. S. Wignall, and E. Barrett-Connor. 1998. "Counterpoint: responding to suppositions and misunderstandings." *American Journal of Epidemiology.* 148:328–33.

Gray, L. E., Jr., J. S. Ostby, and W. R. Kelce. 1997. A dose response analysis of reproductive effects of a single gestational dose of 2,3,7,8-tetrachlorodibenzo-p-dioxin in male Long Evans hooded rat offspring. *Toxicology and Applied Pharmacology* 146:11–20.

Gray, L. E., Jr., C. Wolf, and J. S. Ostby. 1997b. In utero exposure to low doses of 2,3,7,8-tetrachlorodibenzo-p-dioxin alters reproductive development of female Long Evans hooded rat offspring. *Toxicology and Applied Pharmacology* 146: 235–7.

Green Chemistry Institute website. 2002. http://chemistry.org/portal/Chemistry?PID=acsdisplay.html&DOC=greenchemistryinstitute\index.html.

Greenberg, Daniel S. 2001. *Science, Money, and Politics: Political Triumph and Ethical Erosion.* Chicago: University of Chicago Press.

Greenberg, Michael. 2001. Earth Day plus 30 years: Public concern and support for environmental health. *American Journal of Public Health* 91:559–62.

Greenberg Michael, and Daniel Wartenberg. 1991. Communicating to an alarmed community about cancer clusters: A fifty state survey. *Journal of Community Health.* 16:71–81.

Grossman, Daniele, and Seth Shulman. 1993. A case of nerves. *Discover* 14:66–75.

Gudeman, Stephen. 1986. *Economics as Culture: Models and Metaphors of Livelihood.* London, Boston, and Henley: Routledge and Kegan Paul.

Guha, Ranajit. 1989. Dominance without hegemony and historiography. In Ranajit Guha *Subaltern Studies VI: Writings on South Asian History and Society.* Oxford: Oxford University Press.

Gunstone, F. D., ed. 1970. *Topics in Lipid Chemistry.* 3 vols. New York: Wiley-Interscience.

Haley, Robert, Thomas Kurt, and Jim Hom. 1997. Is there a Gulf War Syndrome? Searching for syndromes by factor analysis of symptoms. *Journal of the American Medical Association,* 277:215–222.

Hansen, Anders, ed. 1993. *The Mass Media and Environmental Issues.* Leicester: Leicester University Press.

Hansen, Robert G., and John R. Lott Jr. 1993. Regulating IAQ: The economist's view—indoor air is air that someone owns. *EPA Journal* 19:30–1.

Happe, Kelly E. Forthcoming (anticipated 2002). Genomics and the Social Order: Rhetoric, Media, and the Case of Breast Cancer. Ph.D. dissertation, Department of Communication, University of Pittsburge, Pittsburgh, PA.

Haraway, Donna J. 1985. A Manifesto for Cyborgs: Science, Technology, and Socialist Feminism in the 1980s. *Socialist Review* 80:65–107.

———. 1988. Situated knowledges: The science question in feminism and the privilege of partial perspective. *Feminist Studies* 14: 575–99.

———. 1991. *Simians, Cyborgs, and Women: The Reinvention of Nature.* New York: Routledge.

———. 1997. Modest_Witness@Second_Millenium.FemaleMan©_Meets_*OncoMouse*™. New York: Routledge.

Harnly, Caroline D. 1988. *Agent Orange and Vietnam: An Annotated Bibliography.* Meutchen, NJ and London: Scarecrow Press.

Harootunian, H. 1988. *Things Seen and Unseen. Discourse and Ideology in Tokugawa Nativism.*

———. 1998. Figuring the folk: History, poetics, and representation. In *Mirror of Modernity: Invented Traditions of Modern Japan,* edited by S. Vlastos. Berkeley: University of California Press.

Harper, M. J. K. 1999. The promise of public/private sector collaboration in the development of new contraceptives: The experience of CICCR. *International Journal of Gynecology and Obstetrics.* 67: S23–S30.

Harrison, Mick. 1996. *GreenLaw Preliminary Risk Analysis of the Army Chemical Weapon Incineration Program.* Brea: Kentucky Environmental Foundation.

Harrison, Polly F. 1999. A new model for collaboration: The alliance for microbicide development. *International Journal of Gynecology and Obstetrics.* 67: S39–S53.

Harrison, Polly F., and Allan Rosenfield, eds. 1996. *Contraceptive Research and Development.* Washington, D.C.: National Academy of Sciences.

Hartmann, Betsy. 1998. Cairo consensus stirs new hopes, old concerns. In *Our Bodies, Ourselves for the New Century,* edited by the Boston Women's Health Book Collective. New York: Simon & Schuster.

Hatfield Group website: www.hatfieldgroup.com.

Hashimoto M. 1998. Chihou: Yanagita Kunio's "Japan." In *Mirror of Modernity: Invented Traditions of Modern Japan,* edited by S. Vlastos. Berkeley: University of California Press.

Hayes, Peter. 2001 [1987]. *Industry and Ideology: IG Farben in the Nazi Era.* Cambridge: Cambridge University Press.

Hecht, Sidney M., ed. 1999. *Bioorganic Chemistry: Carbohydrates.* New York: Oxford University Press.

Heidegger, Martin. 1977. *The Question Concerning Technology and Other Essays.* Trans. and Introduction by W. Lovitt. New York: Harper Torchbooks.

Hein, Teri. 2000. *Atomic Farmgirl: The Betrayal of Chief Qualchan, the Appaloosa, and Me.* Golden, Col.: Fulcrum Publishing.

Heise, Lori. (No Date). *Topical Microbicides: New Hope for STI/HIV Prevention.* Takoma Park, MD: Center for Health and Gender Equity.

Heise, Lori L., and Christopher Elias. 1995. Transforming AIDS prevention to meet women's needs: A focus on developing countries. *Social Science and Medicine* 40(7):931–43.

Heise, Lori L., C. Elizabeth McGrory, and Susan Y. Wood. 1998. Practical and ethical dilemmas in the clinical testing of microbicides: A report on a symposium. International Women's Health Coalition, New York.

Hellebust, Rolf. 1997. Aleksei Gastev and the metallization of the revolutionary body. *Slavic Review* 56(3):501–18.

Henriksen, G. L., N. S. Ketchum, J. E. Michalek, and J. A. Swaby. 1997. Serum dioxin and diabetes mellitis in veterans of Operation Ranch Hand. *Epidemiology* 8(3):252–58.

Herrmann, Ann, and Stewart, Abigail, eds. 1994. *Theorizing Feminism.* Boulder, CO: Westview.

Hertzgaard, Mark. 2001. Dioxin studied to death. *The Nation,* May 28.

Hill, Ronald. 1987. State and ideology. In *Khrushchev and Khrushchevism,* edited by Martin McCauley. London: Macmillan Press.

Hirsch, E., and M. O'Hanlon, eds. 1995. *The Anthropology of Landscape.* Oxford: Clarendon Press.

Hoffman, Karen. In progress. Inheriting the wind: industrial pollution and the pursuit of environmental justice. Ph.D. diss., History of Consciousness Board, University of California at Santa Cruz.

Hoffman, Erik, and Robbin Laird. 1985. *Technocratic Socialism: The Soviet Union in the Advanced Industrial Era.* Durham: Duke University Press.

Hogle, Linda F. 2001. Chemoprevention for healthy women: harbinger of things to come? *Health* 5 (3): 299–320.

House of Representatives. 1993. Indoor air pollution: Hearing before the Subcommittee on Health and the Environment of the Committee on Energy and Commerce on H.R. 2919, a bill to amend the Public Health Service Act to authorize a national program to reduce the threat to human health posed by exposure to contaminants in the air indoors. 103rd Cong., 1st Sess., November 1, 1993. Serial No. 103–88. Washington: Government Printing Office. Statements of: Ralph Engel, President, Chemical Specialties Manufacturers Association; The Business Council on Indoor Air; and George Julin III, President, Building Owners and Managers Association.

H.R. 1930, 103rd Cong., 1st Sess. (1993).

H.R. 2919, 103rd Cong., 1st Sess. (1993).

H.R. 2919, 103rd Cong., 2d Sess. (1994). House Rept. 103–719.

H.R. 933, 104th Cong., 1st Sess. (1995).

Hughes, Thomas P. 1969. Technological momentum in history: Hydrogenation in Germany, 1898–1933. *Past and Present* 44 (August): 106–32.

————. 1989. *American Genesis: A Century of Invention and Enthusiasm, 1870–1970.* New York: Viking.

Hunt, S.C., and R.D. Richardson. 1999. Letters: Chronic Multisystem Illness Among Gulf War Veterans. *Journal of the American Medical Association* 282:327–29.

Huu Ngoc. 2002. The first modern scientist of Vietnam. *Vietnam News.* March 4.

Hyams, Kenneth, Stephen Wignall, and Robert Roswell. 1996. War syndromes and their evaluation: From the U.S. Civil War to the Persian Gulf War. *Annals of Internal Medicine*, 125:298–305.

Indoor Environment Connections Online. 2002. http://www.ieconnections.com/iecstaff.htm.

Institute for Global Environmental Studies. 1999. Quality of the environment in Japan 1999: Environmental messages toward sustainable development in the twenty-first century. Kanagawa: Institute for Global Environmental Studies.

Institute of Medicine. 1999. *Veterans and Agent Orange: Update 1998.* Washington, D.C.: National Academy Press.

International Agency for Research (IARC). 1997. IARC monographs on the evaluation of carcinogenic risks to humans. Vol. 69. Polychlorinated dibenzo-para-dioxins and poly-chlorinated dibenzofurans. Lyon, France: International Agency for Research, World Health Organization.

———. 2000. *Gulf War and Health: Volume 1. Depleted uranium, sarin, pyridostigmine bromide, and vaccines.* Washington DC: National Academy Press.

International Women's Health Coalition. Contraceptive technology update: Microbicides. http://www.iwhc.org/micro.html.

———. 1998. News release: Urgent need for women-controlled prevention method galvanizes fifty-five experts from fifteen countries in consensus plan for testing of microbicides. http://www.iwhc.org/12_24_98.htm.

International Working Group on Vaginal Microbicides. 1996. Recommendations for the development of vaginal microbicides. *AIDS 10*: 1–6.

Ivy, M. 1995. *Discourses of the Vanishing: Modernity, Phantasm, Japan.* Chicago: University of Chicago Press.

Jamieson, Neal. 1993. *Understanding Viet Nam.* University of California Press.

Januskevicius, Vytautas. 1971. Darbo Jegos Istekliu Racionalaus Panaudojimo Klausimu Lietuvoje. In *Geografinis Metrastis XI: Lietuvos TSR Gyventojai ir Darbo Istekliai.* Vilnius: Mintis.

Januskevicius, Vytautas and Ona Miliuniene. 1971. "Miestu Ugdymas ir Pramones Isdestymas Tarybu Lietuvoje." In *Geografinis Metrastis XI: Lietuvos TSR Gyventojai ir Darbo Istekliai.* Vilnius: Mintis.

Japan Environment Agency. 1999. Our Intensive Efforts to Overcome the Tragic History of Minamata Disease. Tokyo: Japan Environment Agency.

Jávor, András. 1954. *Az anyagtakarékosság és önköltségcsökkentés műszaki feladatai a vegyiparban.* The technical tasks of material conservation and cost reduction in the chemical industry. Manuscript. Budapest: Felsőoktatási Jegyzetellátó Vállalat.

Jones, James H. 1981. *Bad Blood: The Tuskegee Syphilis Experiment: A Tragedy of Race and Medicine.* New York: Free Press.

Jones, Roger. 1998. Building products made from carbon dioxide and fly ash. Presented at the Second Annual Green Chemistry and Engineering Conference. Washington, D.C. June 30.

KSH (Központi Statisztikai Hivatal—Central Bureau of Statistics). 1988. *Központi fejlesztési programok. A melléktermék- és hulladékhasznosítási program 1987. évi eredményei.* Central development programs. The by-product and waste reuse program. Budapest: Központi Statisztikai Hivatal.

Kalland, A., and G. Persoon. 1995. An anthropological perspective on environmental movements. In *Environmental Movements in Asia*, edited by A. Kalland and G. Persoon. Richmond, Surrey: Curzon.

Kentucky Environmental Foundation. 1998. Public Health and Chemical Weapons Incineration. Brea, KY: Kentucky Environmental Foundation.

Kevles, Bettyann Holtzman. 1997. *Naked to the Bone: Medical Imaging in the Twentieth Century.* Sloan Technology Series. Reading, MA: Addison-Wesley. Originally published by Rutgers University Press.

Kevles, Daniel J. 2000. *The Baltimore Case: A Trial of Politics, Science, and Character.* New York: W. W. Norton.

Keyes, Charles F. 2002. Abstract for Abortions, Agent Orange, and AIDS: Social suffering in Vietnam and Thailand. Panel presentation at annual conference for the Association of Asian Studies, Washington, D.C.

Kinlen, Leo J., and Angela Balkwill. 2001. Infective cause of childhood leukemia and wartime population mixing in Orkney and Shetland, *Lancet*, Vol. 357, Num. 9259, March 17.

Kiran, Erdogan, Pablo G. Debenedetti, and Cor J. Peters. 2000. *Supercritical Fluids: Fundamentals and Applications.* Dordrecht: Kluwer Academic.

Kirby, P. W. 1999a. The architecture of Japanese nature: An anthropological view. *Cambridge Architecture Journal* 11:105–11.

———. 1999b. Simulated natures: Performances of leisure at an artificial beach in Tokyo. *Text, Practice, Performance* 1: 53–65.

———. 2001. Environmental consciousness and the politics of waste in Tokyo: "Nature," health, pollution, and the predicament of toxic Japan. Ph.D. dissertation, University of Cambridge.

———. forthcoming. Getting engaged: Pollution, toxic illness, and discursive shift in a Tokyo community. In *Living Environments: Places, Power, People,* edited by J. Carrier. Oxford: Berg.

Kitriene, Danute, and Antanas Spudulis. 1996. *Chemical Lietuvoje.* Jonava: Naujienu Redakcija.

Klawiter, Maren. 1999a. "Racing for the cure, walking women, and toxic touring: Mapping cultures of action within the Bay Area terrain of breast cancer." *Social Problems* 46 (February): 104–26.

———. 1999b. Reshaping the contours of breast cancer: From private stigma to public actions" Ph.D. dissertaton, Department of Sociology, University of California, Berkeley.

———. 2000. From private stigma to global assembly: Transforming the terrain of breast cancer." In *Global Ethnography: Forces, Connections, and Imaginations in a Postmodern World,* edited by Michael Burawoy. Berkeley: University of California Press.

———. In Press. Risk, prevention and the breast cancer continuum: The NCI, the FDA, health activism and the pharmaceutical industry. *History and Technology* (December 2002).

Kleinman, Arthur. 1988. *The Illness Narratives.* New York: Basic Books.

Kleinman, Arthur, Veena Das, and Margaret Lock. 1997. *Social Suffering.* Berkeley: University of California Press.

Kolata, Gina. 2002. "Looking for the Link." *New York Times.* August 11, 2002. On-line version accessed.

Koplow, David A. 1997. *By Fire and Ice: Dismantling Chemical Weapons While Preserving the Environment.* Amsterdam: Gordon and Breach Publishers.

Krimsky, Sheldon, and Dominic Golding, eds. 1992. *Social Theories of Risk.* Westport: Praeger.

Kroll-Smith, Steve, Phil Brown, and Valerie J. Gunter, eds. 2000. *Illness and the Environment: A Reader in Contested Medicine.* New York: New York University Press.

Kroll-Smith, Steve, and H. Hugh Floyd. 1997. *Bodies in Protest: Environmental Illness and the Struggle over Medical Knowledge.* New York: New York University Press.

Kuletz, Valerie L. 1998. *The Tainted Desert: Environmental and Social Ruin in the American West.* New York: Routledge.

Kuodyte, Dalia et al., 1996. eds. *Laisves Kovu Archyvas.* Kaunas: Lietuvos Politiniu Kaliniu ir Tremtiniu Sajunga.

Kushner, Rose. 1977. "The Politics of Breast Cancer." In *Seizing Our Bodies: The Politics of Women's Health,* edited by Claudia Dreifus. New York: Vintage Books.

Landrigan P. J. 1997. Illness in Gulf War veterans: causes and consequences. *Journal of the American Medical Association* 277:259–61.

Lantsev, Michail S. 1976. *Sotsialnoe Obsepechenie v SSR.* Moscow.

Latour, Bruno. 1987. *Science in Action: How to Follow Scientists and Engineers through Society.* Cambridge: Harvard University Press.

———. 1988. Mixing humans and nonhumans together: The sociology of a door-closer. *Social Problems* 35:298–310.

———. 1991. *We Have Never Been Modern.* Cambridge: Harvard University Press.

———. 1999. *Pandora's Hope: Essays on the Reality of Science Studies.* Cambridge: Harvard University Press.

Latour, Bruno, and Steve Woolgar. 1986 [1979]. *Laboratory Life: The Construction of Scientific Facts.* 2d ed. Princeton: Princeton University Press.

Le Cao Dai. 2000. *Agent Orange in the Viet Nam War, History and Consequences.* Hanoi: Vietnam Red Cross Society.

———. 2000, 2001. Personal communication.

Lee, Charles. 1992. Toxic waste and race in the United States. In *Race and the Incidence of Environmental Hazards: A Time for Discourse,* edited by Bunyan Bryant and Paul Mohai. Boulder: Westview Press.

Lefebvre, H. 1994 [1974]. *The Production of Space.* Oxford and Cambridge, MA: Blackwell.

Lerner, Barron. 2002. "What if Proof Is Elusive?" Newsday.com. August 18, 2002. http://www.newsday.com/news/health/ny-vpler182828983aug18.story.

Lerner, Sharon. 1994. Microbicides: a woman-controlled HIV prevention in the making. *SIECUS Report* 22(5[June/July]): 10–13.

Lewy, Guenter. 1978. *America in Vietnam.* New York: Oxford University Press.

Lietuviskoji Tarybine Enciklopedija. 1985. Vilnius: Vyriausioji Enciklopediju Redakcija.

Lietuvos TSR CSV. 1965. *Tarybu Lietuvai 25 Metai. Statistikos Duomenu Rinkinys.* Vilnius.

———. 1965. *Lietuvos TSR Liaudies Ukis 1966 Metais. Statistiniu Duomenu Rinkinys.* Vilnius.

Lindblom, Charles E. 1977. *Politics and Markets.* New York: Basic Books.

———. 2001. *The market system.* New Haven, CT: Yale University Press.

Lindblom, Charles E., and Edward J. Woodhouse. 1993. *The Policy-Making Process.* 3d ed. Englewood Cliffs, NJ: Prentice Hall.

Lock, M. (1980). *East Asian Medicine in Urban Japan.* Berkeley, Los Angeles, and London: University of California Press.

Locker, David. 1981. *Symptoms and Illness: The Cognitive Organization of Disorder.* London: Tavistock Publications.

Lorde, Audre. 1980. *The Cancer Journals.* San Francisco: Aunt Lute Books.

Lovins, Amory B. 1977. *Soft-Energy Paths: Toward a Durable Peace.* New York: Harper and Row.

Lynch, K. 1960. *The Image of the City.* Cambridge, MA: MIT Press.

MacCormack, C., and M. Strathern. 1980. *Nature, Culture and Gender.* Cambridge: Cambridge University Press.

MacPherson, Myra. 1984. *Long Time Passing: Vietnam and the Haunted Generation.* New York: Doubleday.

Maniusis, Juozas. 1977. *Soviet Lithuania: Achievements and Prospects.* Vilnius: Mintis Publishers.

Markowitz, Gerald, and David Rosner. 2002. *Deceit and Denial: The Deadly Politics of Industrial Pollution.* Berkeley: University of California Press.

Marr, David. 1981. *Vietnamese Tradition on Trial, 1920–1945.* Berkeley: University of California Press.

———. 1987. Vietnamese attitudes regarding illness and healing. In *Death and Disease in Southeast Asia*, edited by Norman G. Owen. Singapore: Oxford University Press. Asian Studies Association of Australia.

Martin, E. 1994. *Flexible Bodies: Tracking Immunity in American Culture—From the Days of Polio to the Age of AIDS.* Boston: Beacon Press.

Marshall, Suzanne. 1996. *Chemical Weapons Disposal and Environmental Justice.* Brea, KY: Kentucky Environmental Foundation.

Marx, Karl. 1964a. Estranged Labor. In *The Economic and Philosophic Manuscripts of 1844,* Edited and introduction by Dirk J. Struik. New York: International Publishers.

———. 1964b. The Power of Money in Bourgeois Society. In *The Economic and Philosophic Manuscripts of 1844,* edited and introduction by Dirk J. Struik. New York: International Publishers.

Masterton, William L., Emil J. Slowinski, and Conrad L. Stanitski. 1985. *Chemical Principles.* 6th ed. Philadelphia: Saunders College Publishing.

Mauskopf, Seymour H. 1993. *Chemical Sciences in the Modern World.* Philadelphia: University of Pennsylvania Press.

Mazoji Lietuviskoji Tarybine Enciklopedija. 1971.Vilnius: Mintis.

McCann, Carole R. 1994. *Birth Control Politics in the United States, 1916–1945.* Ithaca, NY: Cornell University Press.

McCormick, Sabrina, Phil Brown, and Stephen Zavestoski. 2001. The personal is scientific, the scientific is political: The environmental breast cancer movement. Paper presented at the American Sociological Association Annual Meeting. August.

McIlroy, Robert Joseph. 1967. *Introduction to Carbohydrate Chemistry.* London, Butterworths.

McIntosh, C. Alison, and Jason L. Finkle. 1995. The Cairo conference on population and development: A new paradigm? *Population and Development Review* 21(2): 223–60.

McKinlay, John. 2001. A Case for refocusing upstream: The political economy of illness. In *The Sociology of Health and Illness: Critical Perspectives,* edited by Peter Conrad. 6th ed. New York: Worth Publishers.

Meikle, Jeffrey L. 1995. *American Plastic: A Cultural History.* New Brunswick, NJ: Rutgers University Press.

Miller, Mark Crispin. 2001. *The Bush Dyslexicon: Observations on a National Disorder.* New York: W.W. Norton.

Minh Chuyen. 1997. *Di Hoa Chien Tranh.* Hanoi: Nha Xuat Ban Van Hoc.

Ministry of Health and Welfare. 1999. Bonyū-chū no daiokishin-rui ni kansuru chōsa. Dioxin breast milk survey. Tokyo: Ministry of Health and Welfare.

Misiunas, Romulad, and Rein Taagepera. 1983. *The Baltic States: Years of Dependence 1940–1990*. Berkeley: University of California Press.

Monmaney, Terence. 1988. Young Survivors in a Deadly War. *Newsweek*. July 18.

Moore, R., J. Gauna, L. Bird, M. Garza Carcano, W. Ford, V. J. Williamson, Ed. Quintana, L. Granado, J. Risley, C. P. Saunders, J. Gonzalez, A. Carrasco, D. Bunting, Ev. Quintana, R. Contreras, L. R. Pena, and C. Brito. *Letter to Group of Ten Environmental Organizations*. Reprinted in *Not man apart: The newsmagazine of friends of the earth, USA*, 20(2)15.

Morone, Joseph G., and Edward J. Woodhouse. 1989. *The Demise of Nuclear Energy?: Lessons for Democratic Steering of Technology*. New Haven, CT: Yale University Press.

Morris, David B. 1997. About suffering: Voice, genre, and moral community. In *Social Suffering*. edited by A. Kleinman et al. Berkeley: University of California Press.

Morrison, David C. 1991. No easy out: Environmental and grass-roots opposition threatens to upset arms control timetables for eliminating chemical weapons in both the United States and the Soviet Union. *National Journal* 23(19).

Morse, E. 1961. *Japanese Homes and Their Surroundings*. New York: Dover.

Moss, Ralph. 1982. *The Cancer Syndrome*. New York: Grove Press.

Mother's Milk Contains 26 Times New Limit for Dioxins. 1999. *Yomiuri Shimbun*, August 3.

Moyers, Bill. 2002. "October 31, 2001: Which America will we be now?" In *A Just Response: The Nation on Terrorism, Democracy, and September 11, 2001*, edited by Katrina Vanden Heuvel. New York: Thunder's Mouth Press/Nation Books.

Mumford, Lewis. 1934. *Technics and Civilization*. New York: Harcourt, Brace and Co.

Murray, F. J., F. A. Smith, K. D. Nitschke, C. G. Humiston, R. J. Kociba, and B. A. Schwetz. 1979. Three-generation reproduction study of rats given 2,3,7,8-tetrachlorodibenzo-p-dioxin (TCDD) in the diet. *Toxicology and Applied Pharmacology* 50:241–252.

National Cancer Institute. 2002. *Cancer Facts*. Bethesda: National Cancer Institute.

National Cancer Institute, National Institute of Environmental Health Sciences, Office of Resarch on Women's Health, U.S. Public Health Service's Office on Women's Health, Centers for Disease Control and Prevention, eds. 1999. *DES Research Update 1999: Current Knowledge, Future Directions*. Department of Health and Human Services, NIH Pub. No. 00–4722.

National Institutes of Health. 2001. *National Institutes of Health Almanac*. Bethesda, MD. http://www.nih.gov/about/almanac/index.html.

National Research Council. 1989. *Alternative Agriculture*. Washington, D.C.: National Academy Press.

National Toxicology Program (NTP). 2001. Addendum to the ninth report on carcinogens. United States Department of Health and Human Services, Public Health Service, National Toxicology Program. Research Triangle Park, NC.

Neilands, J. B., Gordon H. Orians, E. W. Pfeiffer, Alje Vennema, and Arthur H. Westing. 1972. *Harvest of Death: Chemical Warfare in Vietnam and Cambodia*. New York: The Free Press; London: Collier-Macmillan Limited.

Nelkin, Dorothy. 1985. *The Language of Risk: Conflicting Perspectives in Occupational Health*. Beverly Hills: Sage Publications.

———. 1995. *Selling Science: How the Press Covers Science and Technology*. New York: Freeman.

Nelkin, Dorothy, and Michael S. Brown. 1984. *Workers at Risk: Voices from the Workplace*. Chicago: The University of Chicago Press.

Nelson, Diane. 1999. *Finger in the Wound: Body Politics in Quincentennial Guatemala*. Berkeley: University of California Press.

Nichols, Mary. 1993. "Lessons from radon: Consumers need user-friendly information." *EPA Journal* 19:36–7

Norsigian, Judith. 1996. The women's health movement in the United States. In *Man-Made Medicine*, edited by K. L. Moss. Durham, NC and London: Duke University Press.

Northern California Cancer Center. Breast cancer in the greater Bay Area. *Greater Bay Area Cancer Registry Report* 5 (1994): 1.

Nye, Mary Jo. 1993. *From Chemical Philosophy to Theoretical Chemistry: Dynamics of Matter and Dynamics of Disciplines, 1800–1950*. Berkeley: University of California Press.

OECD (Organization for Economic Cooperation and Development). 2002. Health Data. Washington, D.C.: OECD.

———. 1999. OECD Environmental Data, Compendium 1999. Paris: OECD.

Ohnuki-Tierney, E. 1984. *Illness and Culture in Contemporary Japan: An Anthropological View.* Cambridge: Cambridge University Press.

Ohsako, S., Miyabara, Y., et al. 2001. Maternal exposure to a low dose of 2,3,7,8-tetrachlorodibenzo-p-dioxin (TCDD) suppressed the development of reproductive organs of male rats. *Toxicological Sciences* 60(1):132–43.

Orians, G. H., and E. W. Pfeiffer. 1970. Ecological effects of the war in Vietnam. *Science* 168, 544–554.

Ortner, S., and H. Whitehead. 1981. *Sexual Meanings: The Cultural Construction of Gender and Sexuality.* Cambridge: Cambridge University Press.

Osborne, David, and Peter Pastrik. 1997. *Banishing Bureaucracy: The Five Strategies for Reinventing Government.* Reading, MA: Addison Wesley.

Oudshoorn, Nelly. 1996. The decline of the one-size-fits-all paradigm, or, how reproductive scientists try to cope with postmodernity. In *Between Monsters Goddesses and Cyborgs,* edited by N. Lykke and R. Braidotti. London and Atlantic City, NJ: Zed Books.

Painter Design and Engineering, Inc. Website http://www.painterdesign.com

Palmlund, Ingar. 1992. Social drama and risk evaluation. In *Social Theories of Risk,* edited by Sheldon Krimsky and Dominic Golding. Westport: Praeger.

Pandolfo, S. 1989. Detours of life: space and bodies in a Moroccan village. *American Ethnologist* 16:3–23.

Patai, Daphne. 1991. "U.S. Academics and Third World Women: Is Ethical Research Possible?" In S. B. Gluck and Daphne Patai, eds. *Women's Words: The Feminist Practice of Oral History.* London: Routledge.

Patterson, James. 1987. *The Dread Disease: Cancer and Modern American Culture.* Cambridge, MA: Harvard University Press.

Pazderova-Vejlupkova, J., M. Nemcova, J. Pickova, L. Jirasek, and E. Lukas. 1981. The development and prognosis of chronic intoxication by tetrachlorodibenzo-p-dioxin in men. *Archives of Environmental Health* 36(1): 5–11.

Petchesky, Rosalind P. 1990. *Abortion and Woman's Choice: The State, Sexuality and Reproductive Freedom.* Boston: Northeastern University Press.

———. 1997. Spiraling discourses of reproductive and sexual rights: a post-Beijing assessment of international feminist politics. In *Women Transforming Politics,* edited by C. J. Cohen, K. B. Jones, and J. C. Tronto, 569–87. New York: New York University Press.

Pető, Iván, and Szakács, Sándor. 1985. *A hazai gazdaság négy évtizedének története.* The history of forty years of the domestic economy. Budapest: Közgazdasági és Jogi Könyvkiadó.

Pham Minh Tam, Director of the Committee for the Protection and Care of Children for Thai Binh Province. 2000. Interview.

Pianin, Eric. 2001. Dioxin report by EPA on hold. *Washington Post,* April 12.

Pickering, Andrew, ed. 1992. *Science as Practice and Culture.* Chicago: University of Chicago Press.

Pigman William Ward, and Rudolph Maximilian Goepp. 1948. *Chemistry of the Carbohydrates.* New York: Academic Press.

Poliakoff, Martyn, J. Michael Fitzpatrick, Trevor R. Farren, and Paul T. Anastas. 2002. Green Chemistry: Science and Politics of Change. *Science* 297 (August 2): 807–10.

Population Council, Pacific Institute for Women's Health, International Women's Health Coalition. 1994. Partnership for prevention: A report of a meeting between women's health advocates, program planners, and scientists. New York and Washington, D.C., May 3–12. New York: The Population Council.

Prakash, Gyan. 1999. *Another Reason: Science and Imagination of Modern India.* Princeton: University of Princeton Press.

Price, Richard M. 1997. *The Chemical Weapons Taboo.* Ithaca: Cornell University Press.

Primack, Joel R., and Frank Von Hippel. 1974. *Advice and Dissent: Scientists in the Political Arena.* New York: Basic Books.

Proctor, Richard N. 1995. *Cancer Wars: How Politics Shapes What We Know and Don't Know about Cancer.* New York: Basic Books.

Public Health and Welfare Ministry White Paper, 1997–1999 [CD-ROM]. Tokyo: Gyōsei.

Pulido, Laura. 2000. Rethinking environmental racism: White privilege and urban development in Southern California. *Annals of the Association of American Geographers* 90:12–41.

Raloff, Janet. 1994. Incinerator under fire: safety questions swirl at a facility designed to burn chemical weapons. *Science News* 146:394–6.

Rapp, Rayna. 1999. *Testing Women, Testing the Fetus: The Social Impact of Amniocentesis in America.* New York: Routledge.

Ray, Raka. 1998. Women's movements and political fields: A comparison of two Indian cities. *Social Problems* 45 (1): 21–36.

Raymond, Chris Anne. 1988. Fates of childhood cancer survivors comes under increasing scrutiny. *Journal of the American Medical Association* 260, 22:3246.

———. 1985. Risk in the press: Conflicting journalistic ideologies. In *The language of risk: Conflicting Perspectives in Occupational Health*, edited by DorothyNelkin.Beverly Hills: Sage Publications.

Real Goods. 1997. April 1997 Catalog: Explore the Alternatives. Ukiah, California: Real Goods.

———. 2002. Online catalog listing for Seventh Generation Kitchen Cleaner. Accessed online at http://www.realgoods.com/shop/shop2.cfm?dp=208&ts=2284005.

Reeves, W. C., K. Fukuda, R. Nisenbaum, and W. W. Thompson. 1999. "Letters: Chronic multisystem illness among Gulf War veterans." *Journal of the American Medical Association* 282:327–329.

Reich, Michael. 1991. *Toxic Politics: Responding to Chemical Disasters.* Ithaca, NY: Cornell.

Reiter, R. 1975. *Toward an Anthropology of Women.* New York: Monthly Review Press.

Renn, Ortwin. 1992. Concepts of risk: A classification. In *Social Theories of Risk,* edited by Sheldon Krimsky and Dominic Golding. Westport: Praeger.

Rettig, Richard A. 1977. *Cancer Crusade: The Story of the National Cancer Act of 1971.* Princeton: Princeton University Press.

Reverby, Susan M. 1997. What does it mean to be an expert? A health activist at the FDA. *Advancing the Consumer Interest* 9: 34–6.

Rier, S. E., D. C. Martin, R. E. Bowman, W. P. Dmowski, and J. L. Becker. 1993. Endometriosis in rhesus monkeys (Macaca mulatta) following exposure to 2,3,7,8-tetrachloro-dibenzo-p-dioxin (TCDD). *Fundamentals of Applied Toxicology* 21:433–41.

Riley, Nancy E. 1997. Gender, power, and population change. *Population Bulletin* 52:1.

Robertson, J. 1991. *Native and Newcomer: Making and Remaking a Japanese City.* Berkeley: University of California Press.

Robertson, J. 1998. It takes a village: Internationalization and nostalgia in postwar Japan. In *Mirror of Modernity: Invented Traditions of Modern Japan,* edited by S. Vlastos. Berkeley: University of California Press.

Roe, Emery. 1994. *Narrative Policy Analysis: Theory and Practice.* Durham, NC: Duke University Press.

Rose, Nikolas. 1999. *Powers of Freedom: Reframing Political Thought.* Cambridge: Cambridge University Press.

Rosenberg, Charles E. 1976. *No Other Gods: On Science and American Social Thought.* Baltimore: Johns Hopkins University Press.

Rosenthal, Alon, George M. Gray, and John D. Graham. 1992. Legislating acceptable cancer risk from exposure to toxic chemicals. *Ecology Law Quarterly* 19:269–362.

Rosenthal, Elisabeth. 1997. Maker of cancer drugs to oversee prescriptions at eleven cancer clinics. *New York Times* April 15.

Ross, P. S., R. L. De Swart, P. J. Reijnders, H. Van Loveren, J. G. Vos, and A. D. Osterhaus. 1995. Contaminant-related suppression of delayed-type hypersensitivity and antibody responses in harbor seals fed herring from the Baltic Sea. *Environmental Health Perspectives* 103: 162–67.

Roth, Gabriel. 1999. Not fit to print? Project Censored uncovers the stories that didn't make the news in 1998. *The Guardian,* March 24.

Rubin, James B., and Craig M. V. Tyler. 1998. Partial replacement of Portland cement with fly ashes and kiln dusts using supercritical carbon dioxide processing. Presented at the OECD Workshop on Sustainable Chemistry. Venice. October 15.

Russell, Edmund. 2001. *War and Nature: Fighting Humans and Insects with Chemicals from World War I to Silent Spring.* Cambridge: Cambridge University Press.

Ruzek, Sheryl Burt. 1978. *The Women's Health Movement: Feminist Alternatives to Medical Control.* New York, Praeger Publishers.

Ryan, Charlotte. 1991. *Prime Time Activism.* Boston: South End Press.

S. 656, 103rd Cong., 1st Sess. 1993.

S. 656 103rd Cong., 1st Sess., 139 Cong Rec S 3773. Daily ed. March 25, 1993. Statement of Senator Chaffee.

S. 656, 103rd Cong., 2d Sess. 1994. In the House of Representatives Engrossed House Amendment.

S. 855, 107th Cong, 2d Sess. 2001.

SIPRI (Stockholm International Peace Research Institute). 1980. *Chemical Weapons: Destruction and Conversion.* London: Taylor and Francis Ltd.

Sagers, Matthew J., and Theodore Shabad. 1990. *The Chemical Industry in the USSR: An Economic Geography.* San Francisco: Westview Press.

Saitama Prefecture Declared Safe 1999. *Asahi Shimbun,* February 19.

San Francisco Chronicle. 1997. Editorial: Dioxin Concerns in the East Bay. September 27.

Satchell, Michael. 1993. Death rattle of poison gas: A $billion plan to burn up chemical weapons prompts a huge outcry. *U.S. News and World Report,* September 13.

Savinskij, E. S. 1972. *Khymizatsia NarodnovoKhozeistva i Proportsii Razvitia Khimicheskoi Promishlenosti.* Moscow: Khymia.

Schama, S. 1996. *Landscape and Memory.* London: Fontana Press.

Schantz, S. L., and R. E. Bowman. 1989. Learning in monkeys exposed perinatally to 2,3,7,8-tetrachlorodibenzo-p-dioxin (TCDD). *Neurotoxicology and Teratology* 11:13–9.

Schecter, Arnold. Fall, 2002. E-mail to members of the steering committee, conference on "The Long-term Environmental Consequences of War: Cambodia, Laos and Vietnam." Stockholm, Sweden.

Schecter, Arnold, ed. 1994. *Dioxins and Health.* New York and London: Plenum Press.

Schecter, Arnold, with Le Cao Dai, Olaf Papke, Joelle Prange, John D. Constable, Muneaki Matsuda, Vu Duc Thao, and Amanda Piskac. 2001. Recent Dioxin contamination from Agent Orange in residents of a southern Vietnam city." *Journal of Occupational Environmental Medicine* 43 (5):435–43.

Scheiner, I. 1998. The Japanese village: Imagined, real, contested. In *Mirror of Modernity: Invented Traditions of Modern Japan,* edited by S. Vlastos. Berkeley: University of California Press.

Scheper-Hughes, Nancy. 1992. *Death without Weeping: The Violence of Everyday Life in Brazil.* Berkeley: University of California Press.

Scheper-Hughes, Nancy, and Margaret Lock. 1987. The mindful body: A prolegomenon to future work in medical anthropology. *Medical Anthropology Quarterly,* 1 (1): 6–41.

Schettler, Ted, Gina Solomon, Maria Valenti, and Annette Huddle. 1999. *Generations at Risk: Reproductive Health and the Environment.* Cambridge, MA: MIT Press.

Schierow, Linda-Jo. 1998. Environmental risk analysis: A review of public policy issues. Congressional Research Report for Congress, Environment and Natural Resources Policy Division. 98–618 ENR. Accessed online at http://cnie.org/NLE/CRSreports/Risk/rsk-11a.cfm#Comparative Risk Analysis at EPA

Schneider, Joseph W., and Peter Conrad. 1983. *Having Epilepsy: The Experience and Control of Illness.* Philadelphia: Temple University Press.

Schuck, Peter H. 1986. *Agent Orange on Trial.* Belknap Press (a division of Harvard University Press).

Sclove, Richard. 1995. *Technology and Democracy.* New York: Guilford Press.

Scott, J. C. 1985. *Weapons of the Weak: Everyday Forms of Peasant Resistance.* New Haven: Yale University Press.

Scrip Reports. 1996. *Pharmaceutical Companies Fact File 1996.* U.K.: PJB Publications Ltd.

Sears, Laurie J. 1996. *Shadows of Empire.* Durham and London: Duke University Press.

Senate. 1993. Pending indoor air quality and radon abatement legislation: hearing before the Subcommittee on Clean Air and Nuclear Regulation of the Committee on Environment and Public Works on S. 656, a bill to provide for indoor air pollution abatement, including indoor radon abatement, and for other purposes, and on S. 657, a bill to reauthorize the Indoor Radon Abatement Act of 1988, and for other purposes. 103rd Cong., 1st Sess., May 25, 1993. Washington: Government Printing Office. Statement of Chemical Specialties Manufacturers Association.

Seo, B. W., A. J Sparks, K. Medora, S. Amin, and S. L. Schantz. 1999. Learning and memory in rats gestationally and lactationally exposed to 2,3,7,8-tetrachlorodibenzo-p-dioxin (TCDD). *Neurotoxicology and Teratology* 21:231–9.

Sexton, Ken. 1993. An inside look at air pollution: Complicated public policy issues are at stake. *EPA Journal* 19:9–12.

Seydlitz, Ruth, J. William Spencer, and George Lundskow. 1994. Media presentations of a hazard event and the public's response: An empirical examination. *International Journal of Mass Emergencies and Disasters* 12:279–301.

Shenon, Philip. 1997. Defense secretary vows thorough inquiry on Gulf War illnesses. *New York Times,* March 6.

Shulman, Seth. 1992. *The Threat at Home: Confronting the Toxics Use Legacy of the U.S. Military.*

Skupeika, Antanas. 1971. Lietuvos Chemijos Pramone ir Jos Vystymo Perspektyvos, in *Geografinis Metrastis XI: Lietuvos TSR Gyventojai ir Darbo Istekliai.* Vilnius: Mintis.

Smith, Kirk R. 1993. Taking the true measure of air pollution: We have to look where the people are. *EPA Journal* 19:6–8.

Smithson, Amy E. 1993. *The Chemical Weapons Convention Handbook.* Washington, DC: The Henry L. Stimson Center.

Smoger, Gerson. 2002. Presentation at the Yale Vietnam conference 2002: The ecological and health effects of the Vietnam War. New Haven, Ct. September 13–15.

Snieckus, Antanas. 1970. *Soviet Lithuania on the Road of Prosperity.* Vilnius: Mintis Publishers.

Snow, David, E. Burke Rocheford, Steven Worden, and Robert Benford. 1986. Frame alignment processes, micromobilization, and movement participation. *American Sociological Review.* 51:464–81.

Spector, Malcolm, and John Kitsuse. 1977. *Constructing Social Problems.* Menlo Park, CA: Cummings.

Spencer, J. William, and Elizabeth Triche. 1994. Media constructions of risk and safety: Differential framings of hazard events. *Sociological Inquiry* 64: 199–213.

Spivak, Gayatri Chakravorty. 1988. Can the subaltern speak? In *Marxism and the Interpretation of Culture,* edited by Cary Nelson and Lawrence Grossberg. Champaign: University of Illinois Press.

Stallings, Robert. 1990. Media discourse and the social construction of risk. *Social Problems* 37:80–95.

Star, Susan Leigh. 1991. Power, technologies and the phenomenology of conventions: On being allergic to onions. In *A Sociology of Monsters: Essays on Power, Technology and Domination,* edited by John Law. London: Routledge.

Staudenmeier, John. 1985. *Technology's Storytellers.* Cambridge, MA: MIT Press.

Steinfels, Peter. 1993. The latest advances in cloning challenge bioethicists. *New York Times.*

Steingraber, Sandra. 1993. 'If I live to be 90 still wanting to say something': My search for Rachel Carson. In *Confronting Cancer, Constructing Change: New Perspectives on Women and Cancer,* vol. 2 of the Women/Cancer/Fear/Power series, edited by Midge Stocker. Chicago: Third Side Press.

———. 1997. *Living Downstream: An Ecologist Looks at Cancer and the Environment.* Reading, MA: Addison-Wesley Publishing Company, Inc.

Stellman, Jeanne, Dr. 2000. Presentation to the ad hoc panel convened to assist the NIEHS with developing a preliminary research strategy relating to health and environmental aspects of exposure to dioxin and related compounds in Vietnam. Monterey, California. August eighteenth.

———. 2002. Presentation at the Yale Vietnam conference 2002: The ecological and health effects of the Vietnam War. New Haven, CT September 13–15.

Stengers, Isabelle. 1997. *Power and Invention: Situating Science.* Minneapolis: University of Minnesota Press.

Stephenson, Joan. 2000. Microbicides: Ideas flourish, money to follow? *Journal of the American Medical Association* 283(14): 1811–12.

Stewart, Kathleen. 1996. *A Space on the Side of the Road: Cultural Poetics in an 'Other' America.* Princeton: Princeton University Press.

Stocker, Midge, ed. 1991. *Cancer as a Women's Issue: Scratching the Service.* Vol. 1 of the Women/Cancer/Fear/Power series. Chicago: Third Side Press.

———. 1993. *Confronting Cancer, Constructing Change: New Perspectives on Women and Cancer.* Vol. 2 in the Women/Cancer/Fear/Power series. Chicago: Third Side Press.

Strathern, M. 1980. No nature, no culture: The Hagen case. In *Nature, Culture and Gender,* edited by C. MacCormack and M. Strathern. Cambridge: Cambridge University Press.

Sutton, Paul L. 2002. The history of Agent Orange use in Vietnam—An historical overview from the veteran's perspective. Prepared for the United States Vietnam Scientific Conference on Human Health and Environmental Effects of Agent Orange/Dioxins. Hanoi, March 2002.

Sutton, Paul L., Chair. 2002. National Agent Orange/Dioxin Committee, Vietnam Veterans of America. Presentation at the "Yale Vietnam Conference 2002: The Ecological and Health Effects of the Vietnam War." New Haven, CT: September 13–15.

Szasz, Andrew. 1994. *EcoPopulism: Toxic Waste and the Movement for Environmental Justice.* Minneapolis: University of Minnesota Press.

Szasz, Andrew, and Michael Meuser. 1997. Environmental inequalities: literature review and proposals for new directions in research and theory. *Current Sociology* 45:99–120.

Szász, Károly. 1981. Tüz-és robbanásveszélyes, valamint mérgezö gyógyszeripari hulladékok megsemmisítésével kapcsolatos gondok, problémák. Problems of eliminating inflammable, explosive, and toxic pharmaceutical wastes. In *Tüz- és robbanásveszélyes, valamint mérgezö gyógyszeripari hulladékok megsemmisítésével kapcsolatos gondok, problémák (elöadássorozat).* Problems of eliminating inflammable, explosive and toxic pharmaceutical wastes—lectures, edited by János Nuridsány. Budapest: Magyar Gyógyszeripari Egyesülés.

Tanenbaum, Leora. 2000. "Profit and loss." *Mamm* (March): 50–5.

Tapper, Melbourne. 1999. *In the Blood: Sickle Cell Anemia and the Politics of Race.* Philadelphia: University of Pennsylvania Press.

Thompson, J. 1995. *The Media and Modernity: A Social Theory of the Media.* Cambridge: Polity Press.

Thornton, Joe. 1993. Chlorine, human health and the environment: The breast cancer warning. A Greenpeace report. Washington, D.C.: Greenpeace.

———. 2000. *Pandora's Poison: Chlorine, Health, and a New Environmental Strategy.* Cambridge: MIT Press.

Tonn, K., C. Esser, E. M. Schneider, W. Steinmann-Steiner-Haldenstatt, and E. Gleichmann. 1996. Persistence of decreased T-helper cell function in industrial workers twenty years after exposure to 2,3,7,8-tetrachlorodibenzo-p-dioxin. *Environmental Health Perspectives* 104: 422–26.

Toy, Vivian S. 2002. Long Island study sees no cancer tie to pesticides. *New York Times.* August 6, 2002. On-line version accessed.

Tran, Tini. 2002. Unprecedented Agent Orange conference tackles "ghost" of Vietnam War. Associated Press, March 3.

Tran Van Thuy. 1980s. *Chuyen Tu Te (The story of kindness, or Decency, or How to behave)* Hanoi: Trung Tam Phim Tai Lieu va Khoa Hoc.

Travis, A. S. 1998. *Determinants in the Evolution of the European Chemical Industry, 1900–1936: New Technologies, Political Frameworks, Markets, and Companies.* Dordrecht: Kluwer.

Trinh, T. Minh Ha. 1989. *Woman, Native, Other: Writing Postcoloniality and Feminism.* Bloomington: Indiana University Press.

Trost, Barry M. 1991. The atom economy: A search for synthetic efficiency. *Science* 254 (December 6): 1471–7.

Tsukuba H. 1969. Beishoku, Nikushoku no Bunmei. Rice-eating civilization, meat-eating civilization. Tokyo: Nippon Hōsō Shuppan Kyōkai.

Turner, Bryan S. 1991. Recent developments in the theory of the body. In *The Body: Social Process and Cultural Theory,* edited by Mike Featherstone, Mike Hepworth, and Bryan S. Turner. London: Sage.

———. 1995. *Medical Power and Social Knowledge,* 2d ed. London: Sage Publications.

Turner, T. 1994. Bodies and anti-bodies. In *Embodiment and Experience,* edited by T. J. Csordas. Cambridge: Cambridge University Press.

TV Asahi Admits Part of Report Inappropriate. 1999. *Asahi Shimbun,* February 11.

Uhl, Michael, and Tod Ensign. 1980. *GI Guinea Pigs.* Playboy Press.

U.K. Childhood Cancer Study Investigators. 1999. Exposure to power-frequency magnetic fields and the risk of childhood cancer. *Lancet,* Vol. 354, Issue 9194: 1925.

United Church of Christ Committee for Racial Justice. 1987. Toxic wastes and race in the United States: A national report on the racial and socio-economic characteristics of communities surrounding hazardous waste sites. New York: United Church of Christ.

United Nations. 1994. Report of the International Conference on Population and Development, Cairo, September 5–13. http://www.undp.org/popin/icpd/conference/offeng/poa.html.

United Nations Environment Programme (1999). Dioxin and furan inventories: National and regional emissions of PCDD/PCDF. Geneva: United Nations Environment Programme.

U.S. Congress. 2001. Reinventing government?: The Clinton-Gore Administration's record on paperwork reduction. Hearing before the Subcommittee on National Economic Growth, Natural Resources, and Regulatory Affairs of the Committee on Government Reform, House of Representatives, One Hundred Sixth Congress, second session, April 12, 2000. Washington, DC: Government Printing Office.

U.S. EPA. 1987. Unfinished business: A Comparative assessment of environmental problems. Office of Policy Analysis, Office of Policy, Planning and Evaluation. Washington D.C.: Government Printing Office.

———. 1992a. Environmental equity: reducing risk for all communities. EPA 230-DR-002. Office of Policy, Planning and Evaluation. Washington D.C.: Government Printing Office.

————. 1992b. Indoor air quality and new carpet: What you should know. EPA/560/2–91–003. Washington D.C.: Government Printing Office.

————. 1993. Targeting indoor air pollution: EPA's approach and progress. EPA 400-R-92–012. Office of Air and Radiation, Washington D.C.: Government Printing Office.

————. 1995a. "Current federal indoor air quality activities." EPA 402K-95005. Indoor Air Division, Washington D.C.: Government Printing Office.

————. 1995b. Indoor air quality: Tools for schools—Backgrounder. EPA 402-K-95–001. Indoor Air Division. Washington D.C.: Government Printing Office.

————. 1996. "Environmental Health Threats to Children." EPA 175-F-96–001. Accessed online at http://www.epa.gov/epadocs/child.htm#agenda.

————. 1997. *Special Report on Environmental Endocrine Disruption: An Effects Assessment and Analysis.* Washington, DC: Author.

U.S. EPA (Office of Air and Radiation). 1997. Office of Air and Radiation fiscal year 1997–1998 implementation plan, revised edition. Accessed on-line at http://www.epa.gov/oar/oario.html.

U.S. EPA (Office of Children's Heath Protection). 2002. Website accessed online at http://www.epa.gov/children/mission.htm.

U.S. EPA (Office of Pollution Prevention and Toxics). 1996. The Presidential Green Chemistry Challenge Awards program: Summary of 1996 award entries and recipients. Washington, DC: U.S. Environmental Protection Agency. EPA744-K-96–001.

————. 1998. The Presidential Green Chemistry Challenge: Summary of 1998 Award Entries and Recipients. Washington, D.C.: U.S. Environmental Protection Agency. EPA-744-R-98-001.

U.S. EPA, American Lung Association, Consumer Product Safety Commission, and American Medical Association. 1994. Indoor air pollution: An introduction for health professionals. American Lung Association, Environmental Protection Agency. Consumer Product Safety Commission, American Medical Association, New York, NY, Washington, D.C., Chicago, IL.

U.S. EPA and CPSC. 1995. The inside story: a guide to indoor air quality. EPA 402-K-93–007. Washington D.C.: Government Printing Office.

U.S. EPA, U.S. Public Health Service, and National Environmental Health Association. 1991. Introduction to indoor air quality: a reference manual. EPA/400/3–91/003. Washington D.C.: Government Printing Office.

U.S. GAO. 1983. *Siting of hazardous waste landfills and their correlation with the racial and socio-economic status of surrounding communities.* Washington, D.C.: Government Printing Office.

U.S. GAO. 1991. Indoor air pollution: Federal efforts are not effectively addressing a growing problem. GAO/RCED-92–8. Washington D.C.: Government Printing Office.

U.S. GAO. 1992. Toxic substances: Advantages of and barriers to reducing the use of toxic chemicals. GAO/RCED-92–12. Washington D.C.: Government Printing Office.

van Kammen, Jessika. 1999. Representing users' bodies: The gendered development of anti-fertility vaccines. *Science, Technology and Human Values* 24(3): 307–37.

Vegetables Take Serious Fall. 1999. *Mainichi Shimbun,* February 4.

Vegetables Under Fire. 1999. *Yomiuri Shimbun,* February 5.

Vegyimüvek. 1971. No title. March 1, 1.

Vészi, Endre. 1952. *Gazda Géza Forintjai.* (Géza Gazda's Forints.) Budapest: Népmüvelésügyi Minisztérium.

Vietnam: A Television History (in 13 parts, on 7 cassettes) A co-production of WGBH Boston, Central Independent Television/UK and Antenne-2, France. Copyright 1983 WGBH Educational Foundation.

Vietnam News Agency. 1998. *Vietnam Courier:* Oct. 4–10, 18–24; Nov. 22–28, 29–Dec. 5; Dec. 6–12.

Viscusi, W. Kip. 1983. *Risk By Choice: Regulating Health and Safety in the Workplace.* Cambridge: Harvard University Press.

Visweswaran, Kamala. 1994. *Fictions of Feminist Ethnography.* Minneapolis: University of Minnesota Press.

Vo Quy. 1992. The wounds of war: Vietnam struggles to erase the scars of 30 violent years. *Ceres (the FAO Review)* 24:13–16.

Vostral, Sharra L. 2000. *Conspicuous Menstruation: The History of Menstruation and Menstrual Hygiene Products in America, 1870–1960.* Ph.D. dissertation, Department of History, Washington University.

Wade, L. G., Jr. 1987. *Organic Chemistry.* Englewood Cliffs, NJ: Prentice-Hall.

Wallace, L. A. 1987. *The Total Exposure Assessment Methodology (TEAM) Study: Summary and Analysis: Volume 1.* U.S. Environmental Protection Agency, Office of Research and Development, Washington D.C.: Government Printing Office.

———. 1991. Comparison of risks from outdoor and indoor exposure to toxic chemicals. *Environmental Health Perspectives* 95:7–13.

———. 1993. A Decade of studies of human exposure—what have we learned? *Risk Analysis* 13: 135–9.

Wallace, L. A., E. D. Pellizzari, T. D. Hartwell, V. Davis, L. C. Michael, and R. W. Whitmore. 1989. The Influence of personal activities on exposure to volatile organic compounds. *Environmental Research* 50:37–55.

Ward, Chip. 1999. *Canaries on the Rim: Living Downwind in the West.* London: Verso.

Waste Reduction Comprehensive Planning Office. 1995. Public cleansing services in Tokyo 1994. Tokyo: Waste Reduction Comprehensive Planning Office.

Watsuji T. 1975 [1935]. Fūdo. *Milieus.* Tokyo: Iwanami Shoten.

Webster, Donovan. 1996. *Aftermath: The Remnants of War.* New York: Vintage Books.

Webster, Thomas, and Barry Commoner. 1994. Overview. In *Dioxins and Health,* edited by Arnold Schecter. New York and London: Plenum Press.

Weisel, C. P., and W. J. Chen. 1994. Exposure to chlorination by-products from hot water uses. *Risk Analysis* 14:101–6.

Weisman, Carol S. 2000. Breast Cancer Policymaking. In *Breast Cancer: The Social Construction of an Illness,* edited by Anne S. Kasper and Susan J. Ferguson. New York: St. Martin's Press.

Weitz, Rose. 1996. *The Sociology of Health, Illness and Health Care: A Critical Approach.* Belmont: Wadsworth Publishing Company.

Wells, F. O., Stephen Lock, and M. J. G. Farthing. 2001. *Fraud and Misconduct in Biomedical Research.* 3rd ed. London: BMJ Books.

Westing, Arthur H., ed. 1984. *Herbicides in War: The Long-Term Ecological and Human Consequences.* London and Philadelphia: Taylor and Francis. Stockholm International Peace Research Institute.

Whipple, Chris. 1992. Inconsistent Values in Risk Management. In *Social Theories of Risk.* edited by Sheldon Krimsky and Dominic Golding. Westport: CT: Praeger.

Williams, Gareth. 1984. The genesis of chronic illness: narrative re-construction. In *Sociology of Health and Illness,* Vol. 6, No. 2.

Williams, John R., and Tony Clifford. 2000. *Supercritical Fluid Methods and Protocols.* Totowa, NJ: Humana Press.

Williams, R. 1973. *The Country and the City.* London: Chatto and Windus.

Wilson, James Q. 1984 [1974]. The Politics of regulation. In *The Political Economy: Readings in the Politics and Economics of American Public Policy,* edited by T. Ferguson and J. Rogers. Armonk, New York: M. E. Sharpe, Inc.

Winner, Langdon. 1977. *Autonomous Technology: Technics-Out-of-Control as a Theme in Political Thought.* Cambridge, MA: MIT Press.

Winner, Langdon. 1986. *The Whale and the Reactor: The Search for Limits in an Age of High Technology.* Chicago: University of Chicago Press.

Winnow, Jackie. 1989. Lesbians Working on AIDS: Assessing the Impact on Health Care for Women. *Out/Look: National Lesbian & Gay Quarterly* 2, no.1 (Summer): 10–18.

———. 1991. Lesbians evolving health care: Cancer and AIDS. In *1 in 3: Women with Cancer Confront an Epidemic,* edited by Judy Brady. San Francisco: Cleis Press.

Woodhouse, E. J. 1998. Engineering as a political activity. Technology and Society at a Time of Sweeping Change: Proceedings. Glasgow: IEEE International Symposium on Technology and Society.

Woodhouse, Edward J., and Dean A. Nieusma. 2001. Democratic expertise: Integrating knowledge, power, and participation. In *Knowledge, Power and Participation in Environmental Policy Analysis,* edited by Matthijs Hisschemœller, Rob Hoppe, William N. Dunn, and Jerome Ravetz. Policy Studies Review Annual 12. New Brunswick, NJ: Transaction Publishers.

Woodhouse, Edward, David Hess, Steve Breyman, and Brian Martin. 2002. Science studies and activism: Possibilities and problems for reconstructivist agendas. *Social Studies of Science* 32:297–319.

World Health Organization. 1970. *Health Aspects of Chemical and Biological Weapons.* Geneva: World Health Organization.

World Health Organization. 1999. Dioxins and their effects on human health. World Health Organization fact sheet No. 225. Geneva: World Health Organization.

Yang, J. Z., and W. G. Foster. 1998. Chronic exposure to 2,3,7,8-tetrachlorodibenzo-p-dioxin modulates the growth of endometriosis in the cynomolgus monkey. *Organohalogen Compounds* 37:75.

Yoshino, K. 1992. *Cultural Nationalism in Japan: A Sociological Inquiry.* London and New York: Routledge.

Young, A. L., and G. M. Reggiani. 1988. *Agent Orange and Its Associated Dioxin: Assessment of a Controversy.* Amsterdam, New York, Oxford: Elsevier.

Zakin, Susan. 1997. Doing the Nerve Gas Shuffle. *Sierra* July/August: 26–30.

Zaneveld, Lourens, J. D., Deborah J. Anderson, and Kevin J. Whaley. 1996. Barrier methods. In *Contraceptive Research and Development,* edited by Polly Harrison and Allan Rosenfield. Washington, D.C.: National Academy of Sciences.

Zeitlin, Larry, Richard A. Cone, and Kevin J. Whaley. 1999. Using monoclonal antibodies to prevent mucosal transmission of epidemic infectious diseases. *Emerging Infectious Diseases* 5(1): 54–64.

Zelizer, Viviana A. 1985. *Pricing the Priceless Child: The Changing Social Value of Children.* New York: Basic Books.

Zeneca Patient Education Service. n.d. Zeneca Pharmaceuticals: Bringing Ideas to Life. Wilmington, DE: Zeneca Pharmaceuticals.

List of Contributors

Barbara A. Barnes is a doctoral candidate in sociology at the University of California, Santa Cruz. Her research interests are focused on cultural studies of bodies, movement, space, and performance of risk in modernity. Her previously published work can be found in *Quest: Journal of the National Association for Physical Education in Higher Education.*

Susan E. Bell is A. Myrick Freeman Professor of social sciences, department of sociology and anthropology, Bowdoin College. Her work on women's health, narrative, and the development of medical technology has appeared in *Social Science and Medicine, Qualitative Sociology, Health, Narrative Inquiry, Feminist Studies,* and *Women's Studies International Forum.* A long-time feminist health advocate, she is senior author of "Birth Control" in *The New Our Bodies, Ourselves* (1984, 1992) and *Our Bodies, Ourselves for the New Century* (1998). For the past three years she has organized and run a literature and medicine seminar at Maine General Medical Center (Augusta, Maine) under the auspices of the Maine Humanities Council. She is currently writing a book about the experiences of DES daughters.

Phil Brown is a professor of sociology and environmental studies at Brown University. He is currently examining disputes over environmental factors in asthma, breast cancer, and Gulf War–related illnesses, as well as toxics reduction and precautionary principle approaches that can help avoid toxic exposures. Among his other research interests are gender, race, and class bias in the burden of environmental hazards, health social movements, and community responses to toxic waste contamination. He is co-author of *No Safe Place: Toxic Waste, Leukemia, and Community Action* (Phil Brown and Edwin Mikkelsen) and coeditor of a collection, *Illness and the Environment: A Reader in Contested Medicine.* His third edition of *Perspectives in Medical Sociology* is widely used in colleges. Prior to studying health and the environment, he studied mental health policy, mental patients' rights, and clinical interaction in psychiatric settings. Among his publications from that work are *The Transfer of Care: Psychiatric Deinstitutionalization and Its Aftermath,* and *Mental Health Care and Social Policy* (edited).

Monica J. Casper is an associate professor of sociology at the University of California, Santa Cruz (on leave 2002–2005) and Executive Director of the Intersex Society of North America in Seattle. A medical sociologist and specialist in women's health, she is author of the award-winning book *The Making of the Unborn Patient: A Social Anatomy of Fetal Surgery*. Currently, she is studying the U.S. chemical weapons disposal program, the history and politics of quinacrine sterilization (QS), and the politics and bioethics of surgical "treatment" for intersex conditions. She serves on the Board of Directors of the Institute for Children's Environmental Health.

Diane Niblack Fox is a doctoral candidate in socio-cultural anthropology at the University of Washington. Her interests include postcolonial, environmental, and medical anthropology. From 1991 to 2001 she lived and worked in Vietnam, initially as an English teacher and then as coordinator of volunteer teachers and a study abroad program. She later worked as copyeditor, translator, and writer for the national English language daily and the foreign languages publishing house. Most recently, she has served as a consultant to the Vietnamese Red Cross.

Zsuzsa Gille is an assistant professor of sociology at the University of Illinois at Urbana-Champaign. She specializes in environmental sociology, globalization, ethnography, cultural studies, and Eastern Europe. Her recent publications include articles in *Anthropology of Eastern Europe Review*, the *Annual Review of Sociology*, and *Cultural Studies-Critical Methodologies*, as well as a chapter in *The Politics of Urban Livelihood and Sustainability* (University of California Press, 2001). Presently she is working on a book titled *From the Cult of Waste to the Trash Heap of History: A Social Theory of Waste*.

Karen Hoffman is a graduate student in the History of Consciousness Department at the University of California, Santa Cruz. Her work is on the history of trying to regulate toxic pollutants in the U.S., anti-toxics and environmental justice activism, and social reproduction and change.

Peter Wynn Kirby received his Ph.D. in anthropology at the University of Cambridge. He teaches the anthropology of the environment and the anthropology of cities as an assistant professor at Asia Pacific University in Beppu, Japan. He is also Affiliate Lecturer in Global Environmentalism in the Faculty of Social and Political Sciences, University of Cambridge. In addition to several published articles and essays, he is coediting two collected volumes on space and power and is currently reshaping his doctoral thesis—on the politics of waste in Japan—into a book.

Maren Klawiter is an assistant professor in the School of History, Technology and Society at Georgia Institute of Technology. She received her

Ph.D. in Sociology in 1999 from the University of California, Berkeley and from 1999 to 2001 she was a fellow at the University of Michigan, in the Robert Wood Johnson Foundation Scholars in Health Policy Research Program. She studies health and disease-based activism and is finishing a book, *Reshaping the Contours of Breast Cancer: From Private Stigma to Public Actions*. Her current research focuses on the politics of prevention, the medicalization of risk, direct-to-consumer advertising, and the pharmaceutical industry.

Meadow Linder is a doctoral student in the department of sociology at the University of Michigan. Her research interests include socioeconomic inequalities in health, how organizations, employment, and civic participation shape neighborhood contexts, and the reproduction of inequality across generations.

Brian Mayer is a doctoral student in the department of sociology at Brown University. His interests include environmental and medical sociology, as well as science and technology studies. His recent projects include an investigation of the growth of the precautionary principle as a new paradigm among environmental organizations and a study of social movements addressing environmental health issues.

Sabrina McCormick is a doctoral student in the department of sociology at Brown University. She is a Henry Luce Foundation Fellow through the Watson Institute of International Studies. Her main interests are environmental sociology, medical sociology and the politics of development. As a Luce Fellow, she is engaged in comparing environmentally based movements in the U.S. and Brazil. Additional special interests include the social contestation of environmental illness, the insertion of lay knowledge into expert systems, and the role of social movements in these struggles. She has recent publications by *Ms.* magazine and The National Women's Health Network related to these areas.

Diana Mincyte is a graduate student at the University of Illinois at Urbana-Champaign. She is working in the sociology of science and technology and is interested in relationships between humans and technologies. She is currently exploring the issue of social change in Eastern Europe and how it has been influenced by the development of advanced modern technologies.

Virginia Adams O'Connell is currently assistant professor in the department of sociology and anthropology at Swarthmore College. A recent AAUW Dissertation Fellow and graduate (2001) from the department of sociology at the University of Pennsylvania, her doctoral research examined the effects of the culture of graduate medical education on resident attrition in surgical residency programs. She is author with Charles L. Bosk on a forthcoming chapter in *Society and Medicine: Explorations of the Moral and Spiritual Dimensions* (Transaction Publishers).

Allison Shore earned her M.A. degree in sociology from the University of California, Santa Cruz. She is currently taking a break from academia to focus her energies on environmental justice activism in pollution-plagued southeast San Francisco.

E. J. (Ned) Woodhouse is associate professor of political science in the department of science and technology studies at Rensselaer Polytechnic Institute. His books include *The Demise of Nuclear Energy* and *The Policy-Making Process*. An empirical democratic theorist, he focuses on coping with uncertainty and disagreement as the central problems of technological society. He now is studying nanotechnology, green chemistry, overconsumption by the affluent, and other risky technologies in an attempt to derive general lessons about how technologies can be steered more wisely and fairly.

Stephen Zavestoski is an assistant professor of sociology at the University of San Francisco. His current research examines the role of science in disputes over the environmental causes of unexplained illnesses, the use of the Internet as a tool for enhancing public participation in federal environmental rulemaking, and citizen responses to community contamination. His work appears in journals such as *Science, Technology & Human Values, Journal of Health and Social Behavior, Sociology of Health and Illness,* and in the book *Sustainable Consumption: Conceptual Issues and Policy Problems.*

Index

United States Bureau of Land Management, 258
United States Chemical Weapons Program, 51, 53
United States Congress, 58, 64, 79, 186, 190: and Congressional hearings of, 215
United States Fish and Wildlife Service, 258
United States General Accounting Office (GAO), 26, 46, 49
United States House of Representatives, 209: and Microbicide Development Act, 209
United States House of Representatives Science Committee, 189–190. *See also* United States Congress
United States Institute of Medicine (IOM), 81, 202, 203
United States Public Health Service (PHS), 57: and National Toxicology Program, 82; and syphilis research, 272(n8)
United States Superfund Program, 258, 266(n11)
United States Wetlands Reserve Program, 258
University of Massachusetts Workshop on the Role of Polymer Research in Green Chemistry and Engineering, 181–182: and prediction, 182
unreasonable risk: concept of, 29, 30, 31–32; and language of TSCA, 31; and problems with in TSCA, 31;
Utah, 63, 64: and Bonneville Salt Flats, 59; and Grantsville, 51, 60; and Rush Valley, 51, 59; and Skull Valley, 59, 60; and State Division of Hazardous Waste, 61, 65; and Tooele Army Depot, 60; and Tooele Chemical Stockpile Outreach Office, 51; and Tooele County, xxviii, 51, 52, 53, 59, 60, 63, 65, 66; and Tooele County Emergency Management, 51, 52; and Tooele Chemical Agent Disposal Facility (TOCDF), 55, 59, 60, 61, 62, 67

Veneman, Ann, 259
Veterans Administration (VA), 80, 214, 215: and Agent Orange Projects Office, 80; and compensation benefits, 216
Vietnam, xxviii, xxix, 73, 78, 79, 251, 255: and Agent Orange, xxviii, 73; and Bien Hoa, 81; and Ha Bac province, 81; and interviews in, 84–87; and studies of effects on, 80, 81; and veterans from U.S., 80, 233; and consequences of war, 84–87. *See also* Agent Orange
Vietnam: A Television History, 74
Vietnamese Committee for Protection and Care of Children (CPCC), 82, 84: and Agent Orange, 82
Vietnamese Red Cross, 82, 84
Vilnius 239; and Vilnius University, 249
volatile organic compounds (VOCs), xxviii, 25, 26, 27, 2842, 44, 50, 183; and effects from, 28; and emitters of, 27; and exposure to, 25, 37; and indoors, 41; and indoor chemical pollutants, 27; and products containing, 46; and properties of, 27; and relation to chloroform, 28. *See also* pesticides
Vulcanus, 79
vulnerable: individuals, 111; and populations, 122, 206, 265(n7); and women, 207. *See also* sex workers

Wallace, Lance, 25, 26, 41
War on Cancer, 156
Washington Office of Management and Budget, 186

Washington Post, 215
waste: and cycles of, 16; and disposal of, 3; and hazardous, xvii; and reduction policies, xxix. *See also* hazardous waste
waste incineration, 3, 12, 55; and links with Azuma disease, 20
Water Quality Bureau: of Springfield, 137, 139, 140, 142, 143, 144, 145, 146, 147, 148, 149, 150, 151, 152
West County Toxics Coalition, 162
West Desert Hazardous Industrial Area, 59: and industrial corridor of, 59
West Nile Virus, 217
Western Europe, 198
Western nations, 6: and legal framework of, xxi
White House, 53
Whitman, Governor Christine Todd, 257, 259
Winner, Langdon, 177
Woburn, Massachusetts: and toxic waste, 191
Women, Health and the Environment Community Action Conference, 164–165, 166, 167, 168: and programs of, 165
women's cancer, 165
Women's Cancer Resource Center, 160, 162, 171
Women's Cancer Support Center, 148, 149
Women's Environment & Development Organization (WEDO), 164, 275(n29): and Action for Cancer Prevention Campaign, 164
women's health advocates, 198, 205, 209, 210: and category of scientist, 198
Women's Health Advocates on Microbicides (WHAM), xxxi, 197, 205, 206: and link to the Alliance for Microbicide Development, 208; and collaboration with PC, 197–198, 200, 204, 206, 210; and decision to dissolve, 208; and Statement of Group Principles, 207; and vaginal microbicides, 197
women's health: and movement for, 173–174, 197, 279(n3); and politics of, 197, 198: and tensions of, 199, 205; and transformation, 197, 199
Woodhouse, E.J., viii, xxx, 177
Workers At Risk, 118
World Health Organization (WHO), 81, 135, 164, 202, 204
World Trade Center, 53; *See also* terrorism and "9/11"
World War I, 179
World War II, 64, 179

Yale University: and conference on The Ecological and Health Effects of the Vietnam War, 82
Yanagita, Kunio, 8
Yokkaichi: petrochemical industrial pollution of, 16
Your Guide When the Siren Rings, 52
Yucca Mountain, Nevada, 257; and nuclear waste storage, 257, 259

Zeidenstein, George, 203
Zelizer, Viviana, 122
Zeneca Pharmaceuticals, Zeneca Agrochemicals, and Zeneca Specialties (Zeneca PLC), 163, 164, 170: and AstraZeneca International, 173, 174, 275(n23), 277(n41); and NBCAM and tamoxifen, 163
Zyklon B, xvi